AI in MRI-based Brain Disease Prediction

Editors
Jin Liu
and
Jianxin Wang
School of Computer Science and Engineering
Central South University
Changsha, China
Yi Pan
Shenzhen Institute of Advanced Technology
Chinese Academy of Sciences
Shenzhen, China

CRC Press
Taylor & Francis Group
Boca Raton London New York

CRC Press is an imprint of the
Taylor & Francis Group, an **informa** business
A SCIENCE PUBLISHERS BOOK

Cover credit: Cover image created by Jin Liu, School of Computer Science and Engineering, Central South University, China.

First edition published 2026
by CRC Press
2385 NW Executive Center Drive, Suite 320, Boca Raton FL 33431

and by CRC Press
4 Park Square, Milton Park, Abingdon, Oxon, OX14 4RN

Library of Congress Cataloging-in-Publication Data (applied for)

ISBN: 978-1-032-82871-8 (hbk)
ISBN: 978-1-032-85572-1 (pbk)
ISBN: 978-1-003-51875-4 (ebk)

DOI: 10.1201/9781003518754

Typeset in Times New Roman
by Prime Publishing Services

Preface

The rapid evolution of artificial intelligence (AI) has profoundly transformed the landscape of medical imaging, offering unprecedented advancements in precision, automation, and predictive analytics. Among the various domains of medical imaging, magnetic resonance imaging (MRI)-based brain disease prediction has emerged as a pivotal field, leveraging cutting-edge AI techniques to enhance early diagnosis, treatment planning, and disease progression monitoring.

This book, AI in MRI-based Brain Disease Prediction, comprehensively explores AI-driven methodologies in neuroimaging, bridging the gap between computer science, medical imaging, and neuroscience. It serves as a guiding resource for researchers, clinicians, and students interested in the application of AI to neurological disorders such as Alzheimer's disease, Parkinson's disease, stroke, glioma, and other brain conditions.

The book is structured into multiple sections and begins with an introduction to the fundamental principles of brain anatomy, MRI techniques, and the computational foundations of AI. It then delves into advanced AI methodologies, including deep learning, machine learning, and multimodal data fusion, offering insights into their applications in brain disease prediction. A dedicated section explores the role of AI in fast MRI acquisition and processing, highlighting techniques that optimize scan times while preserving diagnostic accuracy.

The book also addresses the challenges and emerging trends in AI-powered brain disease prediction, such as explainability, model generalization, and clinical integration. With a balanced focus on theoretical foundations and practical applications, we provide real-world case studies and experimental results to illustrate the impact of AI in clinical decision-making and research advancements.

Our objective is to inspire innovation, foster collaboration across disciplines, and contribute to the ongoing efforts to enhance neurological diagnostics and patient care. As AI continues to evolve, we envision a future where AI-empowered

MRI analysis plays a central role in early disease detection, personalized treatment strategies, and precision medicine.

We hope this book is a valuable resource, encouraging further exploration and development in this promising field.

Editors
Jin Liu
Jianxin Wang
Yi Pan
First Edition 2025

Contents

Part 1

Introduction of Brain and Brain MRI

Chapter 1.1

Brain and Magnetic Resonance Brain Imaging

Jin Liu*, Xu Tian and Jianxin Wang
Hunan Provincial Key Laboratory on Bioinformatics,
School of Computer Science and Engineering,
Central South University, Changsha 410083, China

1.1.1 INTRODUCTION

1.1.1.1 The Main Structures of the Brain

The brain is the central organ of the human nervous system, responsible for coordinating and regulating all bodily functions while enabling higher-order cognitive processes such as thought, memory, and language [1]. The brain, which is encased within the skull, works in concert with the spinal cord to form the central nervous system, serving as the control center for the body. Its intricate structure and functionality underscore its critical role in maintaining life and facilitating interaction with the external world.

At the macroscopic level, the brain can be divided into three major components: the cerebral hemispheres, the cerebellum, and the brainstem. The cerebral hemispheres constitute the largest portion of the brain and are divided into left and right hemispheres. They govern higher cognitive functions such as reasoning, decision-making, and voluntary motor control. The cerebellum, located beneath the hemispheres at the back of the brain, is essential for motor coordination, balance, and fine movement control. The brainstem, which connects

*For Correspondence: Jin Liu (liujin06@csu.edu.cn)

DOI: 10.1201/9781003518754-2

the brain to the spinal cord, regulates vital involuntary processes, including breathing, heartbeat, and sleep-wake cycles.

The cerebral cortex is the thin outer layer of the cerebral hemispheres, characterized by its wrinkled appearance. It is organized into four major lobes: the frontal, parietal, temporal, and occipital, each specializing in different functions. The frontal lobe handles executive functions such as planning and motor control, while the parietal lobe processes sensory input, including touch and spatial awareness. The temporal lobe is integral to auditory processing and memory formation, and the occipital lobe is dedicated to visual interpretation. This complex organization allows the brain to process diverse sensory inputs and generate sophisticated responses. Beyond the cortex, the brain houses critical deep structures. The basal ganglia are involved in motor regulation and habit formation, the hippocampus plays a central role in memory and learning, and the amygdala regulates emotional responses such as fear and pleasure. Though smaller in size, these regions are vital to maintaining normal cognitive and behavioral functions.

An intricate network of white matter tracts facilitates communication between different brain regions. One prominent example is the corpus callosum, a thick bundle of nerve fibers that connects the left and right hemispheres, enabling coordinated activity. Functional brain networks, such as the default mode and central executive networks, also play a role in integrating activity across distant areas, supporting both resting and task-oriented cognitive processes.

The brain is surrounded by robust protective mechanisms. The meninges, a three-layered membrane, encase the brain to shield it from physical impacts. Additionally, cerebrospinal fluid (CSF) circulates around and within the brain, providing cushioning and helping to maintain a stable chemical environment. The blood-brain barrier (BBB) is a selective filter, preventing harmful substances in the bloodstream from entering the brain while allowing essential nutrients to pass through.

In summary, the brain's intricate structures and protective systems make it the most vital organ in the human body. It controls every aspect of life, from basic survival functions to complex cognitive and emotional processes, enabling humans to interact with and adapt to their environment. Understanding the brain's anatomy and functions lays the foundation for advancing medical science, particularly in diagnosing and treating neurological disorders.

1.1.1.2 Brain Regions and Their Functions

Brain regions are functional and anatomical units of the brain, each contributing to specific cognitive, sensory, motor, or regulatory tasks [2]. Researchers use standardized atlases and templates that segment the brain into regions based on anatomy, connectivity, or functional activity to facilitate systematic exploration of brain functions. These tools have become indispensable in neuroimaging, offering consistent references for comparing data across studies and individuals.

Numerous brain atlases and spatial templates have been developed to define and study brain regions. Below is a detailed introduction to commonly used atlases:

- **MNI152 (Montreal Neurological Institute 152):** Initiated by the Montreal Neurological Institute, MNI152 is a standardized brain template created by averaging the MRI scans of 152 healthy individuals. The template provides a symmetrical, normalized representation of the human brain, enabling researchers to map brain activity and anatomical features in a consistent spatial framework. Its computational foundation involves linear and nonlinear transformations to align individual brains to a common space, making it one of the most widely used references in neuroimaging.
- **AAL (Automated Anatomical Labeling Atlas):** Developed by Tzourio-Mazoyer and colleagues, the AAL atlas divides the brain into 116 anatomical regions based on structural landmarks identified from MRI data. Each region corresponds to a known gyri or subcortical structure. AAL is primarily used for structural analysis and functional connectivity studies due to its detailed anatomical labeling.
- **CC200 (Craddock Atlas):** Proposed by Craddock and colleagues, this atlas segments the brain into 200 regions using functional connectivity clustering methods. It analyzes resting-state fMRI data to identify areas with correlated activity patterns, making it ideal for studying functional networks.
- **Harvard-Oxford Atlas:** Developed by researchers at Harvard and Oxford, this probabilistic atlas segments the brain into cortical and subcortical regions based on anatomical landmarks. It is frequently used in fMRI studies for both structural and functional localization.
- **Yeo's 7/17 Networks Atlas:** Created by Yeo and colleagues, this atlas divides the brain into 7 or 17 large-scale functional networks, such as the default mode network and visual network. The segmentation is based on the clustering of resting-state fMRI data and is widely used in functional connectivity studies.
- **Talairach Atlas:** Based on the work of Jean Talairach and colleagues, this atlas was one of the earliest coordinate-based systems for the human brain. It provides a reference for identifying brain regions using a stereotaxic coordinate system, though MNI-based methods have largely replaced it.

These atlases offer distinct advantages based on their segmentation methods, spatial resolution, and application focus, enabling researchers to choose the most appropriate tool for their specific study needs. These atlas are cornerstones in neuroimaging research, offering a detailed representation of the brain's anatomical features and a consistent spatial framework for mapping brain activity. Below, five brain regions are described with their spatial locations, anatomical structures, surrounding connections, and key functions.

- **Precentral Gyrus:** The precentral gyrus, located in the posterior portion of the frontal lobe along the central sulcus, is part of the primary motor cortex. It spans the lateral surface of the brain, with its medial boundary being the central sulcus and its lateral boundary merging into the premotor cortex. This region plays a crucial role in voluntary motor control, with its neurons organized somatotopically, representing different body parts. It connects extensively with the premotor cortex and subcortical motor pathways, ensuring precise execution of motor commands.

- **Postcentral Gyrus:** Adjacent to the precentral gyrus, the postcentral gyrus lies in the anterior part of the parietal lobe and corresponds to the primary somatosensory cortex. It processes sensory inputs such as touch, pain, and proprioception. Positioned posterior to the central sulcus, it receives afferent input from the thalamus and strongly connects with the parietal association areas. Its somatotopic organization mirrors the precentral gyrus, emphasizing its role in sensory-motor integration.
- **Hippocampus:** The hippocampus, a prominent structure in the medial temporal lobe, curves around the thalamus and forms part of the limbic system. It is integral to memory consolidation, spatial navigation, and emotional regulation. Anatomically, it is surrounded by the parahippocampal gyrus and amygdala, with dense connections to the prefrontal cortex, thalamus, and hypothalamus. The hippocampus's role in forming long-term memories and its vulnerability to neurodegeneration make it a key area of interest in Alzheimer's research.
- **Amygdala:** Deeply embedded in the medial temporal lobe, anterior to the hippocampus, the amygdala is a small, almond-shaped structure essential for emotional processing and memory. It receives sensory inputs from the thalamus and sensory cortices, integrating these to generate emotional responses such as fear and pleasure. Its connections with the prefrontal cortex, hippocampus, and hypothalamus enable it to influence behavior, autonomic responses, and memory formation under emotionally charged conditions.
- **Superior Temporal Gyrus:** The superior temporal gyrus (STG) lies in the lateral aspect of the temporal lobe, running parallel to the lateral sulcus. This region is central to auditory processing, language comprehension, and social cognition. It is connected to the auditory cortices, Wernicke's area, and frontal lobe regions through the arcuate fasciculus. Damage to the STG can lead to deficits in language comprehension and auditory processing disorders.

The evolution of brain imaging research has marked a significant shift from studying the brain as a whole to focusing on its distinct regions and their specific functions. This regional approach has deepened our understanding of how localized neural activity contributes to cognition, emotion, and behavior. Advanced neuroimaging techniques and standardized atlases and templates have been instrumental in this progress. By providing precise spatial and functional mapping, brain imaging has enabled researchers to explore the intricate roles of individual brain regions, uncover connectivity patterns, and identify region-specific biomarkers for neurological and psychiatric disorders. This transition from a whole-brain perspective to a region-focused paradigm represents a major leap forward, offering more targeted insights into brain function and its clinical implications.

1.1.1.3 Common Brain Disorders

The brain's intricate structure and function make it susceptible to various disorders that result from abnormalities in specific brain regions [3]. These conditions often lead to disruptions in cognitive, motor, or sensory functions, profoundly affecting an individual's quality of life. Advances in neuroimaging have played a critical role in understanding these disorders, providing insights into their origins, symptoms, and structural or functional alterations in the brain. This section explores some of the most well-known brain disorders, including Alzheimer's disease, Parkinson's disease, autism spectrum disorder, and stroke, highlighting their distinct characteristics and neuroimaging findings.

Alzheimer's disease is a progressive neurodegenerative disorder primarily affecting the elderly. The condition originates from the accumulation of amyloid-beta plaques and tau protein tangles in the brain, which lead to neuronal loss and brain atrophy. Early symptoms include memory impairment, especially for recent events, which gradually progress to difficulties with language, problem-solving, and daily activities. Neuroimaging studies, particularly MRI, reveal significant atrophy in the hippocampus and medial temporal lobe, regions critical for memory and learning. PET scans using amyloid or tau tracers further show the deposition of pathological proteins, aiding in early diagnosis and monitoring disease progression.

Parkinson's disease is a movement disorder caused by the degeneration of dopaminergic neurons in the substantia nigra, a structure within the basal ganglia. This degeneration leads to a dopamine deficit, disrupting motor control. The hallmark symptoms include bradykinesia (slowness of movement), resting tremors, muscle rigidity, and postural instability. Advanced cases may also involve non-motor symptoms such as cognitive decline and depression. Neuroimaging, particularly diffusion MRI, shows reduced connectivity within the basal ganglia circuits, while PET and single-photon emission computed tomography (SPECT) highlight reduced dopamine transport activity in the striatum. These imaging modalities are invaluable for diagnosing PD and differentiating it from other parkinsonian syndromes.

Autism spectrum disorder is a neurodevelopmental condition characterized by deficits in social communication, restricted interests, and repetitive behaviors. The exact origins of ASD remain unclear, but it is believed to involve a combination of genetic and environmental factors that disrupt early brain development. Structural MRI studies frequently show alterations in brain volume, particularly in the frontal and temporal lobes, which are critical for social and language processing. Functional MRI (fMRI) reveals atypical connectivity pat- terns in networks such as the default mode network and salience network, which are involved in social cognition and sensory integration. These findings provide a window into the neural underpinnings of ASD and help identify potential biomarkers for diagnosis and intervention. A stroke is a sudden interruption of blood flow to the brain, resulting in localized brain damage. It can be ischemic, caused by a blockage in a blood vessel, or hemorrhagic, resulting from bleeding in or around the brain. The symptoms depend on the affected region but often include sudden weakness or numbness, difficulty speaking, vision disturbances, and impaired coordination. Imaging techniques such as CT and MRI are crucial for stroke diagnosis. CT is commonly used to detect hemorrhagic strokes, while diffusion-weighted imaging (DWI) in MRI is highly sensitive for detecting ischemic strokes in the early stages. Perfusion imaging helps evaluate the extent of blood flow disruption, guiding decisions about therapeutic interventions like thrombolysis or thrombectomy.

These brain disorders exemplify how localized dysfunction in specific regions can manifest as systemic impairments. From progressive neurodegeneration in Alzheimer's and Parkinson's diseases to developmental abnormalities in autism and acute damage in stroke, each condition reveals unique structural or functional alterations. Neuroimaging has become indispensable in understanding these disorders, providing insights into their pathophysiology, aiding early diagnosis, and guiding treatment decisions. By mapping the brain's vulnerabilities, imaging plays a pivotal role in advancing research and improving clinical outcomes for individuals affected by these conditions.

1.1.2 FOUNDATION OF BRAIN IMAGE

1.1.2.1 Brain Imaging Technology

Brain imaging technology has revolutionized our understanding of the human brain, offering detailed insights into its structure, function, and pathology [4]. These technologies capture brain images through various mechanisms, such as detecting differences in tissue density, measuring electromagnetic signals, or tracking biochemical activity. Depending on the modality, imaging may require contrast agents, such as gadolinium in MRI or radioactive tracers in PET, to enhance visibility and specificity. For example, CT scans rely on X-rays to measure tissue density, while MRI uses magnetic fields and radiofrequency waves to map hydrogen atoms in tissues. On the other hand, PET imaging tracks positrons emitted by radioactive isotopes to visualize metabolic and functional processes. These principles form the foundation of brain imaging, which has evolved significantly over the past century. By tracing this evolution, we can appreciate the transformative contributions of key modalities like CT, MRI, and PET to neuroscience and clinical practice.

The quest to visualize the brain began in the early 20th century, driven by the need to understand neurological diseases. Early methods, such as pneumoencephalography, involved invasive procedures where air was injected into the cerebrospinal fluid to create contrast in X-ray images. While these methods were groundbreaking then, they were highly uncomfortable and posed significant risks to patients. A major leap occurred with the advent of X-ray imaging, pioneered by Wilhelm Roentgen in 1895. Although X-rays provided a basic outline of skull and brain structures, they lacked the resolution and specificity to capture detailed brain anatomy or function. The limitations of these early methods set the stage for developing more advanced imaging technologies.

The introduction of CT in the early 1970s marked a turning point in brain imaging. Invented by Godfrey Hounsfield and Allan Cormack, CT technology combined X-ray imaging with computer algorithms to generate cross-sectional images of the brain. CT scans provided detailed anatomical views, enabling the identification of tumors, hemorrhages, and other structural abnormalities with unprecedented clarity. CT rapidly became a cornerstone of clinical neuroimaging due to its non-invasive nature, quick acquisition time, and ability to differentiate between soft tissues and bone. While CT remains widely used today, particularly in emergency settings such as stroke diagnosis, its reliance on ionizing radiation highlighted the need for alternative methods with improved safety and functional imaging capabilities.

In the 1980s, MRI emerged as a transformative technology for brain imaging. Based on principles of nuclear magnetic resonance, MRI uses powerful magnetic fields and radiofrequency pulses to produce detailed images of brain structures without ionizing radiation. Early pioneers, including Raymond Damadian and Paul Lauterbur, contributed to the development of this technology, which soon became the gold standard for neuroimaging. MRI offered exceptional resolution and contrast, allowing the visualization of fine anatomical details. Over time, specialized MRI techniques, such as functional MRI (fMRI) and DWI, expanded its capabilities. fMRI enabled researchers to map brain activity by detecting changes in blood oxygenation, while DWI became critical for identifying acute ischemic strokes. MRI's versatility and safety have made it indispensable for both research and clinical applications. The 1990s saw the rise of PET, which introduced molecular imaging to the field of brain imaging. PET uses radioactive tracers that emit positrons, enabling the visualization of metabolic activity and neurotransmitter function. This technique provided unique insights into brain disorders at the molecular level, such as amyloid-beta deposition in Alzheimer's disease and dopaminergic dysfunction in Parkinson's disease. PET imaging requires cyclotrons to produce short-lived isotopes, which initially limited its accessibility. However, its ability to study the brain's biochemistry and detect early pathological changes has solidified its role in research and specialized clinical settings. Combined PET-MRI scanners, developed more recently, integrate the strengths of both modalities, offering simultaneous structural, functional, and molecular imaging.

Today, brain imaging technologies continue to evolve, focusing on combining modalities to provide comprehensive insights. Hybrid systems such as PET-MRI and advanced techniques like resting-state fMRI, quantitative susceptibility mapping (QSM), and connectome mapping are pushing the boundaries of neuroscience and clinical diagnostics. Integrating artificial intelligence and machine learning further enhances image analysis, enabling faster and more accurate interpretations.

The historical development of brain imaging technology reflects a journey of innovation and discovery. From the rudimentary and invasive methods of the early 20th century to today's sophisticated multimodal imaging systems, each technological breakthrough has deepened our understanding of the brain. CT, MRI, and PET represent pivotal milestones in this evolution, shaping how we study and treat brain disorders. As technology advances, the future of brain imaging holds even greater promise for unraveling the complexities of the human brain.

1.1.2.2 Computed Tomography

The introduction of computed tomography (CT) in the early 1970s marked a significant advancement in medical imaging, allowing for detailed cross-sectional visualization of the brain [5]. Unlike traditional X-ray imaging, which produces overlapping two-dimensional projections, CT scanning captures multiple X-ray projections from different angles and reconstructs them into a three-dimensional representation of the brain. This was made possible through the pioneering work of Godfrey Hounsfield and Allan Cormack, who developed the technique to reconstruct internal structures mathematically based on X-ray attenuation measurements.

The ability to differentiate soft tissues, bone, and cerebrospinal fluid with high precision made CT a crucial tool for diagnosing conditions such as stroke, tumors, and traumatic brain injuries. Its rapid acquisition time and non-invasive nature further solidified its role in emergency and clinical settings. CT imaging is based on the principle of X-ray attenuation, which describes how different tissues absorb or transmit X-ray photons. As an X-ray beam passes through the brain, the intensity of the transmitted radiation is reduced according to the tissue's density and composition. This attenuation follows the Lambert-Beer law, which mathematically models the exponential decrease in X-ray intensity as it travels through matter. The transmitted intensity is given by the equation:

$$I = I_0 e^{-\int_0^L \mu(x)dx}, \tag{1}$$

where I_0 represents the initial X-ray intensity, I is the transmitted intensity after passing through the tissue, $\mu(x)$ is the linear attenuation coefficient at a given location, and L is the total path length of the X-ray beam. This equation is fundamental in CT imaging, as it allows the system to calculate how much X-ray energy is absorbed by different tissues and subsequently construct an image based on these differences in attenuation.

In order to generate a full cross-sectional image, CT scanners collect projection data from multiple angles around the patient's head. This process is described mathematically by the Radon Transform, which integrates the attenuation values along straight paths through the brain. The projection data, called the sinogram, represents how X-rays are absorbed across different angles. Image reconstruction is then performed using an inverse Radon Transform, which converts these projections into a two-dimensional slice. Early CT scanners used iterative reconstruction methods, but modern systems predominantly employ a technique known as filtered back-projection. This method first applies a convolution filter in the frequency domain to remove artifacts and enhance edge detection before integrating the data across all angles to reconstruct the final image:

$$\mu(x,y) = \int_0^{\pi} R_\theta(t) * H(f)\, d\theta, \tag{2}$$

where $\mu(x, y)$ represents the attenuation coefficient at a given point in the image, $R_\theta(t)$ is the projection data at angle θ, and $H(f)$ is the high-pass filter applied in the frequency domain to enhance the reconstructed image. This technique ensures that CT images maintain high spatial resolution while minimizing blurring artifacts, providing clinicians with clear anatomical details.

Clinically, CT imaging has become an essential diagnostic tool, particularly in acute neurological conditions. It is the first-line imaging modality for evaluating stroke, as it quickly differentiates between ischemic and hemorrhagic strokes, guiding immediate treatment decisions. In trauma cases, CT effectively detects skull fractures, intracranial hemorrhages, and cerebral edema. Additionally, it plays a crucial role in the diagnosis and monitoring of brain tumors, hydrocephalus, and structural abnormalities. While CT imaging provides exceptional anatomical detail and rapid scanning times, it exposes patients to ionizing radiation, necessitating careful consideration, particularly for repeated scans or pediatric patients.

Despite the emergence of alternative imaging techniques such as MRI and PET, CT remains indispensable due to its speed, availability, and diagnostic accuracy. Advances in technology, including multi-slice CT and dual-energy CT, continue to enhance image quality and expand its applications. As neuroimaging evolves, CT remains a cornerstone in the field, offering a reliable and efficient method for examining brain structure and pathology.

1.1.2.3 Magnetic Resonance Imaging

Magnetic resonance imaging (MRI) represents one of the most significant advancements in neuroimaging, offering unparalleled soft tissue contrast and the ability to visualize anatomical structures and brain function without the use of ionizing radiation [6]. Developed from nuclear magnetic resonance (NMR), MRI emerged as a revolutionary imaging modality in the 1980s, with key contributions from researchers such as Paul Lauterbur and Peter Mansfield, who pioneered techniques for spatial encoding and rapid image acquisition. Unlike CT, which relies on X-ray attenuation, MRI exploits the magnetic properties of hydrogen nuclei (protons) within water molecules to generate high-resolution images. The ability to produce detailed brain images has made MRI an indispensable tool for diagnosing neurological disorders, mapping brain function, and studying microstructural properties.

MRI operates by placing the subject inside a powerful magnetic field, typically between 1.5 and 7 Tesla, which aligns hydrogen protons along the field direction.

A radiofrequency (RF) pulse is then applied to excite these protons, temporarily altering their alignment. When the RF pulse is turned off, the protons return to equilibrium, releasing energy through electromagnetic signals. The time it takes for the protons to realign with the magnetic field, known as relaxation time, varies depending on the tissue type. These relaxation characteristics, described by the longitudinal relaxation time (T1) and the transverse relaxation time (T2), form the basis for MRI contrast:

$$M_z(t) = M_0(1 - e^{-t/T_1}), \tag{3}$$

$$M_{xy}(t) = M_0 e^{-t/T_2}, \tag{4}$$

where M_z and M_{xy} represent the magnetization components along and perpendicular to the main magnetic field, respectively. T_1 relaxation reflects how quickly protons realign with the magnetic field, while T_2 relaxation represents how quickly transverse magnetization decays due to local magnetic field inhomogeneities. By adjusting imaging parameters, MRI scans can be optimized to highlight different tissue properties, making it possible to distinguish gray matter, white matter, and cerebrospinal fluid with remarkable clarity.

One of the key strengths of MRI is its versatility, with multiple imaging techniques designed to capture different aspects of brain structure and function. Structural MRI (sMRI) is the most commonly used variant, providing high-resolution images of brain anatomy for detecting tumors, neurodegeneration, and structural abnormalities. T_1-weighted scans offer excellent contrast for anatomical details, while T_2-weighted and fluid-attenuated inversion recovery (FLAIR) images are particularly useful for identifying lesions in conditions like multiple sclerosis and stroke.

Beyond structural imaging, MRI has evolved to include functional and microstructural imaging techniques. Functional MRI (fMRI) measures brain activity by detecting changes in blood oxygenation levels, known as the blood oxygenation level-dependent (BOLD) signal. This technique allows researchers to map neural activity during cognitive tasks and at rest, providing insights into functional connectivity and brain disorders. The BOLD signal is governed by changes in local deoxyhemoglobin concentration, which alters magnetic susceptibility and influences MR signal intensity. The fundamental equation describing BOLD signal change over time can be expressed as:

$$\Delta S = S_0 \left(1 - e^{-\frac{t}{T_2^*}} \right), \tag{5}$$

where ΔS represents the signal change, S_0 is the baseline signal intensity, and T_2* is the effective transverse relaxation time influenced by blood flow and oxygenation.

Another powerful MRI variant is diffusion tensor imaging (DTI), which measures the movement of water molecules in brain tissue to map white matter tracts. Since water diffusion is anisotropic in myelinated fibers, DTI captures directional movement patterns, revealing the structural connectivity of the brain. The diffusion process is described by the diffusion tensor equation:

$$S = S_0 e^{-bD}, \tag{6}$$

where S is the diffusion-weighted signal, S_0 is the baseline signal, b is the diffusion weighting factor, and D represents the diffusion coefficient. By analyzing diffusion properties, DTI provides valuable insights into white matter integrity, aiding in studying neurodegenerative diseases, traumatic brain injury, and psychiatric disorders.

MRI has become the gold standard for brain imaging due to its high spatial resolution, ability to image multiple tissue contrasts, and lack of radiation exposure. It is widely used in diagnosing neurological conditions such as Alzheimer's disease, epilepsy, and brain tumors, as well as in cognitive neuroscience research. However, MRI has certain limitations, including its longer scan times compared to CT, higher costs, and sensitivity to motion artifacts. Additionally, the presence of metal implants or claustrophobia in patients can pose challenges. Despite these limitations, MRI remains the most comprehensive imaging technique for studying the brain. With continuous advancements, including ultra-high-field MRI, real-time imaging, and machine learning-based image processing, MRI continues to push the boundaries of neuroimaging. While MRI excels in anatomical and functional imaging, it does not directly measure biochemical processes, an area where positron emission tomography (PET) provides unique advantages by enabling molecular imaging of brain metabolism and neurotransmitter activity.

1.1.2.4 Positron Emission Tomography

PET is a molecular imaging technique that provides unique insights into brain function by detecting metabolic and biochemical activity rather than structural details [7]. Unlike CT and MRI, which primarily visualize anatomical features, PET allows researchers and clinicians to study physiological processes, such as glucose metabolism, neurotransmitter activity, and protein aggregation. This capability has made PET a powerful tool in neuroscience, particularly for diagnosing neurodegenerative disorders, psychiatric conditions, and brain tumors. PET imaging, developed in the 1970s, was built on the principles of positron-emitting radiotracers, which decay to produce gamma rays that can be detected to create functional brain maps. Over the years, advancements in radiopharmaceuticals and imaging technologies have significantly enhanced PET's specificity and diagnostic accuracy.

The fundamental principle of PET imaging involves the injection of a biologically active molecule labeled with a positron-emitting radionuclide, such as fluorine-18 (^{18}F), carbon-11 (^{11}C), or oxygen-15 (^{15}O). These isotopes undergo beta-plus (β^+) decay, emitting a positron that travels a short distance before colliding with an electron. This annihilation event results in the production of two gamma photons, each traveling in opposite directions at 511 keV energy. These photons are detected by a ring of scintillation detectors, and their point of origin is computed using the principles of coincidence detection. The fundamental equation governing the annihilation event follows:

$$e^{+} + e^{-} \rightarrow 2\gamma \text{ (511 keV each)}, \tag{7}$$

where a positron (e^{+}) and an electron (e^{-}) annihilate to produce two gamma photons.

In order to reconstruct the PET image, the scanner records the detected photon pairs and applies the inverse Radon transform, similar to CT imaging, but modified to account for the three- dimensional nature of PET emission data. The projection data are processed using iterative reconstruction algorithms, such as maximum likelihood expectation maximization (MLEM) and ordered-subset expectation maximization (OSEM), refining the image quality by iteratively estimating the most probable radiotracer distribution. The mathematical formulation of the likelihood function in MLEM reconstruction is expressed as:

$$P(N \mid \lambda) = \prod_{i=1}^{N} e^{-\lambda_i} \frac{\lambda_i^{n_i}}{n_i!}, \tag{8}$$

where λ_i represents the expected photon count in a given detector bin, and n_i is the observed photon count. This iterative approach improves spatial resolution and reduces noise in PET images, enabling more accurate quantification of metabolic activity.

A major strength of PET imaging lies in its ability to use different radiotracers to target specific biological processes. Fluorodeoxyglucose (^{18}F-FDG) is the most widely used tracer, measuring glucose metabolism and providing insights into brain energy consumption. Since many neurodegenerative diseases, such as Alzheimer's disease, involve metabolic decline in specific brain regions, FDG-PET is a key diagnostic tool for detecting early-stage pathology. In contrast, dopaminergic tracers, such as 18F-DOPA and 11C-Raclopride, are employed to study the dopamine system, making PET essential for diagnosing Parkinson's disease and other movement disorders.

Beyond metabolic imaging, PET has enabled significant breakthroughs in neurodegeneration research by using specialized tracers to visualize amyloid-beta and tau protein accumulation, hallmarks of Alzheimer's disease. ^{18}F-Florbetapir and ^{18}F-Flutemetamol selectively binds to amyloid plaques while ^{18}F-Flortaucipir targets tau neurofibrillary tangles, providing crucial biomarkers for early diagnosis and disease progression monitoring. Similarly, PET tracers for neuroinflammation, such as ^{11}C-PK11195 allows researchers to study the role of microglial activation in neurodegenerative diseases and psychiatric disorders.

Despite its advantages, PET imaging has limitations. The use of radioactive tracers requires strict regulatory controls and access to a cyclotron for isotope production, making PET less widely available than CT or MRI.

Additionally, PET has lower spatial resolution compared to MRI, making it less suitable for detailed anatomical assessments. However, PET-MRI hybrid systems have emerged as a powerful solution, combining MRI's high anatomical resolution with PET's functional specificity, enabling comprehensive brain imaging with reduced radiation exposure.

As neuroimaging advances, PET continues to be a crucial technique for studying brain function at the molecular level. Its ability to track neurotransmitter dynamics, detect early disease biomarkers, and monitor therapeutic responses makes it an invaluable tool for both research and clinical practice. While PET excels in functional imaging, MRI remains the dominant modality for structural assessments, and their complementary nature highlights the growing trend of multimodal imaging approaches in modern neuroscience.

1.1.3 ADVANCEMENTS AND TRENDS IN BRAIN IMAGE STUDIES

1.1.3.1 Process and Steps of Brain Image Processing

Brain imaging processing plays a crucial role in neuroimaging research and clinical applications by refining raw imaging data to extract meaningful information [8]. Brain images, whether obtained through MRI, CT, or PET, often contain artifacts, misalignments, and noise that must be corrected to ensure accurate analysis. The necessity of processing arises from the complexity of brain structures and the need for precise comparisons across subjects and imaging sessions. For example, in longitudinal studies tracking disease progression, small anatomical changes must be detected reliably. Similarly, differences in scanner hardware and acquisition parameters must be normalized in multi-center studies to enable consistent analysis. Processing techniques such as image registration, brain region segmentation, and intensity normalization help achieve these objectives by ensuring spatial alignment, structural delineation, and signal standardization across datasets.

Brain image processing involves several essential steps that prepare the data for subsequent analysis. Preprocessing typically includes noise reduction, bias field correction, and skull stripping to remove non-brain tissues. Registration (image alignment) is a fundamental step that aligns images from different subjects, time points, or modalities into a common coordinate system, facilitating cross-subject comparisons. Segmentation is another critical step that partitions brain images into different anatomical regions, such as gray matter, white matter, cerebrospinal fluid, or functionally distinct areas based on standardized atlases. These steps provide the foundation for subsequent analysis tasks, including statistical comparisons, disease classification, and functional connectivity assessments.

Brain Image Registration

Brain image registration is a fundamental process in brain imaging that aligns images from different subjects, time points, or modalities into a common spatial framework [9]. The necessity of registration arises from the inherent variability in brain anatomy across individuals, as well as positional differences due to patient movement or variations in acquisition protocols. In longitudinal studies, where subtle changes in brain structures must be tracked over time, precise alignment is critical to distinguishing actual physiological changes from image distortions. Similarly, in multimodal imaging, such as integrating MRI with

PET, accurate spatial correspondence ensures that anatomical and functional information can be meaningfully combined for better clinical interpretation. Without robust registration, comparisons across individuals or within the same subject over different time points would be unreliable, leading to inaccuracies in functional mapping, statistical analysis, and disease diagnosis. The process of image registration involves several key steps that systematically transform a moving image to match a fixed reference image. First, a transformation model is defined, which determines how the spatial coordinates of one image are mapped onto another. Depending on the complexity of the registration task, the transformation can be rigid, affine, or nonlinear. Rigid transformations involve only translations and rotations, preserving distances and shapes, making them suitable for intra-subject alignment in the same imaging modality. Affine transformations extend this by allowing scaling and shearing, providing additional flexibility for aligning images with slight distortions. In contrast, nonlinear transformations introduce complex, smooth deformations to accommodate anatomical differences across subjects, which is essential for inter-subject registration and cross-modal comparisons. Once the transformation model is chosen, a similarity metric is used to quantify how well the transformed moving image aligns with the fixed image. For unimodal registration, where images originate from the same modality, simple intensity-based metrics such as mean squared error (MSE) or normalized cross-correlation (NCC) are effective. However, for multimodal registration, where intensity distributions differ significantly, mutual information (MI) is widely used, as it measures statistical dependence rather than direct intensity differences:

$$MI(I_f, I_m) = \sum_{i,j} p_{ij} \log \frac{p_{ij}}{p_i p_j}, \tag{9}$$

where p_{ij} represents the joint probability distribution of pixel intensities between the fixed image I_f and the moving image I_m, while p_i and p_j denote their respective marginal distributions. After defining the similarity metric, an optimization algorithm iteratively refines the transformation parameters to maximize alignment. Methods such as gradient descent and Powell's method are commonly employed, adjusting parameters based on local or global similarity gradients. Finally, the transformed image is resampled onto the fixed image's coordinate grid using interpolation techniques to ensure smooth and artifact-free alignment.

Several registration algorithms have been developed to optimize spatial alignment in neuroimaging, each with advantages and limitations. The Demons algorithm, introduced by Thirion in 1998, is a nonlinear, optical flow-based method that estimates deformation fields by computing forces between image intensity gradients. It is computationally efficient and well-suited for small deformations but is sensitive to intensity variations and local minima, leading to inaccurate registration in highly heterogeneous brain structures. The Symmetric Normalization (SyN) algorithm, proposed by Avants et al. (2008), employs a diffeomorphic transformation model that ensures invertibility and topology preservation. SyN has become a gold standard in inter-subject registration, particularly in large-scale neuroimaging studies, due to its ability to capture smooth yet complex deformations. However, its computational cost is significantly higher than simpler methods, making it less suitable for time-sensitive applications. Another widely used approach is Elastix and ANTs registration, which combines rigid, affine, and nonlinear methods hierarchically. These frameworks offer high flexibility and accuracy but require careful parameter tuning to avoid overfitting or excessive deformation. The choice of algorithm depends on the specific requirements of the imaging study, with rigid methods being sufficient for intra-subject alignment, while non-linear approaches provide superior accuracy for inter-subject comparisons and cross-modal fusion.

A representative example of a registration algorithm is the Symmetric Normalization (SyN) method, implemented in the widely used ANTs framework. SyN models registration as an optimization problem where the goal is to find a smooth, invertible transformation $\phi(x)$ that maps the moving image onto the fixed image while preserving anatomical topology. The transformation is parameterized as:

$$\phi(x) = x + u(x), \tag{10}$$

where $u(x)$ is the displacement field that defines local deformations. The optimization process minimizes an energy function composed of a similarity metric and a regularization term:

$$E(\phi) = D(I_f, I_m \circ \phi) + \lambda R(\phi), \tag{11}$$

where D represents the similarity measure, such as mutual information, and R is a regulaization term enforcing smoothness constraints.

The SyN algorithm is iterative, refining the transformation field through an optimization loop. Below is a pseudo-code representation of the SyN method:

Algorithm 1 Symmetric Normalization (SyN)

Require: Fixed image I_f, Moving image I_m
Ensure: Registered image

Initialize deformation fields $\phi_{fm} - Id$, $\phi_{mf} - Id$ (identity mapping)
for each iteration **do**
  Compute update fields:
    $u_{fm} = \text{Grad}\ (I_f) \cdot (I_f - I_m \circ \phi_{fm})$
    $u_{mf} = \text{Grad}\ (I_m) \cdot (I_m - I_f \circ \phi_{mf})$
    Smooth update fields using Gaussian filter
    Update deformation fields:
  $\phi_{fm} = \phi_{fm} \circ \exp(u_{fm})$
  $\phi_{mf} = \phi_{mf} \circ \exp(u_{mf})$
end for
return Registered image:
$I'_m = I_m \circ \phi_{fm}$

By iteratively refining the displacement field and applying smooth regularization, SyN achieves accurate, topology-preserving alignment. This makes it particularly effective for cross-subject registration, where anatomical differences are more pronounced.

Image registration is a crucial step in brain imaging, ensuring spatial consistency across subjects, time points, and modalities. The process involves defining a transformation model, selecting a similarity metric, optimizing parameters, and resampling the transformed image. Different algorithms provide trade-offs between accuracy, computational efficiency, and robustness to intensity variations. Due to its ability to produce smooth, invertible deformations, the SyN algorithm has become a standard in neuroimaging studies, particularly in longitudinal and population-based analyses. As neuroimaging datasets grow in complexity, future advancements will likely focus on integrating deep learning-based registration methods to learn complex spatial mappings from large datasets, further enhancing speed and accuracy.

Brain Region Segmentation

Brain region segmentation is a fundamental task in neuroimaging that aims to partition the brain into meaningful anatomical or functional regions [10]. This step is critical for studying brain structure, mapping functional activity, and diagnosing neurological disorders. Segmentation allows for quantifying brain volume, cortical thickness, and tissue composition, which are essential for understanding neurodegenerative diseases, brain development, and individual variability. Additionally, segmentation is necessary for accurate feature extraction in machine learning-based disease prediction and for improving multimodal image fusion.

Brain region segmentation is closely tied to brain atlases and templates, such as the MNI152 space, AAL atlas, and Yeo's functional networks, which provide standardized references for defining brain regions. These atlases facilitate inter-subject comparisons and enable automated labeling of brain structures. However, due to anatomical variations and imaging artifacts, direct alignment with a standard atlas is insufficient, necessitating advanced segmentation methods to delineate individual brain regions accurately. Over the years, segmentation techniques have evolved from traditional rule-based methods to machine learning and, more recently, deep learning approaches.

Early segmentation methods primarily relied on intensity-based and atlas-based techniques. One of the simplest approaches is thresholding, where brain tissues are classified based on intensity values in MRI or CT images. For example, a binary thresholding function for segmenting gray matter *GM* can be expressed as:

$$S(x) = \begin{cases} 1, & \text{if } T_1 \le I(x) \le T_2 \\ 0, & \text{otherwise,} \end{cases} \quad (12)$$

where $I(x)$ is the intensity at voxel x, and T_1 and T_2 are manually defined intensity thresholds. While thresholding is computationally efficient, it lacks robustness to intensity variations and does not consider spatial relationships.

More sophisticated methods, such as Gaussian Mixture Models (GMM), assume that different brain tissues follow distinct intensity distributions. GMM models the probability distribution of intensities as a weighted sum of Gaussian components:

$$p(x|\theta) = \sum_{k=1}^{K} \pi_k \mathcal{N}(x|\mu_k, \Sigma_k), \tag{13}$$

where π_k is the mixing weight, π_k and Σ_k are the mean and covariance of the k-th Gaussian component. The parameters are optimized using the Expectation-Maximization (EM) algorithm, iteratively refining the classification. However, GMM does not incorporate spatial information, leading to noisy segmentations.

To overcome this limitation, Markov Random Fields (MRF) introduce spatial constraints by modeling the segmentation as a probabilistic graph. The segmentation label S at voxel x is estimated by minimizing an energy function:

$$E(S) = \sum_{x} D(x) + \lambda \sum_{x,y} V(S_x, S_y), \tag{14}$$

where $D(x)$ is the data term derived from intensity distributions, $V(S_x, S_y)$ is a smoothness term penalizing abrupt label changes, and λ controls the balance between data fidelity and smoothness. MRF-based methods significantly improve segmentation consistency but remain computationally intensive and sensitive to parameter tuning.

With the advent of machine learning, segmentation shifted towards supervised and unsupervised learning approaches, leveraging statistical models to improve accuracy. Random Forests (RF) and Support Vector Machines (SVMs) became popular due to their ability to learn complex decision boundaries. A Random Forest classifier for voxel-wise segmentation aggregates multiple decision trees, where the prediction for a voxel x is given by:

$$S(x) = \frac{1}{N} \sum_{i=1}^{N} T_i(x), \tag{15}$$

where $T_i(x)$ is the label predicted by the i-th decision tree, and N is the total number of trees. RF-based segmentation methods improved robustness to intensity variations and could incorporate texture and spatial features.

Another influential method is Active Shape Models (ASM), which incorporates prior shape knowledge for robust segmentation. ASM optimizes segmentation by minimizing a shape energy function:

$$E(S) = E_{data} + \alpha E_{shape}, \tag{16}$$

where E_{data} ensures alignment with intensity features and E_{shape} enforces anatomical constraints. ASM is particularly effective for segmenting highly structured regions like the hippocampus and ventricles, though it requires extensive manual annotation for training.

While machine learning methods improved segmentation accuracy, they relied heavily on handcrafted features, limiting their ability to generalize across diverse datasets. This challenge led to the rise of deep learning-based segmentation, which automatically learns feature representations from raw imaging data.

Deep learning has revolutionized brain region segmentation by enabling end-to-end learning of complex spatial and intensity patterns. One of the most widely used architectures is U-Net, a fully convolutional network (FCN) designed for biomedical image segmentation. U-Net follows an encoder-decoder structure, where the encoder extracts hierarchical features, and the decoder reconstructs the segmentation mask using upsampling layers. The segmentation output is refined through skip connections, preserving fine-grained spatial details. The key segmentation loss function used in U-Net is the Dice coefficient, defined as:

$$\mathcal{L}_{Dice} = 1 - \frac{2|P \cap G|}{|P| + |G|}, \tag{17}$$

where P is the predicted segmentation, and G is the ground truth.

Recently, transformers have been introduced into medical image segmentation to capture global contextual information. Swin-Transformer, a hierarchical vision transformer, replaces convolutional layers with self-attention mechanisms, allowing long-range dependencies to be modeled. The self-attention operation is computed as:

$$\text{Attention}(Q, K, V) = \text{softmax}\left(\frac{QK^T}{\sqrt{d_k}}\right)V, \tag{18}$$

where Q, K, V are query, key, and value matrices, and d_k is the dimension of the key vector. By leveraging self-attention, Swin-Transformer can segment brain regions more effectively than traditional CNNs, particularly in complex anatomical structures.

Another emerging method is Segment Anything Model (SAM), a foundation model trained on large-scale datasets to enable generalizable segmentation. Unlike previous deep learning approaches requiring extensive labeled data, SAM can segment new brain regions with minimal manual input using prompt-based learning.

Brain region segmentation is essential for neuroimaging, enabling quantitative analysis and disease assessment. Traditional methods, such as Gaussian Mixture Models and Markov Random Fields, provided early solutions but struggled with robustness. Machine learning techniques, including Random Forests and Active Shape Models, improved segmentation through statistical learning but required extensive feature engineering. Deep learning approaches, particularly U-Net, and Transformers, have set new benchmarks in segmentation accuracy by learning complex spatial and intensity relationships directly from data. As segmentation techniques continue to advance, future research is expected to focus on self-supervised learning and foundation models like SAM, which could further improve segmentation performance across diverse datasets and imaging modalities.

Advanced Techniques in Brain Image Processing

As neuroimaging technology continues to evolve, advanced image-processing techniques are required to extract meaningful insights from increasingly complex data [11]. Two major frontiers in brain image processing include the development of novel imaging modalities, such as Quantitative Susceptibility Mapping (QSM), and the fusion of multimodal imaging data, particularly the integration of MRI and PET. These advancements address critical challenges in neuroimaging by providing improved contrast for specific tissue properties and enabling comprehensive analyses that combine structural, functional, and metabolic information. Efficient processing of these advanced imaging modalities requires specialized algorithms that enhance image reconstruction, alignment, and analysis while preserving biological fidelity.

Quantitative Susceptibility Mapping (QSM) is an emerging MRI technique that precisely measures magnetic susceptibility variations in brain tissues. Unlike conventional MRI sequences, which rely on T1 or T2 contrast, QSM derives information from phase images acquired in gradient-echo sequences. This makes QSM highly sensitive to iron content, calcium deposits, and myelin density, enabling the study of neurodegenerative diseases such as Parkinson's disease, Alzheimer's disease, and multiple sclerosis. However, QSM processing presents unique challenges due to the ill-posed nature of susceptibility reconstruction. The core processing pipeline for QSM involves phase unwrapping, background field removal, and susceptibility inversion. The raw phase image from MRI is affected by phase wrapping artifacts, which must be corrected using unwrapping algorithms such as the Laplacian-based phase unwrapping method:

$$\phi_{unwrapped} = Laplacian^{-1}(\phi_{wrapped}). \tag{19}$$

After phase unwrapping, the next step is background field removal to eliminate non-local susceptibility sources, such as air-tissue interfaces. Techniques such as Sophisticated Harmonic Artifact Reduction for Phase Data (SHARP) and Projection onto Dipole Fields (PDF) are widely used. The final step, susceptibility inversion, reconstructs the magnetic susceptibility $\chi(x)$ from the observed local field $B_z(x)$ by solving the ill-posed dipole equation:

$$B_z(\mathbf{r}) = d(\mathbf{r}) * \chi(\mathbf{r}), \tag{20}$$

where $d(\mathbf{r})$ is the dipole kernel. Since direct inversion of this equation amplifies noise and artifacts, regularized methods such as Bayesian QSM and deep-learning-based QSM are employed:

$$\chi(\mathbf{r}) = \mathcal{F}^{-1}\left(\frac{\mathcal{F}\left(B_z(\mathbf{r})\right)}{\mathcal{F}\left(d(\mathbf{r})\right)} + \lambda R)(\chi)\right), \tag{21}$$

where $R(\chi)$ is a regularization term enforcing smoothness or sparsity constraints. Recent deep learning approaches, such as QSMnet, leverage convolutional neural networks (CNNs) to learn the inverse mapping from phase images to susceptibility maps, significantly improving accuracy and robustness. The ongoing development of QSM processing methods is expanding its clinical applications, providing a valuable tool for studying neurodegenerative and psychiatric disorders.

The fusion of multimodal imaging data has become an essential technique in neuroimaging, as no single imaging modality can provide a complete picture of brain function and pathology. Among multimodal techniques, integrating Magnetic Resonance Imaging (MRI) and Positron Emission Tomography (PET) has gained particular interest, as MRI provides high-resolution anatomical and functional data, while PET offers metabolic and molecular insights. Processing and fusing MRI-PET images requires sophisticated alignment and synthesis algorithms to achieve accurate spatial correspondence and complementary information extraction. A key challenge in MRI-PET fusion is image alignment, as MRI and PET are acquired using different physics principles, resulting in variations in resolution, contrast, and geometric distortions. Traditional methods use rigid or affine transformations followed by intensity-based similarity optimization. However, nonlinear deformable registration techniques, such as the Diffeomorphic Demons algorithm, have been employed to improve spatial alignment. The transformation function is computed by minimizing an energy function:

$$E(T) = D(I_{PET}, I_{MRI} \circ T) + \lambda R(T), \tag{22}$$

where $D(I_{PET}, I_{MRI} \circ T)$ measures intensity similarity, and $R(T)$ enforces spatial smoothness. Beyond spatial alignment, advanced fusion methods focus on cross-modal image synthesis, either enhancing PET images using MRI priors or generating synthetic PET images from MRI. One approach, known as DeepMR-PET, employs Generative Adversarial Networks (GANs) for PET image synthesis:

$$\min_{G} \max_{D} \mathbb{E}_{x \sim p_{\text{data}}(x)}\left[\log D(x)\right] + \mathbb{E}_{z \sim p_z(z)}\left[\log\left(1 - D(G(z))\right)\right], \tag{23}$$

where G is the generator producing synthetic PET images from MRI inputs, and D is the discriminator distinguishing real from synthesized images. By learning the underlying mapping between MRI and PET, DeepMR-PET allows functional information to be inferred from anatomical images, reducing the need for PET scans in certain clinical scenarios. Another advanced technique in MRI-PET fusion is Graph Convolutional Networks (GCNs), which model multimodal relationships using graph representations of brain connectivity. In GCN-based fusion, each brain region is treated as a node, and multimodal features are aggregated through spectral convolution:

$$H^{(l+1)} = \sigma\left(\tilde{D}^{-1/2}\tilde{A}\tilde{D}^{-1/2}H^{(l)}W^{(l)}\right), \tag{24}$$

where $H^{(l)}$ represents the feature matrix at layer l, $\tilde{A}$ is the adjacency matrix encoding multimodal relationships and $W^{(l)}$ is the learnable weight matrix. This method has been particularly useful in studying brain disorders like Alzheimer's, where structural and metabolic alterations co-occur.

Advanced brain image processing techniques are crucial for extracting meaningful information from novel imaging modalities and multimodal datasets. The processing of QSM has provided new insights into brain tissue composition by mapping magnetic susceptibility, yet its ill-posed nature requires sophisticated inversion techniques such as Bayesian regularization and deep learning-based QSM. Meanwhile, MRI-PET fusion has enabled more comprehensive analyses by integrating structural, functional, and metabolic data with methods ranging from deformable registration to GAN-based image synthesis. These advancements underscore the ongoing shift towards more integrative and data-driven approaches in neuroimaging, where machine learning and deep learning will continue to play a transformative role in improving image processing and analysis. As the field progresses, further innovations in multimodal fusion and novel image reconstruction will enhance our ability to diagnose and study neurological diseases with unprecedented precision.

1.1.3.2 Trends and Frontiers in Brain Imaging Analysis

Brain imaging analysis has become an essential tool for understanding neurological disorders, aiding clinical diagnosis and research. Advances in neuroimaging techniques have provided unprecedented insights into the structural, functional, and molecular characteristics of the brain, leading to significant progress in disease detection, progression monitoring, and personalized treatment strategies. The primary applications of brain imaging analysis include the diagnosis of neurodevelopmental disorders such as Autism Spectrum Disorder (ASD), neurodegenerative diseases like Alzheimer's Disease (AD) and Parkinson's Disease (PD), and brain tumors such as gliomas and glioblastomas. In ASD, brain imaging examines differences in brain connectivity and structural abnormalities that underlie social and cognitive impairments. In AD, neuroimaging biomarkers, including hippocampal atrophy and amyloid plaque deposition, have enabled early diagnosis and disease staging. In oncology, imaging analysis of brain tumors using MRI and PET has facilitated tumor grading, surgical planning, and treatment response assessment. Beyond disease-related applications, brain imaging is also employed in cognitive neuroscience, brain-computer interfaces (BCI), and mental health research, broadening its impact in medical and technological domains.

As brain imaging analysis continues to evolve, emerging trends in artificial intelligence, multi-modal data integration, and individualized biomarker discovery are shaping the future of the field.

Autism Spectrum Disorder Diagnosis

Autism Spectrum Disorder (ASD) is a neurodevelopmental condition characterized by deficits in social interaction, communication difficulties, and restricted or repetitive behaviors [12]. The heterogeneity of ASD poses significant challenges for early diagnosis and individualized treatment. While the exact etiology of ASD remains unclear, numerous studies have demonstrated that it is associated with altered brain connectivity rather than localized structural abnormalities. This suggests that ASD is a connectopathy, where disruptions in functional and structural networks contribute to cognitive and behavioral impairments. Functional Magnetic Resonance Imaging (fMRI) has emerged as a powerful tool for studying these atypical connectivity patterns, enabling researchers to map large-scale brain networks and identify ASD-related alterations in neural communication.

Functional MRI (fMRI) measures brain activity by detecting fluctuations in blood oxygenation level-dependent (BOLD) signals, which reflect neural activity indirectly. Since ASD is primarily linked to disruptions in functional brain networks, fMRI provides a crucial window into how different brain regions interact. The study of resting-state functional connectivity (rs-fMRI) has been particularly valuable in ASD research, as it allows for the examination of intrinsic brain activity in the absence of task-based stimulation.

In order to analyze functional connectivity, the brain is typically parcellated into distinct regions based on an anatomical or functional atlas (e.g., AAL, Harvard-Oxford, or Yeo's 7-network atlas). The time series extracted from each region is then used to compute pairwise connectivity measures, forming a brain connectivity matrix W, where each element W_{ij} represents the functional connection strength between regions i and j. A common approach is to use Pearson's correlation coefficient to quantify functional connectivity:

$$W_{ij} = \frac{\mathrm{cov}(X_i, X_j)}{\sigma_{X_i}\sigma_{X_j}}, \quad (25)$$

where X_i and X_j are the time series of brain regions i and j, and σ_{X_i}, σ_{X_j} are their respective standard deviations. Alternative connectivity metrics include mutual information (MI), wavelet coherence, and partial correlation, which capture different aspects of inter-regional relationships. In ASD research, studies have consistently reported disruptions in long-range connectivity, particularly in the default mode network (DMN), salience network (SN), and executive control networks, reflecting altered social cognition, sensory processing, and executive function.

Graph theory provides a powerful framework for analyzing the topological organization of brain networks in ASD. In this approach, the brain is modeled as a graph, where nodes represent brain regions, and edges correspond to functional or structural connections between them. Several key graph metrics are used to quantify network properties:

- Degree Centrality (k_i) measures the number of direct connections a node has:

$$k_i = \sum_j W_{ij};$$

- Clustering Coefficient (C_i) captures the tendency of a node's neighbors.

$$C_i = \frac{1}{k_i(k_i - 1)} \sum_{j,k} W_{ij} W_{jk} W_{ki};$$

- Global Efficiency (E_g) reflects the network's overall integration and information transfer efficiency:

$$E_g = \frac{1}{N(N-1)} \sum_{i \neq j} \frac{1}{d_{ij}};$$

where d_{ij} is the shortest path length between nodes i and j. ASD studies utilizing graph theory have identified reduced long-range connectivity and increased local clustering, leading to weaker global integration and stronger local segregation. This suggests that individuals with ASD exhibit hyper-connectivity within localized brain regions but disrupted communication across distant regions, potentially explaining their difficulties in integrating complex social and sensory information.

Given the complexity of brain networks, interpreting their role in ASD diagnosis requires advanced explainability techniques. Machine learning models trained on connectivity features have demonstrated strong classification performance in distinguishing ASD from neurotypical individuals. However, to improve clinical applicability, network explainability techniques such as Graph Attention Networks (GATs) and SHAP (Shapley Additive Explanations) have been employed to highlight the most discriminative brain connections. One approach is to apply node importance ranking based on classification contribution:

$$\text{Importance}\,(i) = \sum_j W_{ij} \cdot \alpha_j, \tag{26}$$

where α_j represents the learned importance weight of region j in a predictive model. Studies using these techniques have identified key ASD-related brain connections, particularly between the prefrontal cortex, posterior cingulate cortex, and temporal lobe, which are crucial for social cognition and executive function.

Brain imaging analysis for ASD has greatly benefited from advancements in fMRI-based network modeling and graph theory, providing deeper insights into the altered connectivity patterns associated with autism. The application of functional connectivity analysis and graph-based metrics has revealed widespread network disruptions, with reduced long-range connectivity and increased local clustering as prominent features of ASD. Furthermore, explainability techniques have facilitated the identification of key brain region interactions, offering potential biomarkers for improved ASD diagnosis. As neuroimaging data expands, future research will likely leverage deep learning models and large-scale multi-site datasets to refine ASD diagnostics further, ultimately contributing to more effective therapeutic strategies.

Alzheimer's Disease Diagnosis

Alzheimer's Disease (AD) is a progressive neurodegenerative disorder and the leading cause of dementia worldwide [13]. The disease is characterized by gradual neuronal loss, brain atrophy, and cognitive decline, particularly affecting memory, executive function, and spatial navigation. Pathologically, AD is associated with the accumulation of amyloid-beta (Aβ) plaques and tau protein neurofibrillary tangles, which trigger neuroinflammation and synaptic dysfunction, ultimately leading to widespread brain tissue degeneration. These pathological processes cause profound changes in brain structure, notably in the hippocampus, entorhinal cortex, posterior cingulate cortex, and precuneus, regions crucial for memory consolidation. The progression of AD follows a characteristic trajectory, starting with mild cognitive impairment (MCI) and advancing to severe dementia. Early detection of structural alterations in the brain is critical for identifying high-risk individuals and developing timely interventions. Structural Magnetic Resonance Imaging (sMRI) is a primary neuroimaging technique used for detecting and monitoring AD-related brain atrophy. Compared to other imaging modalities, sMRI provides high-resolution anatomical details, making it particularly effective for quantifying cortical thinning, ventricular enlargement, and hippocampal atrophy, all of which serve as structural biomarkers of AD progression. Advanced computational methods have been developed to extract meaningful features from sMRI for automated AD diagnosis and disease staging, ranging from traditional imaging biomarkers to deep learning-based approaches.

Early computational approaches for AD diagnosis relied on radiomics and image-based feature extraction. These methods involve quantifying morphological changes in brain structures, such as gray matter volume (GMV), cortical thickness, and hippocampal atrophy, as well as texture-based features capturing tissue heterogeneity. A commonly used metric for measuring hippocampal atrophy is volumetric analysis, where the volume of a brain region V_{ROI} is normalized relative to the total intracranial volume V_{TIV}:

$$\text{Atrophy Index} = \frac{V_{\text{ROI}}}{V_{\text{TIV}}}. \tag{27}$$

Machine learning classifiers, such as Support Vector Machines (SVMs), Random Forests, and Logistic Regression, have been extensively applied to these imaging features to classify individuals into AD, mild cognitive impairment (MCI), and cognitively normal (CN) groups. The classification function in an SVM model is typically defined as:

$$f(x) = \text{sign}\,(\mathbf{w}^T\mathbf{x} + b), \tag{28}$$

where $\mathbf{x}$ represents the feature vector, $\mathbf{w}$ is the learned weight vector, and b is the bias term. While these traditional methods have provided valuable insights, they require manual feature engineering and may fail to capture complex spatial relationships in brain atrophy patterns. The advent of deep learning has significantly improved AD diagnosis by enabling auto mated feature extraction from raw sMRI data. Convolutional Neural Networks (CNNs) have been particularly effective in capturing subtle structural changes across different brain regions. A typical CNN for AD diagnosis consists of multiple convolutional layers extracting hierarchical spatial features:

$$h_l = f(W_l * h_{l-1} + b_l), \tag{29}$$

where W_l represents the convolutional kernel at layer l, h_{l-1} is the feature map from the previous layer, and f is a non-linear activation function (e.g., ReLU). Recently, Vision Transformers (ViTs) have emerged as powerful alternatives to CNNs for AD classification, leveraging self-attention mechanisms to capture long-range dependencies in brain imaging data. The self-attention mechanism in a Transformer is defined as:

$$\text{Attention}\,(Q, K, V) = \text{softmax}\left(\frac{QK^T}{\sqrt{d_k}}\right)V, \tag{30}$$

where Q, K, V are query, key, and value matrices, and dk is the dimension of the key vector. Transformers have demonstrated superior performance in identifying subtle, spatially distributed atrophy patterns in AD, making them a promising tool for early disease detection. AD is a multi-factorial disease influenced by genetic, biochemical, and neurophysiological factors. Consequently, integrating multi-modal biomedical data has become an essential strategy for improving diagnostic accuracy. One key approach is MRI-PET fusion, which combines the high-resolution anatomical information of MRI with the metabolic and molecular insights from PET imaging. The fusion process involves deformable image registration to align MRI and PET scans, followed by feature extraction and joint classification:

$$F_{\text{fused}} = \alpha F_{\text{MRI}} + (1-\alpha) F_{\text{PET}}, \tag{31}$$

where α is a weighting parameter that balances structural and functional information. In addition to image fusion, feature-level fusion integrates imaging biomarkers with non-imaging data, such as genetic markers (APOE genotype), cerebrospinal fluid (CSF) biomarkers (Aβ and tau levels), and cognitive test scores. A common feature fusion strategy is concatenation-based fusion, where multimodal features $F_1, F_2, \ldots, F_n$ are combined into a unified representation:

$$F_{\text{multi-modal}} = [F_1, F_2, \ldots, F_n]. \tag{32}$$

Recent advancements have also explored decision-level fusion, where multiple classifiers trained on different modalities generate independent predictions, which are then aggregated using ensemble learning techniques like weighted voting or stacking. These multi-modal approaches have significantly improved the ability to predict early-stage AD (prodromal AD) and differentiate between Alzheimer's and other forms of dementia.

Given the complexity of AD pathology, ensuring that AI-driven diagnostic models are interpretable and clinically meaningful is crucial. Explainability techniques such as Gradient-weighted Class Activation Mapping (Grad-CAM) and SHAP (Shapley Additive Explanations) are commonly used to highlight the most informative brain regions contributing to AD classification. These methods assign importance scores to different brain regions, allowing researchers to identify key neuroimaging biomarkers associated with disease progression:

$$\text{SHAP importance} = \sum_{S \subseteq N \setminus \{i\}} \frac{|S|!\left(|N|-|S|-1\right)!}{|N|!}\left(f\left(S \cup \{i\}\right) - f\left(S\right)\right), \tag{33}$$

where $f(S)$ represents the predictive model's output based on a subset of features S.

Multi-modal biomarker analysis has identified hippocampal atrophy, increased amyloid deposition in the precuneus and posterior cingulate cortex, and disrupted functional connectivity in the default mode network (DMN) as critical indicators of AD progression. The discovery of these multi-modal biomarkers has significantly enhanced early AD detection and individualized risk assessment, paving the way for precision medicine approaches in dementia research.

The diagnosis of Alzheimer's Disease has greatly benefited from advancements in neuroimaging analysis, particularly through structural MRI-based atrophy quantification and deep learning-driven feature extraction. Traditional methods, such as radiomics and machine learning classifiers, have provided valuable diagnostic frameworks, but deep learning approaches like CNNs and Transformers have significantly improved accuracy by capturing subtle, spatially distributed atrophy patterns. Given the complex and multi-factorial nature of AD, integrating multi-modal biomedical data through MRI-PET fusion, genetic analysis, and cerebrospinal fluid biomarkers has further enhanced diagnostic precision. Explainability techniques have provided crucial insights into AD-related biomarkers, supporting early detection and personalized treatment strategies. As neuroimaging research advances, integrating deep learning, multi-modal fusion, and explainable AI will continue to drive innovation in AD diagnostics, ultimately improving clinical decision-making and patient outcomes.

Glioma Diagnosis

Gliomas are a group of primary brain tumors that arise from glial cells, which provide support and nourishment to neurons [14]. They are among the most common and aggressive types of brain tumors, with glioblastoma multiforme (GBM) being the most malignant form. Gliomas are characterized by rapid growth, infiltration into surrounding brain tissue, and poor prognosis. They are classified based on their histopathological features and malignancy grade, with glioblastoma being a grade IV tumor marked by the presence of necrosis and microvascular proliferation. Diagnosing gliomas involves both anatomical imaging to define tumor boundaries and functional imaging to assess the tumor's metabolic activity, tissue characteristics, and infiltrative behavior.

Gliomas differ significantly from neurodegenerative diseases and developmental disorders, such as Alzheimer's or autism, because they involve localized neoplastic growth, often with significant disruption to surrounding brain regions. Given the heterogeneity of gliomas and their variable progression, early diagnosis, precise tumor segmentation, and predicting prognosis are critical for determining the best treatment strategy, particularly since treatment plans can vary significantly based on tumor size, location, and genetic factors. This section discusses the two major diagnostic tasks in glioma management: tumor segmentation and prognostic prediction.

The segmentation of gliomas in brain imaging is a crucial step for accurate tumor de-lineation, which is necessary for surgical planning, radiation therapy, and post-treatment monitoring. Accurate segmentation of gliomas ensures that the tumor is correctly identified and its boundaries are distinguished from healthy tissue, which is essential for evaluating tumor response to treatment and detecting recurrence. Glioma segmentation has traditionally been performed manually, but due to the time-consuming and subjective nature of this approach, automated segmentation methods using machine learning and deep learning have become increasingly popular.

A common deep learning-based approach for glioma segmentation is using U-Net, a fully convolutional network that is particularly well-suited for medical image segmentation. U-Net's architecture consists of an encoder-decoder structure with skip connections that preserve high-resolution spatial features, which are crucial for identifying tumor boundaries. The loss function typically used for segmentation tasks in glioma is the Dice coefficient:

$$\mathcal{L}_{Dice} = 1 - \frac{2|P \cap G|}{|P| + |G|}, \tag{34}$$

where P represents the predicted tumor mask, and G is the ground truth. U-Net has been widely used for segmenting gliomas into distinct components, such as the core tumor, peritumoral edema, and the necrotic region, allowing for detailed analysis of tumor volume and response to therapy. In addition to U-Net, 3D convolutional neural networks (3D CNNs) have also been employed to process volumetric MRI data, which is beneficial for capturing three-dimensional tumor structures and spatial relationships.

Another emerging technique for glioma segmentation is Transformer-based models, such as Swin-Transformer, which leverage self-attention mechanisms to capture global context and long-range dependencies within the image. These models outperform CNNs in complex tasks, especially when dealing with heterogeneous tissue types and irregular tumor shapes. This approach allows the model to dynamically focus on critical regions of the glioma while preserving surrounding tissue information, improving segmentation accuracy for more complex glioma shapes, and variably enhancing the delineation of the tumor's interface with normal brain tissue.

In addition to precise tumor segmentation, predicting the prognosis of gliomas is another crucial task for guiding treatment and improving patient outcomes. Glioma prognosis involves predicting both the likelihood of tumor recurrence and distinguishing it from pseudoprogression, which is a common phenomenon where the tumor appears to enlarge temporarily after treatment due to radiation-induced inflammation rather than actual tumor growth. Ac- curate prognostic predictions can help clinicians decide on the most appropriate treatment strategies, such as chemotherapy, radiation therapy, or surgery.

Recent studies have shown that combining structural MRI, functional MRI, and PET can provide important insights into glioma prognosis. For example, PET imaging, using tracers such as 18F-FDG (fluorodeoxyglucose), can reveal areas of high metabolic activity associated with tumor recurrence, while MRI can highlight areas of tumor necrosis and edema. Machine learning techniques, including random forests and support vector machines (SVMs), have been applied to integrate these multimodal imaging features alongside clinical factors (such as patient age and Karnofsky performance status) to predict glioma recurrence and distinguish it from pseudoprogression.

A common approach to predict glioma recurrence involves training a classifier on a combination of radiomic features (e.g., texture, shape, and intensity) extracted from MRI and PET data. SVM is a popular classifier that can be formulated as:

$$f(x) = \text{sign}(\mathbf{w}^T\mathbf{x} + b), \tag{35}$$

where $\mathbf{x}$ is the feature vector of multimodal data, $\mathbf{w}$ is the weight vector learned by the SVM, and b is the bias term. Based on the learned features, these classifiers are trained to differentiate between recurrence and pseudoprogression.

Recently, deep learning models have also been used for prognostic prediction. Deep neural networks (DNNs) and CNNs are applied to multi-modal data (MRI, PET) to automatically learn discriminative features for recurrence prediction. In particular, multimodal fusion networks are trained to integrate MRI and PET data directly during the learning process, improving the robustness of predictions by leveraging complementary information from both modalities. These models can automatically extract high-level features and predict recurrence with high accuracy.

Glioma diagnosis involves complex tasks that require accurate segmentation of tumor regions and reliable prognostic predictions to guide treatment decisions. Tumor segmentation is facilitated by deep learning models, particularly U-Net and Transformer-based architectures, which can handle the heterogeneous nature of gliomas. Prognostic prediction, focusing on recurrence and pseudoprogression, benefits from multimodal imaging data fusion, integrating MRI and PET features with clinical information. Using machine learning classifiers, such as SVM and DNN, enables improved differentiation between recurrence and pseudoprogression, offering significant potential for personalized treatment. As glioma imaging analysis continues to evolve, integrating advanced deep learning models and multi-modal data will continue to push the boundaries of diagnosis and treatment planning, leading to better outcomes for patients with this challenging disease.

REFERENCES

[1] Maria Ayub and Antonello Mallamaci. 2023. An Introduction: Overview of Nervous System and Brain Disorders. pp 1–24. *In*: A. Imran and G. Hussain (eds). The Role of Natural Antioxidants in Brain Disorders. Food Bioactive Ingredients. Springer, Cham.

[2] Christopher D. Smyser, Abraham Z. Snyder and Jeffrey J. Neil. 2011. Functional connectivity MRI in infants: Exploration of the functional organization of the developing brain. NeuroImage. 56(3): 1437–1452.

[3] Keiichiro Minatohara, Mika Akiyoshi and Hiroyuki Okuno. 2016. Role of immediate-early genes in synaptic plasticity and neuronal ensembles underlying the memory trace. Frontiers in Molecular Neuroscience. 8: 78.

[4] Chiahui Yen, Chia-Li Lin and Ming-Chang Chiang. 2023. Exploring the frontiers of neuroimaging: A review of recent advances in understanding brain functioning and disorders. Life. 13(7): 1472.

[5] Geoffrey D. Rubin. 2014. Computed tomography: Revolutionizing the practice of medicine for 40 years. Radiology. 273(2S): S45–S74.

[6] Reda, Rodolfo, Alessio Zanza, Alessandro Mazzoni, Andrea Cicconetti, Luca Testarelli and Dario Di Nardo. 2021. An update of the possible applications of

magnetic resonance imaging (MRI) in dentistry: A literature review. Journal of Imaging. 7(5): 75.

[7] Johannes Schwenck, Dominik Sonanini, J.M. Cotton, Hans-Georg Rammensee, Christian la Fougère, Lars Zender, et al. 2023. Advances in PET imaging of cancer. Nature Reviews Cancer. 23(7): 474–490.

[8] Tal Yarkoni, Russell A. Poldrack, Thomas E. Nichols, David C. Van Essen and Tor D. Wager. 2011. Large-scale automated synthesis of human functional neuroimaging data. Nature Methods. 8(8): 665–670.

[9] Mark Jenkinson, Christian F. Beckmann, Timothy E.J. Behrens, Mark W. Woolrich, Stephen M. Smith. 2012. FSL. NeuroImage. 62(2): 782–790.

[10] Ivana Despotović, Bart Goossens and Wilfried Philips. 2015. MRI segmentation of the human brain: challenges, methods, and applications. Computational and Mathematical Methods in Medicine. 2015(1): 450341.

[11] Christos Davatzikos. 2019. Machine learning in neuroimaging: Progress and challenges.

[12] H.K. Hughes, R.J. Moreno and P. Ashwood. 2023. Innate immune dysfunction and neuroinflammation in autism spectrum disorder (ASD). Brain, Behavior, and Immunity. 108: 245–254.

[13] Amir Abbas Tahami Monfared, M.J. Byrnes, Leigh Ann White and Quanwu Zhang. 2022. Alzheimer's disease: epidemiology and clinical progression. Neurology and Therapy. 11(2): 553–569.

[14] Michael Weller, Martin van den Bent, M. Preusser, Emilie Le Rhun, Jörg C. Tonn, Giuseppe Minniti, et al. 2021. EANO guidelines on the diagnosis and treatment of diffuse gliomas of adulthood. Nature Reviews Clinical Oncology. 18(3): 170–186.

Chapter **1.2**

Technical Foundations

Jin Liu*, Mengshen He and Jianxin Wang
Hunan Provincial Key Laboratory on Bioinformatics,
School of Computer Science and Engineering,
Central South University, Changsha 410083, China

1.2.1 INTRODUCTION

1.2.1.1 Supervised and Unsupervised Learning

Supervised learning and unsupervised learning are two essential paradigms in the field of machine learning, each serving distinct purposes and employing different methodologies. They address diverse types of problems and have significant applications in a wide range of domains. Supervised learning represents a fundamental paradigm in machine learning that aims to establish a mapping function between input features and their corresponding target outputs through labeled training data. This methodology is particularly effective for tasks with well-defined outcomes, such as classification and regression problems. The learning process involves optimizing a model's parameters by minimizing the discrepancy between predicted and actual outputs, ultimately enabling the model to generalize to unseen data.

Core supervised learning algorithms include:

- **Support Vector Machines (SVM):** A sophisticated classification algorithm that constructs an optimal hyperplane to maximize the margin between classes. For a binary classification problem, the decision function is given by:

*For Correspondence: Jin Liu (liujin06@csu.edu.cn)

DOI: 10.1201/9781003518754-3

$$f(x) = \text{sign}\left(\sum_{i=1}^{n} \alpha_i y_i K(x_i, x) + b\right) \quad (1)$$

where

- $y_i \in \{+1, -1\}$ represents the class labels
- α_i are the Lagrange multipliers obtained through optimization
- $K(x_i, x)$ is the kernel function measuring similarity between input x and support vector x_i
- b is the bias term
- sign is the signum function which returns +1, 0, or –1, though 0 is typically not used in binary classification.

Common kernel functions include:

- Linear: $K(x_i, x) = x_i^T x$
- Polynomial: $K(x_i, x) = (\gamma x_i^T x + r)^d$
- Radial Basis Function (RBF): $K(x_i, x) = \exp(-\gamma \|x_i - x\|^2)$

- **Random Forests:** An ensemble method combining multiple decision trees. The final prediction for classification is:

$$\hat{y} = \text{mode}\left\{h_k(x) : k = 1, \ldots, K\right\} \quad (2)$$

where $h_k(x)$ represents the prediction of the k-th tree, and K is the total number of trees.

- **Logistic Regression:** A probabilistic classification model that estimates the probability of class membership using the logistic function:

$$P(y = 1 \mid x) = \frac{1}{1 + e^{-(\beta_0 + \beta^T x)}} \quad (3)$$

where β_0 is the intercept and β are the feature coefficients.

- **Multilayer Perceptron (MLP):** A versatile architecture modeling complex non-linear relationships. For a single neuron:

$$y = \sigma\left(\sum_{i=1}^{n} w_i x_i + b\right) \quad (4)$$

where σ is the activation function, w_i are weights, and b is the bias.

Supervised learning has numerous real-world applications, including:

- **Image Classification:** Training models on labeled image data to identify objects or scenes automatically.
- **Disease Prediction:** Building predictive models for medical diagnostics using labeled healthcare data.
- **Sentiment Analysis:** Using labeled text data to classify the sentiment (e.g., positive or negative) of written content.

Unsupervised learning focuses on discovering hidden patterns and structures in unlabeled data. Unlike supervised learning, it does not rely on predefined output labels but instead learns the intrinsic properties of the data. This paradigm is widely applied to clustering, dimensionality reduction, and anomaly detection tasks.

Key unsupervised learning algorithms include:

- **Clustering Algorithms:** Group similar data points together, revealing natural groupings within data.
  - **K-Means:** Partitions data into K clusters by minimizing the within-cluster sum of squares:

$$J = \sum_{j=1}^{k} \sum_{x_i \in C_j} \| x_i - \mu_j \|^2 \tag{5}$$

  where C_j represents the set of data points in cluster j, and μ_j is the center of cluster j.
  - **Hierarchical Clustering:** Creates a tree-like structure by calculating distances between clusters. Common distance metrics include complete linkage (maximum distance), single linkage (minimum distance), and average linkage (average distance), providing a multi-scale view of the data.
- **Dimensionality Reduction Algorithms:** Reduce data dimensions while preserving key information, aiding visualization and complexity reduction.
  - **Principal Component Analysis (PCA):** Achieves linear dimensionality reduction by projecting onto orthogonal directions of maximum variance. The method first computes eigenvectors of the data covariance matrix, then projects data onto eigenvectors corresponding to the largest eigenvalues, effectively extracting the main directions of variation.
  - **Independent Component Analysis (ICA):** Separates mixed signals into statistically independent components, commonly used for blind source separation. ICA assumes observed signals are linear mixtures of independent source signals and estimates mixing and unmixing matrices to recover the original signals, which are widely applied in EEG and audio signal processing.

Unsupervised learning has diverse applications, such as:

- **Data Clustering:** Grouping customers in marketing for targeted campaigns using clustering algorithms.
- **Feature Extraction:** Reducing the complexity of high-dimensional datasets by identifying key features.
- **Anomaly Detection:** Identifying outliers in data distributions is critical for fraud detection or fault monitoring.

In summary, supervised and unsupervised learning are the two foundational paradigms that underpin machine learning. While supervised learning focuses on predictive modeling using labeled data, unsupervised learning emphasizes discovering patterns and structures in unlabeled data. Together, they provide the theoretical and practical basis for addressing a wide variety of machine-learning problems [1, 2].

1.2.1.2 Classification, Regression, and Clustering Methods

Classification, regression, and clustering constitute the three primary task types in machine learning, each addressing distinct problem domains and playing a critical role in various applications. These methods are widely employed due to their ability to handle diverse data characteristics and achieve specific objectives.

Classification methods aim to predict discrete labels by learning the relationship between input features and predefined categories. In other words, classification tasks aim to assign data points to one of a set of distinct classes. Such methods are widely used in applications like disease diagnosis, spam detection, and image recognition.

Classification models predict discrete labels by establishing a mapping between input features and predefined categories, commonly implemented through sophisticated algorithms such as SVM, Random Forests, and MLP. These models are extensively applied in medical diagnosis, text categorization, and image recognition, effectively addressing complex classification challenges. Performance evaluation for classification tasks is fundamentally derived from confusion matrix elements [True Positives (TP), True Negatives (TN), False Positives (FP), and False Negatives (FN)], which form the basis for comprehensive metrics, including accuracy, precision, recall, and F1-score, providing quantitative criteria for model selection and optimization.

Regression methods are designed to predict continuous output variables by modeling the relationship between input features and target values, commonly applied in scenarios where numerical predictions are required, such as forecasting housing prices, stock trends, or clinical scores. Common regression algorithms include Linear Regression (a simple method that assumes a linear relationship between input and output variables), Support Vector Regression (SVR) (a regression extension of SVM that can handle non-linear relationships), and Gradient Boosting Regression (a powerful ensemble method capable of capturing complex non-linear patterns). These algorithms each have their own characteristics and can be selected based on data complexity and application requirements, providing effective predictive capabilities for solving real-world problems.

The performance of regression models is evaluated using error metrics between predicted values and actual values, which quantify the prediction accuracy across the dataset. Common evaluation metrics include Mean Squared Error (MSE), which measures the average of squared differences between predictions and actual values; Mean Absolute Error (MAE), which calculates the average of absolute differences between predictions and actual values; and Coefficient of Determination (R^2) which measures the proportion of variance in the dependent variable explained by the model. These metrics offer complementary advantages in different application scenarios, providing essential criteria for model selection and optimization.

Clustering is an unsupervised learning method to discover natural groupings or structures within data. Unlike classification, clustering does not rely on predefined labels but instead identifies groups based on similarities in the data. Clustering is widely used in fields such as market segmentation, image segmentation, and anomaly detection.

The performance of clustering methods is typically evaluated using the following metrics:

- **Silhouette Coefficient:** A measure of how similar a data point is to its cluster compared to other clusters.
- **Clustering Purity:** Evaluates the alignment between clustering results and true categories.

In summary, classification, regression, and clustering represent the three main task types in machine learning, each suited for discrete label prediction, continuous value prediction, and data grouping, respectively. In practical applications, these methods are often combined with specific evaluation metrics and validation strategies to ensure their reliability and generalization capabilities [3–5].

1.2.1.3 Feature Engineering and Data Preprocessing

Feature engineering and data preprocessing are fundamental steps in the machine learning pipeline, directly influencing model performance, generalization ability, and computational efficiency. These stages aim to improve data quality, extract meaningful information, and ensure machine learning models can effectively learn from the data.

Data preprocessing focuses on improving the quality, consistency, and comparability of data through a series of systematic operations. Key steps include:

- **Data Cleaning:** Addressing issues such as missing values, outliers, and duplicate entries to ensure data integrity and accuracy.
- **Standardization and Normalization:** Transforming data to a uniform scale to eliminate the effects of differing feature magnitudes, which helps models converge faster and perform better.
- **Denoising:** Removing random noise from the data using filtering or other noise reduction techniques to enhance signal quality.
- **Batch Transformation:** Adjusting data distributions for imbalanced datasets to ensure fair representation of all classes and improve model training.

The primary goal of preprocessing is to ensure high-quality data as the foundation for feature engineering and subsequent model training. Feature engineering involves designing, extracting, and selecting the most discriminative features that maximize the data's utility for the target task. It is a critical step in improving model accuracy and interpretability. Key aspects include:

- **Feature Extraction:** Deriving meaningful features from raw data. For example, common features in image data include morphological features, statistical features, and texture features.

- **Feature Selection:** Identifying and retaining the most relevant features while discarding redundant or irrelevant ones. This can be achieved using filter methods, wrapper methods, or embedded methods.
- **Feature Construction:** Creating new features by combining or transforming existing ones to capture underlying patterns in the data.

The primary objective of feature engineering is to enhance the model's ability to learn meaningful patterns and relationships within the data.

Dimensionality reduction techniques are frequently used in feature engineering to reduce the number of features, mitigate the curse of dimensionality, and improve computational efficiency. Common methods include:

- **t-Distributed Stochastic Neighbor Embedding (t-SNE):** A non-linear dimensionality reduction method that preserves local relationships between data points in the reduced space.
- **Linear Discriminant Analysis (LDA):** A supervised dimensionality reduction approach aims to maximize the separation between classes by optimizing the ratio of between-class variance to within-class variance.

Dimensionality reduction not only reduces computational complexity but also helps improve model robustness and interpretability by eliminating redundant or noisy features.

In summary, feature engineering and data preprocessing are essential components of the machine learning pipeline. They are pivotal in improving data quality, extracting key patterns, and reducing computational complexity. By carefully designing and implementing these steps, machine learning models can achieve superior performance and generalization capabilities in real-world applications [6].

1.2.2 DEEP LEARNING FOUNDATIONS

As a pivotal branch of machine learning, deep learning has achieved breakthrough advancements in brain image analysis through its powerful feature learning and representation capabilities. Compared to traditional machine learning approaches, deep learning can automatically extract hierarchical feature representations, thereby more effectively capturing complex patterns and high-level semantic information within brain imaging data.

This section systematically introduces key deep learning technologies in brain image analysis, encompassing fundamental network architectures such as Artificial Neural Networks (ANN), Convolutional Neural Networks (CNN), Graph Neural Networks (GNN), Recurrent Neural Networks (RNN), Generative Adversarial Networks (GAN), and Vision Foundation Models, along with optimization strategies and representative application scenarios. These deep learning methodologies provide more sophisticated solutions for brain image analysis, demonstrating significant advantages, particularly in processing large-scale, high-dimensional medical imaging datasets.

1.2.2.1 Artificial Neural Networks

Artificial Neural Networks constitute the foundation of deep learning, drawing inspiration from the structure and function of biological neural systems. These networks consist of multiple interconnected layers of neurons that adaptively adjust their parameters through a learning process to perform complex pattern recognition and data mapping. The essential components and operational principles of neural networks include:

- **Neuron Model:** The fundamental computational unit comprises inputs, weights, biases, and activation functions that perform weighted summation and non-linear transformation.
- **Network Architecture:** Consisting of input, hidden, and output layers, each extracting features at different levels of abstraction.
- **Forward Propagation:** The process by which information flows from the input layer through hidden layers to the output layer, generating predictions.
- **Backpropagation:** The optimization process of calculating gradients and updating network parameters based on loss functions, forming the core learning mechanism.

In brain image analysis, artificial neural networks demonstrate powerful modeling capabilities by learning hierarchical features from complex neuroimaging data, enabling tasks such as brain structure segmentation, disease classification, and prognosis prediction [7, 8].

1.2.2.2 Convolutional Neural Networks (CNN)

Convolutional Neural Networks represent one of the most successful deep learning architectures for processing image data, with their specialized network structure particularly well-suited for brain imaging data with inherent spatial structures. Through local connectivity, weight sharing, and hierarchical feature extraction, CNNs effectively learn spatial hierarchical features in images, enabling high-precision visual tasks. Core components of CNNs include:

- **Convolutional Layers:** Extract local features through convolution kernels, effectively capturing spatial patterns and structural information in brain images while preserving spatial topological relationships.
- **Pooling Layers:** Downsample feature maps to reduce computational complexity, enhance feature robustness, and expand the receptive field.
- **Fully Connected Layers:** Integrate spatial features to complete final classification or regression tasks, mapping high-dimensional features to target output spaces.

In brain image analysis, CNNs are widely applied to lesion detection, tissue segmentation, disease classification, and prediction tasks, typically outperforming traditional image processing methods. For instance, CNNs demonstrate exceptional accuracy and reliability in early diagnosis of Alzheimer's disease, precise segmentation of brain tumors, and classification of neuropsychiatric disorders [9–12].

1.2.2.3 Graph Neural Networks (GNN)

Graph Neural Networks are specialized deep learning models designed for processing graph-structured data, offering unique advantages in brain network analysis. Unlike traditional neural networks, GNNs can learn directly on irregular topological structures, preserving relational information between nodes and making them particularly suitable for analyzing structural and functional connectivity patterns in the brain.

Key features of GNNs in brain network analysis include:

- **Node Representation:** Learning vector representations of brain regions that capture both local and global topological information, reflecting the role and importance of each region within the overall network
- **Edge Features:** Modeling connection strength and functional relationships between brain regions, characterizing interaction patterns and information transfer between neuronal populations
- **Graph Convolution:** Information propagation and feature aggregation on graph structures, enabling hierarchical feature extraction from local connections to global brain network properties

GNNs demonstrate powerful modeling capabilities in brain functional network analysis and disease diagnosis tasks. For instance, by learning about brain connectivity graphs constructed from functional MRI (fMRI) or diffusion tensor imaging (DTI), GNNs can identify abnormal connection patterns in neuropsychiatric disorders such as autism spectrum disorder and schizophrenia, providing new computational tools for early diagnosis and intervention [13–15].

1.2.2.4 Recurrent Neural Networks (RNN)

Recurrent Neural Networks are specialized deep learning architectures designed for processing sequential data, playing a crucial role in dynamic brain image analysis. Unlike feedforward neural networks, RNNs maintain internal hidden states that preserve historical information, enabling them to capture temporal dynamics and evolutionary patterns in brain activity. Core components and characteristics of RNNs include:

- **Recurrent Structure:** Processing sequential data through recurrent connections in hidden states, where each time step's output depends on both current input and previous hidden states
- **Long Short-Term Memory (LSTM):** Addressing the vanishing gradient problem in traditional RNNs through gating mechanisms that selectively retain and update information

- **Gated Recurrent Unit (GRU):** A simplified variant of LSTM that achieves similar functionality with fewer parameters, offering greater computational efficiency for certain tasks
- **Bidirectional RNNs:** Considering both past and future information simultaneously, enhancing contextual understanding and feature extraction capabilities

In brain image analysis, RNNs are widely applied to functional MRI (fMRI) time series analysis, epileptic seizure prediction, monitoring progression of neurodegenerative diseases, and analyzing resting-state functional network dynamics, offering new research perspectives for understanding the temporal dynamics of the brain and disease mechanisms [16, 17].

1.2.2.5 Generative Adversarial Networks (GAN)

Generative Adversarial Networks provide a novel research paradigm for brain image analysis through adversarial learning between generator and discriminator. GANs consist of two neural networks: a generator that creates realistic images and a discriminator that attempts to distinguish between real and generated images. This competitive mechanism drives continuous improvement in the generator, ultimately producing high-quality synthetic images. Core design elements and working principles of GANs include:

- **Adversarial Training:** Generator and discriminator are trained through a zero-sum game, forming a dynamic equilibrium that enhances overall system performance
- **Latent Space Representation:** Encoding key features of brain images in a low- dimensional latent space, enabling efficient image generation and manipulation
- **Conditional Generation:** Producing brain images based on specific conditions (such as disease labels or patient information), enhancing controllability
- **Cycle Consistency:** Maintaining content consistency in image translation tasks, ensuring preservation of semantic information before and after transformation

In brain image analysis, GANs are widely applied to image enhancement (improving brain image quality, reducing noise and artifacts), data augmentation (generating synthetic samples to expand training datasets, addressing data scarcity), and cross-modal translation (achieving conversion between different imaging modalities, such as mapping from MRI to CT), providing powerful technical support for brain disease research and clinical diagnosis [18, 19].

1.2.2.6 Vision Foundation Models

Vision Foundation Models (such as Transformer, ViT) represent the latest advancements in deep learning, demonstrating enormous potential in brain image analysis. These models transcend the limitations of traditional convolutional neural networks through self-attention mechanisms and large-scale pre-training, introducing new analytical paradigms and performance enhancements to brain imaging. Core characteristics and technical advantages of Vision Foundation Models include:

- **Self-attention Mechanism:** Capturing long-range dependencies in brain images, enabling global context modeling, and effectively identifying distant associations between anatomical structures and functional connections
- **Pre-training Strategies:** Acquiring universal visual representations through large-scale data pre-training, establishing powerful feature extractors that provide rich semantic and structural knowledge for downstream tasks
- **Transfer Learning:** Applying pre-trained models to specific brain image analysis tasks, significantly reducing the demand for annotated data and enhancing few-shot learning capabilities
- **Multimodal Integration:** Combining different modalities of brain data for more comprehensive analysis and understanding, mining cross-modal common features and complementary information

In brain imaging research, Vision Foundation Models have been successfully applied to brain tumor segmentation, neurodegenerative disease diagnosis, brain age prediction, and other tasks, demonstrating exceptional performance and generalization ability. These models excel in processing high-dimensional brain images with complex structures, more accurately capturing anatomical features and pathological changes, and providing powerful technical support for precision medicine and personalized diagnosis and treatment [20, 21].

REFERENCES

[1] Komal Sharma, Akwinder Kaur and Shruti Gujral. 2014. Brain tumor detection based on machine learning algorithms. International Journal of Computer Applications. 103(1): 7–11.

[2] Toufique A. Soomro, L. Zheng, A.J. Afifi, A. Ali, S. Soomro, M. Yin, et al. 2022. Image segmentation for MR brain tumor detection using machine learning: a review. IEEE Reviews in Biomedical Engineering. 16: 70–90.

[3] Evangelia I. Zacharaki, S. Wang, S. Chawla, D. Soo Yoo, R. Wolf, E.R. Melhem, et al. 2009. Classification of brain tumor type and grade using MRI texture and shape in a machine learning scheme. Magnetic Resonance in Medicine: An Official Journal of the International Society for Magnetic Resonance in Medicine. 62(6): 1609–1618.

[4] Zaixu Cui and Gaolang Gong. 2018. The effect of machine learning regression algorithms and sample size on individualized behavioral prediction with functional connectivity features. NeuroImage. 178: 622–637.

[5] Govindaraj Vishnuvarthanan, M.P. Rajasekaran, P. Subbaraj and A. Vishnuvarthanan. 2016. An unsupervised learning method with a clustering approach for tumor identification and tissue segmentation in magnetic resonance brain images. Applied Soft Computing. 38: 190–212.

[6] Sahan M. Vijithananda, Mohan L. Jayatilake, Badra Hewavithana, Teresa Gonçalves, Luis M. Rato, Bimali S. Weerakoon, et al. 2022. Feature extraction from MRI ADC images for brain tumor classification using machine learning techniques. Biomedical Engineering Online. 21(1): 52.

[7] Vincent A. Magnotta, Dan Heckel, N.C. Andreasen, T. Cizadlo, Patricia W. Corson, James C. Ehrhardt, et al. 1999. Measurement of brain structures with artificial neural networks: Two-and three-dimensional applications. Radiology. 211(3): 781–790.

[8] Fabian Isensee, Marianne Schell, Irada Pflueger, G. Brugnara, David Bonekamp, Ulf Neuberger, et al. 2019. Automated brain extraction of multisequence MRI using artificial neural networks. Human Brain Mapping. 40(17): 4952–4964.

[9] Jose Bernal, Kaisar Kushibar, Daniel S. Asfaw, S. Valverde, A. Oliver, R. Martí, et al. 2019. Deep convolutional neural networks for brain image analysis on magnetic resonance imaging: A review. Artificial Intelligence in Medicine. 95: 64–81.

[10] Nyoman Abiwinanda, Muhammad Hanif, S. Tafwida Hesaputra, Astri Handayani and Tati Rajab Mengko. 2019. Brain tumor classification using convolutional neural network. World Congress on Medical Physics and Biomedical Engineering 2018. Prague, Czech Republic 1: 183–189. Springer.

[11] Jeremy Kawahara, Colin J. Brown, Steven P. Miller, Brian G. Booth, Vann Chau, Ruth E. Grunau, et al. 2017. BrainNetCNN: Convolutional neural networks for brain networks; towards predicting neurodevelopment. NeuroImage. 146: 1038–1049.

[12] Sérgio Pereira, Adriano Pinto, Victor Alves and Carlos A. Silva. 2016. Brain tumor segmentation using convolutional neural networks in MRI images. IEEE Transactions on Medical Imaging. 35(5): 1240–1251.

[13] Alaa Bessadok, Mohamed Ali Mahjoub and Islem Rekik. 2022. Graph neural networks in network neuroscience. IEEE Transactions on Pattern Analysis and Machine Intelligence. 45(5): 5833–5848.

[14] Xiaoxiao Li, Yuan Zhou, Nicha Dvornek, Muhan Zhang, Siyuan Gao, Juntang Zhuang, et al. 2021. Braingnn: Interpretable brain graph neural network for fMRI analysis. Medical Image Analysis. 74: 102233.

[15] Hejie Cui, Wei Dai, Yanqiao Zhu, Xuan Kan, Antonio Aodong Chen Gu, Joshua Lukemire, et al. 2022. Braingb: A benchmark for brain network analysis with graph neural networks. IEEE Transactions on Medical Imaging. 42(2): 493–506.

[16] Eric Z. Chen, Puyang Wang, Xiao Chen, Terrence Chen and Shanhui Sun. 2022. Pyramid convolutional RNN for MRI image reconstruction. IEEE Transactions on Medical Imaging. 41(8): 2033–2047.

[17] Ruoxuan Cui, Manhua Liu and Alzheimer's Disease Neuroimaging Initiative. 2019. RNN-based longitudinal analysis for diagnosis of Alzheimer's disease. Computerized Medical Imaging and Graphics. 73: 1–10.

[18] Changhee Han, Leonardo Rundo, Kohei Murao, T. Noguchi, Yuki Shimahara, Zoltán Ádám Milacski, et al. 2021. MADGAN: Unsupervised medical anomaly detection GAN using multiple adjacent brain MRI slice reconstruction. BMC Bioinformatics. 22: 1–20.

[19] Hazrat Ali, Md. Rafiul Biswas, Farida Mohsen, Uzair Shah, Asma Alamgir, Osama Mousa, et al. 2022. The role of generative adversarial networks in brain MRI: A scoping review. Insights Into Imaging. 13(1): 98.

[20] Yue Sun, Limei Wang, Gang Li, Weili Lin and Li Wang. 2024. A foundation model for enhancing magnetic resonance images and downstream segmentation, registration and diagnostic tasks. Nature Biomedical Engineering. 1–18.

[21] Joseph Cox, Peng Liu, Skylar E. Stolte, Yunchao Yang, Kang Liu, Kyle B. See, et al. 2024. BrainSegFounder: Towards 3D foundation models for neuroimage segmentation. Medical Image Analysis. 97: 103301.

Chapter 1.3

AI-Empowered Fast Magnetic Resonance Imaging

Shanshan Wang[1*], Ruoyou Wu[1,2], Jing Yang[1,2], Wenxin Fan[1,2], Xinrui Ma[1,2], Hongming Wang[1] and Hongru Liu[1,2]

[1]Shenzhen Institutes of Advanced Technology, Chinese Academy of Sciences, Shenzhen 518055, China

[2]University of Chinese Academy of Sciences, Beijing 100049, China

1.3.1 AI-BASED STRUCTURAL MAGNETIC RESONANCE IMAGING

1.3.1.1 Introduction

Structural magnetic resonance imaging (sMRI) is a classic technique that uses magnetic resonance imaging to obtain the anatomical structures inside the human body. It is primarily used to observe the structure of the brain and other organs. It utilizes the behavior of hydrogen nuclei when they are excited by radiofrequency pulses in a strong magnetic field to generate data [1]. sMRI is a non-invasive imaging technique that can reveal different characteristics of underlying anatomical structures [2]. In clinical applications, sMRI is commonly used to detect and evaluate tumors [3], cerebral infarctions [4], cerebral hemorrhages [5], and other pathologies. With high-resolution images, it can accurately locate and assess the size, shape, and impact of lesions on surrounding tissues. Structural magnetic resonance imaging can provide clear anatomical images, aiding in detailed study and diagnosis. It also allows for obtaining images from multiple angles (axial, coronal, and sagittal), providing comprehensive structural information.

---

*For Correspondence: Shanshan Wang (ss.wang@siat.ac.cn)

DOI: 10.1201/9781003518754-4

Additionally, since it does not involve ionizing radiation, it is relatively safe for patients. However, compared to other imaging modalities, its data acquisition time is relatively long. This extended scanning time significantly limits the spatial and temporal resolution of MRI data and can also lead to motion artifacts. This has prompted research into various techniques to accelerate the MRI data acquisition process. Traditional methods for accelerating MRI data acquisition have primarily undergone three stages: fast sequence design [6], parallel imaging (PI) [7, 8], and compressed sensing (CS) [9]. With the rapid development of artificial intelligence, neural networks have found widespread applications in computer vision, medical image processing, speech recognition, and other fields [10]. Inspired by this progress, methods based on deep learning for accelerating structural magnetic resonance imaging have rapidly advanced [11–17]. Neural networks first utilize offline data for model training, enabling subsequent online reconstruction. Compared to traditional methods for accelerating magnetic resonance imaging, these deep learning-based approaches offer superior reconstruction quality and faster reconstruction speeds [11]. Based on the degree of reliance on fully sampled data during the training phase, these deep learning-based magnetic resonance imaging methods have roughly undergone a paradigm shift from supervised learning to semi-supervised learning and then to unsupervised learning. In order to provide readers with a comprehensive understanding of the entire process, this section first introduces three different learning paradigms: supervised learning, semi-supervised learning, and unsupervised learning. It then discusses research advancements in accelerating magnetic resonance imaging using these learning paradigms.

1.3.1.2 Three Learning Paradigms

Deep learning is a branch of machine learning capable of modeling and understanding complex patterns and representations in data. It has achieved significant success in some fields, such as computer vision, medical image processing, and speech recognition [10]. Compared to traditional methods, it has stronger feature extraction and learning capabilities. Based on reliance on fully sampled data, deep learning can be roughly divided into three paradigms: supervised, semi-supervised, and unsupervised.

Supervised Learning

Supervised learning is a fundamental paradigm that learns a mapping from inputs to targets using paired data. This means that the input data and labels in each training sample are paired. The target of supervised learning is to enable the model to learn the mapping between input data and model output to predict new or unseen samples correctly [18]. It has been widely applied in various fields, such as image and speech recognition, medical diagnosis, and natural language processing. The process of supervised learning includes steps such as data collection, data preprocessing, model selection, training, validation, hyperparameter tuning, and prediction. Once the model is trained, it can predict the corresponding target for new input data. In the supervised learning paradigm, given a paired dataset $\boldsymbol{D}_n = ((\boldsymbol{b}_1, \boldsymbol{x}_1), \ldots, (\boldsymbol{b}_n, \boldsymbol{x}_n)) \in (\mathcal{B} \times \mathcal{X})^n$, our target is to learn a function $f : \mathcal{B} \to \mathcal{X}$ such that all $f(b_i)$ approximate x_i. This is achieved by minimizing the following loss function:

$$R_{emp}(f_\theta) = \frac{1}{n} \sum_{i=1}^{n} L(f_\theta(\boldsymbol{b}_i), \boldsymbol{x}_i) \tag{1}$$

Here, θ represents the parameters or weights of the model f, and $L(\cdot)$ denotes the loss function used to characterize the difference between $f_\theta(b_i)$ and x_i, with commonly used loss functions including l_1 and l_2 losses. By various optimization algorithms, such as stochastic gradient descent (SGD), the loss function can be minimized. For structural MRI, supervised learning methods are one of the most classic learning paradigms, which typically learn the nonlinear mapping relationship between undersampled input and fully sampled data.

Semi-Supervised Learning

Semi-supervised learning, as a branch of machine learning, primarily leverages a small amount of labeled data and a large amount of unlabeled data to address certain learning tasks. Positioned conceptually between supervised and unsupervised learning, it leverages a large amount of unlabeled data alongside a smaller labeled dataset [19, 20]. In general, semi-supervised learning improves the performance of one of the tasks by utilizing information related to another task. For example, in a classification task, other samples with unknown labels might be used to assist the classification process. For semi-supervised learning, it includes three assumptions: the first is the smoothness assumption, which states that if two input points $b \in B$ and $b' \in B$ are close to each other in the input space, then their corresponding labels x and x' should be similar. The smoothness assumption can be applied transitively to unlabeled data. The second assumption is the low-density assumption, suggesting that the classifier's decision boundary ideally traverses low-density regions in the input space. In simpler terms, the decision boundary should avoid passing through high-density regions. The low-density assumption and the smoothness assumption are closely related to each other; the former can be viewed as a counterpart to the smoothness assumption for the underlying data distribution. The third assumption is the manifold assumption, which posits that sample points located on the same low-dimensional manifold should share the same label. In general, in semi-supervised learning, we have a dataset that includes a small labeled dataset $\{(b_i, x_i)\}$ and a large unlabeled dataset $\{b_j\}$. The learning objective is to use the labeled data to assist in the learning of the unlabeled data, which can be represented using the following combined loss function:

$$\min_\theta \sum_i L(f_\theta(\boldsymbol{b}_i, \boldsymbol{x}_i)) + \sum_j U(f_\theta(\boldsymbol{b}_j)), \tag{2}$$

where θ represents the parameters of the model, $L(\cdot)$ denotes the loss on the labeled data, and $U(\cdot)$ denotes the loss on the unlabeled data. In structural magnetic resonance imaging, semi-supervised learning methods can effectively utilize a large amount of undersampled data with only a small amount of fully sampled data.

Unsupervised Learning

Unsupervised learning is an important class of learning algorithms in machine learning that helps reveal inherent patterns or structures within data without external supervision. Typical objectives of unsupervised learning primarily include discovering similarities within a set of examples, determining data distributions, or performing dimensionality reduction [21]. Self-supervised learning can be considered a branch of unsupervised learning that utilizes the input data as supervision. Its characteristics include two aspects: one involves a "semi-automatic" process to obtain "labels" from the data itself. The other aspect involves predicting parts of the data from other parts. Specifically, the "other parts" referred to may be incomplete, deformed, or distorted [22]. Mathematically, the objective of unsupervised learning is to learn representations of data without explicit labels, often achieved by optimizing generative models that capture the underlying distribution of the data. Given a dataset $\boldsymbol{D}_n = \{\boldsymbol{b}_1, \boldsymbol{b}_2, \ldots, \boldsymbol{b}_n\}$ without labels, we aim to learn a model $p(\boldsymbol{b})$ that approximates the true data distribution $p_{data}(b)$. This can be achieved by optimizing the following objective function:

$$\max_{\theta} \sum_{i} \log p_{\theta}(\boldsymbol{b}_i), \tag{3}$$

where θ represents the parameters of the generative model, adjusting these parameters maximizes the likelihood of the data. In structural magnetic resonance imaging, training the model using only undersampled data is particularly suitable for scenarios where full-sampled data is limited.

1.3.1.3 Applications

Since Wang et al. [11] introduced deep learning into the field of magnetic resonance imaging, deep learning-based structural magnetic resonance imaging has developed rapidly. These methods have roughly shifted from supervised learning to semi-supervised learning and finally to unsupervised learning. Different learning paradigms have varying data requirements, and by reducing data dependency and increasing domain knowledge, the applicability of the models can be improved. This section will specifically introduce the applications of these methods in structural magnetic resonance imaging.

Supervised Learning for Fast sMRI

In structural magnetic resonance imaging, supervised learning methods are the most commonly used, relying on pairs of undersampled and fully sampled data. We have pairs of k-space data and corresponding image data $\{(b_i, x_i)\}_{i=1}^{n}$. First, we construct a neural network f, which is parameterized by θ. Then, we use the encoding matrix E_Ω to undersample the k-space data, obtaining the network's input. The network's output $f_\theta(b_\Omega, E_\Omega)$ and the fully sampled data x are used to compute the loss. The network model is optimized by minimizing the following objective function:

$$\min_\theta \frac{1}{n}\sum_{i=1}^{n} \ell\left(f_\theta\left(\boldsymbol{b}_\Omega^i, \boldsymbol{E}_\Omega^i\right), \boldsymbol{x}^i\right), \tag{4}$$

where Ω represents the undersampling matrix, and θ represents the model parameters. Supervised learning methods are mainly divided into two categories: data-driven methods and model unrolling-based methods. Data-driven methods primarily utilize extensive training data and powerful deep-learning techniques to learn mapping relationships and features from the data directly. They typically involve offline training, followed by online inference using the learned knowledge to recover clear images from undersampled k-space data [11, 23–41]. For example, Wang et al. [11] first trained a neural network in an end-to-end manner to learn the nonlinear mapping between undersampled magnetic resonance imaging and fully sampled acquisitions. Han et al. [23] designed a U-shaped network to recover high-resolution magnetic resonance imaging by reducing radial sampling and addressing data constraints using domain adaptation. Zhu et al. [28] proposed a unified framework called AUTOMAP, which utilizes manifold learning and sparse convolutional filters to address generalized reconstruction problems.

Although data-driven methods can perform better than traditional approaches, their model interpretability tends to be lower, often requiring large amounts of annotated data. Model unrolling-based methods are a technique that combines physical models with deep learning. They unfold the computational process of the physical model into a multi-step iterative procedure, mapping these iterative steps into layers of a deep neural network. This approach aims to enhance the performance of image reconstruction [42–53]. For example, Yang et al. [52] proposed an ADMM-Net model, the first application to compressive sensing magnetic resonance imaging using an unfolded iterative optimization algorithm. By introducing variables ADMM alternatively optimizes the following three subproblems:

$$\begin{cases} \boldsymbol{x}^{(k+1)} = \arg\min\limits_{x} \frac{1}{2}\left\|A\boldsymbol{x} - \boldsymbol{b}\right\|_2^2 - \sum\limits_{l=1}^{L}\left\langle \alpha_l^{(k)}, \boldsymbol{z}_l^{(k)} - D_l\boldsymbol{x}\right\rangle + \sum\limits_{l=1}^{L}\frac{\rho_l}{2}\left\|\boldsymbol{z}_l^{(k)} - D_l\boldsymbol{x}\right\|_2^2 \\ \boldsymbol{z}^{(k+1)} = \arg\min\limits_{z} \sum\limits_{l=1}^{L}\lambda_l g(z_l) - \sum\limits_{l=1}^{L}\left\langle \alpha_l^{(k)}, z_l - D_l\boldsymbol{x}^{(k+1)}\right\rangle + \sum\limits_{l=1}^{L}\frac{\rho_l}{2}\left\|z_l - D_l\boldsymbol{x}^{(k+1)}\right\|_2^2, \\ \alpha^{(k+1)} = \arg\min\limits_{\alpha} \sum\limits_{l=1}^{L}\left\langle \alpha_l, D_l\boldsymbol{x}^{(k+1)} - \boldsymbol{z}_l^{(k+1)}\right\rangle \end{cases} \tag{5}$$

where $k \in [1, 2,..., n]$ denotes the k-th iteration, $\alpha = \{\alpha_i\}$ denotes Lagrangian multipliers and $\rho = \{\rho_i\}$ denotes penalty parameters. For simplicity, let $\beta_i = \frac{\alpha_i}{\rho_i}(i \in [1, 2, \ldots, L])$ and $A = PF$, P is a under-sampling matrix, F is a Fourier transform. The three subproblems have the following solutions:

$$\begin{cases} X^{(k)} : \boldsymbol{x}^{(k)} = F^T\left[P^TP + \sum_{l=1}^{L} \rho_l F D_l^T D_l F^T\right]^{-1}\left[P^T\boldsymbol{y} + \sum_{l=1}^{L} \rho_l F D_l^T (\boldsymbol{z}_l^{(k-1)} - \beta_l^{(k-1)})\right] \\ Z^{(k)} : \boldsymbol{z}_l^{(k)} = h(D_l\boldsymbol{x}^{(k)} + \beta_l^{(k-1)}; \lambda_l/\rho_l), \\ M^{(k)} : \beta_l^{(k)} = \beta_l^{(k-1)} + \eta_l\left(D_l\boldsymbol{x}^{(k)} - \boldsymbol{z}_l^{(k)}\right) \end{cases} \tag{6}$$

where $h(;)$ is a nonlinear shrinkage function, and the parameter η_i is an update rate. The authors subsequently improved the ADMM algorithm and proposed Generic-ADMM-CSNet for compressed sensing imaging [53], which provides a new idea for MRI reconstruction. Model unrolling-based methods unfold known physical models, ensuring that the reconstruction results adhere to physical principles, thereby enhancing the model's reliability and physical consistency. However, unlike purely data-driven methods, model unrolling-based approaches require higher computational resources.

In supervised learning methods, various network architectures are used for undersampled structural magnetic resonance imaging. Among them, generative adversarial networks (GANs) are a popular choice. For example, Quan et al. [31] proposed a CS-MRI method that uses a residual convolutional GAN with cycle consistency loss during training to enforce data consistency. In addition to GANs, other network architectures such as ResNet, Transformer, recurrent neural networks (RNNs), diffusion models, and others have been studied to improve the reconstruction performance of structural MRI. Wu et al. [54] proposed a volumetric layer-wise deep ResNet to enhance feature sparsity and increase receptive field. In addition, uncertainty estimation is also an important research direction. For example, Schlemper et al. [55] introduced Bayesian deep learning techniques to model reconstruction uncertainty. They further designed a heteroscedastic loss to reduce model uncertainty and improve reconstruction performance. Supervised learning methods have significant advantages in structural magnetic resonance imaging, improving the accuracy of image reconstruction. However, these methods rely on large amounts of annotated data and computational resources.

Semi-Supervised Learning for Fast sMRI

Although supervised learning methods outperform traditional methods and provide the best results in many aspects, fully sampled data is difficult to obtain in many medical scenarios, and the available data is often insufficient for large deep-learning models. Semi-supervised learning is one of the classic learning paradigms in machine learning, primarily using a small amount of labeled data and a large amount of unlabeled data to perform specific tasks. It includes both supervised and unsupervised learning components, with the corresponding objective function as follows:

$$\min_{\theta} \frac{1}{n}\sum_{i=1}^{n}\ell_1\left(f_\theta(\boldsymbol{b}_\Omega^i, \boldsymbol{E}_\Omega^i), \boldsymbol{x}^i\right), \tag{7}$$

$$\min_{\theta} \frac{1}{m} \sum_{j=1}^{m} \ell_2\left(f_\theta(\boldsymbol{b}_\Omega^j, \boldsymbol{E}_\Omega^j), \hat{\boldsymbol{x}}^j \right), \tag{8}$$

where n and m represent the sample sizes used for supervised and unsupervised learning, respectively. Generally, n is much smaller than m, and $\hat{x}$ represents the pseudo-labels generated by the model trained through supervised learning.

Semi-supervised learning primarily employs three strategies to accelerate structural MRI image reconstruction: noise suppression [56], interpolation and filtering [57], and contrast image synthesis [58]. For example, Desai et al. [56] proposed a Noise2Recon method for joint reconstruction and denoising. Based on the smoothness assumption of semi-supervised learning, the model can adapt to perturbations in local inputs, implying that when small perturbations are applied to input data, the model's predictions should remain similar to those without perturbations. The objective function of Noise2Recon can be expressed as:

$$\min_{\theta} \mathbb{E}\left[\mathcal{L}_{sup}\left(f_\theta(\Omega \boldsymbol{b}^{(s)}), \boldsymbol{x}^{(s)} \right) \right] + \lambda \mathbb{E}\left[\mathcal{L}_{unsup}\left(f_\theta(\boldsymbol{b}^{(u)} + \varepsilon), f_\theta(\boldsymbol{b}^{(u)}) \right) \right], \tag{9}$$

where $x^{(s)}$ is the image space counterpart of $b^{(s)}$, Ω denotes undersampling mask, λ denotes a weighting coefficient, ε denotes a randomly generated masked noise map. Noise2Recon addresses the issue of the lack of labeled data in certain application environments and achieves joint reconstruction and denoising of MRI. Another work in this area is VORTEX, proposed in [59], which incorporates physics-driven data augmentation into a semi-supervised consistency training framework, enabling high-quality reconstruction even with a small amount of labeled data.

MRI imaging has various modalities, each playing a different role in clinical practice. However, a single case may only contain a few of these modalities, and some modalities are relatively difficult to obtain. Synthesizing modalities that are difficult to obtain from other commonly available modalities becomes one approach to solve this issue. For example, in reference [60], a new semi-supervised deep generative model called ssGAN is proposed to address the problem of multi-contrast MRI synthesis. An SSA-CGAN model was proposed [61], which learns from unpaired data points using adversarial loss. The cyclic loss enforces consistent reconstruction mapping, while another adversarial loss utilizes paired data points to address the issue of limited paired data. In general, semi-supervised learning provides an intriguing option for assisting MRI reconstruction despite relatively fewer studies conducted in this area.

Unsupervised Learning for Fast sMRI

The structural MRI image reconstruction methods based on supervised learning and semi-supervised learning use all or a small amount of fully sampled data as reference data for the model. However, obtaining fully sampled data in the MRI imaging field is challenging due to various constraints, and prolonged scanning can cause discomfort to patients. In this situation, studying how to optimize deep learning models without fully sampled data. Therefore, adopting unsupervised learning methods to address this issue is a good choice. These methods are primarily based on self-supervised learning approaches [62–74] and generative model methods [75–79]. Self-supervised learning methods primarily involve constructing reference data from the undersampled data to enable network training without fully sampled data. The corresponding loss function can be expressed as follows:

$$\min_{\theta} \frac{1}{n} \sum_{i=1}^{n} \ell\left(\boldsymbol{b}_{\Lambda}^{i}, \boldsymbol{E}_{\Lambda}^{i}\left(f_{\theta}(\boldsymbol{b}_{\Psi}^{i}, \boldsymbol{E}_{\Psi}^{i})\right)\right), \tag{10}$$

where the undersampled data is divided into two parts Ψ and Λ, and Ψ is used for model reconstruction, while Λ is used to calculate the loss function.

There have been studies utilizing self-supervised learning for structural magnetic resonance image reconstruction. For example, Yaman et al. [62] first introduced self-supervised learning into magnetic resonance image reconstruction and proposed the SSDU model. In this model, the original undersampled data is divided into two parts, with one part used for the DC layer of the model and the other part used for calculating the loss. This seminal work in self-supervised magnetic resonance image reconstruction inspires subsequent self-supervised learning methods. Although this approach achieves performance close to supervised learning methods, the reduction in learnable data due to data partitioning decreases model performance at high acceleration rates. To address this, the authors improved the original SSDU model and proposed a multi-mask SSDU method [65]. This method retrospectively divides Ω multiple times into disjoint sets Ψ and Λ. For each object i, let each segmentation $\Omega_i = \Psi_j \cup \Lambda_j$, $j = 1,\ldots,K$ represent the number of segmentations. Furthermore, $\Theta_j = \Omega \backslash \Lambda_j$, $j = \{1,\ldots,K\}$. The corresponding objective function is as follows:

$$\min_{\theta} \frac{1}{N \cdot K} \sum_{i=1}^{N} \sum_{j=1}^{K} \mathcal{L}\left(\boldsymbol{b}_{\Lambda_j}^{i}, \boldsymbol{E}_{\Lambda_j}^{i}\left(f_{\theta}\left(\boldsymbol{b}_{\Theta_j}^{i}, \boldsymbol{E}_{\Theta_j}^{i}\right)\right)\right), \tag{11}$$

The multi-mask method effectively leverages the measurement data by ensuring that the parts of the model input and loss calculation contain more low-frequency and high-frequency components. In addition, some studies incorporate Bayesian methods into solving inverse problems. Pang et al. [70] proposed a self-supervised deep learning recovery method that is implemented on a Bayesian deep network. This method predicts the uncertainty of the image by training the network with random weights. These methods provide a certain level of reliability guarantee for the reconstructed images.

Furthermore, unsupervised learning methods based on generative models have also been used in structural magnetic resonance imaging. These models primarily rely on Generative Adversarial Networks to generate corresponding target data using random distributions or undersampled data as inputs. For instance, Xia et al. [80] introduced a super-resolution algorithm based on conditional GANs for high-resolution and isotropic cardiac cine imaging. This algorithm combines optical flow components to generate auxiliary images that guide image synthesis, enabling the synthesis of three-dimensional isotropic, anatomically plausible, and slice-consistent cardiac MR images. Additionally, Lei et al. [81] employed WGAN for unpaired adversarial training and evaluated the quality of reconstructed images based on Wasserstein distance, effectively addressing the issue of model instability. Moreover, fractional diffusion models have been used to progressively accelerate the data distribution fitting in MRI [82]. The recent popularity of diffusion models has also brought new vitality to this field [83]. With the powerful capabilities of generative models, these methods have achieved excellent results. In addition to the methods mentioned above, other approaches, such as manifold learning and deep subspace learning, address the network training problem in the absence of fully sampled data. For instance, Zou et al. [84] proposed a variational manifold method for accelerating dynamic MRI. In recent years, there have been rapid developments in unsupervised learning-based techniques for fast structural magnetic resonance imaging. These techniques have achieved performance comparable to supervised learning, effectively reducing the reliance on fully sampled data.

1.3.1.4 Summary

In summary, deep learning-based methods for structural magnetic resonance imaging have experienced rapid development and yielded promising results. These methods have undergone a paradigm shift from supervised learning to semi-supervised learning and finally to unsupervised learning. While these methods offer powerful learning capabilities, they lack strong guidance from traditional iterative algorithms. Combining traditional compressive sensing with deep learning techniques will facilitate the development of more versatile and interpretable models, leading to improved performance. However, there are challenges to address, such as performance evaluation, model stability, generalization, and privacy preservation. Through further research in the future, these issues will gradually be resolved.

1.3.2 AI-BASED QUANTITATIVE MAGNETIC RESONANCE IMAGING

1.3.2.1 Introduction of qMRI

Quantitative magnetic resonance imaging (qMRI) is a powerful non-invasive imaging technique that enables precise quantification of various biophysical and biochemical properties of tissues [85]. These properties include:

Diffusion Characteristics: Quantifies the microscopic diffusion of water molecules within tissues and is sensitive to the integrity and organization of tissue microstructures, such as cell membranes, fibers, and extracellular matrix.

Relaxation Times: The qMRI can measure the transverse (spin-spin) relaxation time constant T2 and the longitudinal (spin-lattice) relaxation time constant T1, which are influenced by the chemical environment, tissue microstructure, and macromolecular content of the tissue, providing insights into tissue composition and pathological changes.

Myelin Water Fraction: The qMRI techniques, such as multicomponent T2 relaxometry, can non-invasively quantify the myelin content in the central nervous system by measuring the fraction of water protons trapped within the myelin sheaths surrounding axons.

Perfusion: The qMRI perfusion imaging techniques, like arterial spin labeling, can quantify tissue blood flow and blood volume without the need for exogenous contrast agents, enabling the assessment of tissue metabolism and vascular integrity.

A key strength of qMRI is its ability to generate quantitative parametric maps [86], where the measured physical quantities are expressed in standardized units (e.g., diffusion coefficients in mm^2/s, relaxation times in ms, perfusion in ml/100g/min), and these calibrated, reproducible measurements across different MRI scanners and institutions are crucial for enabling objective disease diagnosis, treatment monitoring, and multicenter research studies.

Traditionally, qMRI data reconstruction follows a two-step process. First, multiple contrast images are generated from the acquired k-space data using different acquisition parameters, such as repetition time, diffusion weighting, or echo time. These parameters lead to reconstructed images with varying contrasts. In the second step, a signal model is applied to these images to estimate the qMRI parameters. These parameters reflect the biophysical and biochemical properties of the tissue, including water diffusion, relaxation times, myelin water fraction, and perfusion. This process yields quantitative, calibrated, and reproducible measurements essential for accurate disease diagnosis, treatment monitoring, and multicenter research studies.

The traditional process of acquiring multiple contrast images for qMRI reconstruction typically requires extensive scan times, limiting its clinical use. Reducing these scan times has become a significant research priority. One strategy to achieve this is by undersampling the k-space, capturing only a fraction of the full k-space data for each contrast image. However, significant undersampling can cause ill-posed inverse problems for the individual contrast images, leading to artifacts in the final reconstructed images. This trade-off between scan time reduction and image quality has been an ongoing challenge in the field of qMRI, necessitating the development of advanced image reconstruction and parameter estimation techniques that can accurately estimate the qMRI parameters from the undersampled k-space data without incurring significant image degradation [87].

1.3.2.2 AI-based Fast Quantitative Magnetic Resonance Imaging

Recently, artificial intelligence (AI) has shown significant potential for reconstructing undersampled magnetic resonance (MR) data, especially deep learning methods [88], which are particularly relevant for the field of quantitative magnetic resonance imaging where the acquisition of multiple contrast images with complete k-space coverage is time-consuming and often impractical in a clinical setting. Artificial intelligence reconstruction methods have demonstrated the ability to effectively handle the ill-posed inverse problem arising from the undersampling of k-space data, leveraging the powerful representation learning capabilities of deep neural networks to learn complex relationships between the undersampled k-space measurements and the desired fully-sampled contrast images. By training these artificial intelligence models on large datasets of paired undersampled and fully-sampled MR data, they can learn to accurately predict the missing k-space information and reconstruct high-quality contrast images, which can then be used for the subsequent estimation of qMRI parameters, thereby allowing for substantial reductions in scan time without compromising the quantitative accuracy and reproducibility that is crucial for clinical diagnosis and research applications.

AI-based fast quantitative magnetic resonance imaging techniques can be broadly classified into direct qMRI and indirect qMRI [87]. The indirect qMRI approach, analogous to traditional qMRI methods, entails reconstructing multiple-contrast magnetic resonance images, which are subsequently used to estimate quantitative parameters via physical or computational models. We will discuss these methods in more depth in the following sections.

Indirect Reconstruction

This part primarily discusses the two-stage approach, wherein image reconstruction is first performed to generate contrast images, followed by the estimation of quantitative magnetic resonance imaging parameters by fitting signal models to the reconstructed images, thereby enabling the extraction of biophysically meaningful parameters that characterize the underlying tissue properties.

Image Reconstruction

AI-based image reconstruction employs neural networks trained to produce images free from artifacts. This section examines research that utilizes the redundant information found in contrast images during the neural network training phase. In this approach, AI-based reconstruction is treated as an advanced artifact removal task. The network is fed aliased images generated using Fourier transform methods, allowing it to learn complex patterns for effective artifact reduction and high-quality image reconstruction. A neural network $\mathcal{H}(\check{\boldsymbol{Z}}|\theta)$, parameterized by $\boldsymbol{\theta}$, is designed to take aliased contrast images $\check{\boldsymbol{Z}}$ as model input and produce artifact-free contrast images $\hat{\boldsymbol{I}}$ as model output [89–91]:

$$\hat{\boldsymbol{I}} = \mathcal{H}(\check{\boldsymbol{Z}}|\theta) \tag{12}$$

The network parameters $\boldsymbol{\theta}$ are determined through a training phase prior to image reconstruction, which can be formulated as:

$$\hat{\theta} = \arg\min_{\theta} \sum \mathcal{L}\left(\boldsymbol{W}_t, \mathcal{H}(\boldsymbol{Z}_t \,|\, \boldsymbol{\theta})\right), \tag{13}$$

where $\mathcal{L}$ represents the corresponding loss function, $\boldsymbol{W}_t$ and $\boldsymbol{Z}_t$ represent the datasets used for model training. Specifically, $\boldsymbol{Z}_t$ is used for network input, corresponding to low-quality data. W_t represents reference data corresponding to high-quality data, which can be fully sampled image domain data or k-space data, depending on the specific application scenario. For instance, a classical loss function, such as the sum of squared differences, can be employed when training with fully sampled k-space data [92]:

$$\hat{\theta} = \arg\min_{\theta} \sum_{t} \left\| W_t - \varepsilon \mathcal{H}(Z_t \mid \theta) \right\|_2^2, \tag{14}$$

The iterative reconstruction framework can also be integrated into the neural network model [93–96]. In this scenario, the optimization problem can be expressed as:

$$\hat{I} = \arg\min_{I} \left\| Y - \varepsilon I \right\|_2^2 + \sum_{i}^{n^i} \lambda_i \left\| \phi_i(I) \right\|_l, \tag{15}$$

where ε is modified to a generative neural as a regularizer:

$$\hat{I} = \arg\min_{I} \left\| Y - \varepsilon I \right\|_2^2 + \lambda \left\| \mathcal{H}(\hat{Z} \mid \theta) - I \right\|_l. \tag{16}$$

The neural network can be trained on various types of datasets [97, 98], including previously acquired datasets, synthetic datasets [99], or a combination of both [91]. Additionally, training can be performed on image patches rather than the entire image. Even with limited training data, this approach can yield neural network models with good performance [100]. Furthermore, self-supervised learning is also an effective method that does not rely on fully sampled data [90]. The input data typically consists of real-valued images [100–103]. In addition, complex neural networks have also been explored to utilize the phase information fully to improve subsequent parameter estimation. These methods explore the correlation between the real and imaginary parts of complex images by using complex convolution inspired by complex multiplication [97].

A range of neural network architectures have been explored for image reconstruction, including U-NET, which has been successfully applied in various image reconstruction tasks [101, 104]. Fully connected convolutional neural networks have demonstrated promising results in image denoising and reconstruction [103, 105]. Multiscale residual networks have been shown to capture multiscale features effectively in images [100]. Deep cascades of residual dense networks have been employed to leverage the strengths of both residual and dense connections [99]. Deep, complex residual networks have been designed to handle complex-valued images and exploit the correlations between real and imaginary components [97].

Parameter Estimation

AI-based estimation techniques employ neural networks to approximate the inverse of the qMRI model function, enabling the reconstruction of high-quality and high-fidelity parameter maps from low-quality contrast images generated during input images reconstruction step. A neural network $\mathcal{H}(\hat{Z} \mid \theta)$ is utilized, where the network outputs estimated parameter maps: $\widehat{X} = \mathcal{H}(\widehat{\boldsymbol{Z}} \mid \theta)$ [104, 106–113]. The model's training process is similar to that in Equation 13, but with Z_t representing input images with artifact and W_t representing the artifact-free parameter maps.

Various loss functions have been developed to enhance the performance of neural networks. For example, some loss functions use the mean squared error of each estimate, first normalizing it using the corresponding Cramér-Rao bound (CRB) and then averaging across all estimated parameter maps and training samples [114]. Additionally, total variation regularization can be combined with mean squared error to create a composite loss function, which results in smoother reconstructed parameter maps [115]. Complex-valued contrast images are also used for training neural network models, effectively enhancing the accuracy of parameter quantification [116, 117]. Additionally, random forest regression [118] and kernel regression [119] methods have also been used to estimate artifact-free quantitative parameter maps from contrast images, though these images may contain undersampling artifacts. Additionally, deep learning frameworks have also been used to accelerate multi-parameter estimation [120]. Additionally, explainable neural network frameworks for parameter matching that leverage the advantages of attention mechanisms have also been studied [121].

Direct Reconstruction

Direct Model-based Reconstruction

Methods within the direct model-based reconstruction subcategory leverage the inherent redundancies in the data by incorporating a physics-based signal model or physical prior knowledge into the reconstruction process, thereby enabling the exploitation of domain-specific information to constrain the solution space and improve the accuracy of the estimated quantitative magnetic resonance imaging parameters [122–126].

(1) In model-based synthetic parameter images via AI in qMRI, a significant challenge arises from the disturbances introduced by imperfections in real scans, such as B_0 inhomogeneities, particularly in non-Cartesian sampling trajectories, which can substantially compromise quantitative accuracy [127]. In order to mitigate these disturbances, the conventional approach involves acquiring a large number of images, typically exceeding the number of unknowns in the physical model, thereby rendering the problem overdetermined. However, this approach comes at the cost of prolonged scan times, making qMRI a time-consuming process. Therefore, developing methods capable of accurately estimating parameter maps from fewer acquired images is of paramount importance.

Recently, deep neural networks have been explored for mapping fewer acquired images to parameter maps, but these networks often require substantial training data and can be prone to instability [128, 129]. In order to overcome these limitations, two primary strategies have been proposed. The first strategy focuses on predicting missing images through a replenishment network. This network learns the physics-based relationships among images, exploiting the fact that missing and acquired images reside within the same manifold represented by a physical model. The second approach involves utilizing a correction network to remove disturbances, thereby enhancing the overall quality of the images. Both methods leverage the principles of physics to learn the connections implicitly between generated and acquired images. Additionally, parameter maps can be estimated from the output images of the network using either conventional parameter fitting or network fitting. This section demonstrates two exemplary applications of this approach: quantitative magnetization transfer (qMT) imaging and diffusion tensor imaging (DTI).

Quantitative magnetization transfer imaging seeks to provide a quantitative measurement of the macromolecular content of tissue, exploiting the magnetization transfer effect. Conventional qMT protocols involve acquiring multiple images at various off-resonance frequencies for subsequent parameter fitting, which unfortunately leads to prolonged scan times. Recently, the qMTNet architecture was proposed to generate 2D qMT parameter maps from a reduced number of four off-resonance images by leveraging a missing image generation strategy [129]. The qMTNet framework comprises two subnetworks: qMTNet-acq, which generates eight missing off-resonance images from the four acquired images, and qMTNet-fit, which subsequently processes the complete set of 12 images to estimate the qMT parameters. Notably, a direct fitting network that operates on the four off-resonance images was also evaluated, but its performance was found to be less stable compared to the qMTNet architecture, which incorporates a generation module to augment the input data.

Diffusion tensor imaging is a noninvasive technique that allows for the evaluation of tissue microstructure and structural connectivity within the human brain. The DTI model estimates a 3×3 symmetric diffusion tensor matrix, denoted as $\mathbf{D}$, which comprises six unknown parameters. In theory, the estimation of the diffusion tensor requires only one nondiffusion image (the b0 image) and six diffusion-weighted images (DWIs). However, in practical applications, a larger number of DWIs are typically acquired to compensate for the inherently low signal-to-noise ratio (SNR) associated with the images. Consequently, this leads to longer scan times. In order to overcome this limitation, deep learning-based approaches have been proposed. These methods aim to estimate diffusion parameters using a reduced set of six DWIs and one b0 image for 2D DTI [128, 130]. One example of a method addressing this challenge is DeepDTI [130]. It begins by carefully selecting six diffusion-weighted images with optimized diffusion encoding directions. These directions are determined by minimizing the condition number of the diffusion tensor transformation matrix and maximizing uniformity. Next, a convolutional neural network (CNN) is utilized to enhance the quality of the DWIs. This CNN takes both the DWIs and an anatomical T1-weighted image as inputs. Then, traditional tensor fitting methods can be used to estimate the corresponding diffusion tensors from the improved DWI images, thereby enhancing the accuracy of the estimates.

(2) In most AI-based quantitative magnetic resonance imaging techniques, the model-integrated regularization term and loss function are designed such that the predominant loss measures the disparity between the estimated parameter maps and their corresponding parameter labels. By exploiting the physical and

imaging models, it becomes possible to generate synthetic contrast images and synthetic k-space data based on the estimated maps. The discrepancies between these input and synthetic data can be incorporated as a supplementary loss term within the network. This additional term serves the purpose of enforcing data consistency (DC) and preserving model fidelity.

$$\begin{cases} \mathcal{L} = \lambda_1 \mathcal{L}_1 + \lambda_2 \mathcal{L}_2 \\ \mathcal{L}_1 = \left\| \hat{\mathbf{x}} - \mathbf{x} \right\|_F^2 \\ \mathcal{L}_2 = \left\| \hat{\rho}_t - \rho_t \right\|_F^2 \quad \text{or} \quad \left\| \hat{\mathbf{B}}_t - \widehat{\mathbf{B}_t} \right\|_F^2 \end{cases}, \tag{17}$$

The optimization problem is formulated as a trade-off between two terms with λ_1 and λ_2 serving as regularization parameters that balance the contributions of each term. The network estimates the parameter $\hat{\mathbf{x}}$, and $\hat{\rho}_t = \mathbf{A}(\hat{\mathbf{x}}, t)$ and $\widehat{\mathbf{B}}_t = \mathbf{E}\hat{\rho}_t$ represent the synthetic contrast images and k-space data, respectively.

This approach opens up the possibility of training a qMRI network without requiring labeled parameter maps. Specifically, a network can be trained solely using the $\mathcal{L}_2$ loss term, eliminating the need for the $\mathcal{L}_1$ loss term, which relies on the labeled parameter maps in Equation (17). The discrepancies between the synthetic and input data are utilized to enforce network "self-supervision," enabling self-supervised or unsupervised learning. Additionally, additional regularization terms that don't rely on labeled data can be integrated into the $\mathcal{L}_2$ loss term to further improve reconstruction performance.

The Magnetization Transfer Contrast Mapping using Magnetic Resonance Fingerprinting (MTC-MRF) approach employs a deep neural network to estimate magnetization transfer-related parameters, but this supervised learning method necessitates a large amount of labeled training data and considerable time for training. In order to address these limitations, an unsupervised learning architecture [131] was designed to tackle the complex nonlinear inverse mapping problem in 3D MTC-MRF.

Subsequently, these network outputs, along with additional acquired T2 maps and MRF scan parameters, were utilized to generate synthetic MTC-MRF images through the two-pool Bloch-McConnell simulation. The loss function can be expressed as:

$$\mathcal{L} = \| \hat{\rho}_t - \rho_t \|_F^2 , \tag{18}$$

where $\hat{\rho}_t$ represents the machine-acquired data, and ρ_t denotes the synthesized MTC-MRF data. Compared to traditional non-deep learning methods, this approach requires only a small amount of unlabeled data for training and can reduce training time by approximately 1,000 times.

(3) Iterative model consistency network design

As formulated in Equations 19 and 20,

$$\hat{\mathbf{x}} = \arg\min_{\mathbf{x} \in \mathbb{C}^{N \times N_p}} \frac{1}{2} \| \mathbf{A}(\mathbf{x}, t) - \rho_t \|_F^2 + \mathcal{R}(\mathbf{x}), \tag{19}$$

$$\hat{\mathbf{x}} = \arg\min_{\mathbf{x}\in\mathbb{C}^{N\times N_p}} \frac{1}{2} \| \mathbf{EA}(\mathbf{x}, t) - \mathbf{B}_t \|_F^2 + \mathcal{R}(\mathbf{x}; \rho_t), \tag{20}$$

where $\mathbf{x}$ represents the vectorized parameter map, and N_p represents the number of parameters to be estimated; $\mathbf{A}(\mathbf{x}, t) = [\mathbf{A}(\mathbf{x}, t_1), \mathbf{A}(\mathbf{x}, t_2), \ldots, \mathbf{A}(\mathbf{x}, t_L)]$, $\rho_t = [\rho_{t_1}, \rho_{t_2}, \ldots, \rho_{t_L}]$, L represents the total number of samples, $\boldsymbol{B}_t = [\boldsymbol{b}_{t_1}, \boldsymbol{b}_{t_2}, \boldsymbol{b}_{t_L}]$, represents the acquired k-space data. $\mathbf{E}$ denotes the forward encoding operator and $\mathcal{R}(\mathbf{x}; \rho_t)$ indicates the joint regularization of the parameter maps and images.

The fast qMRI problem can be formulated as an optimization task, with the parameter map considered an unknown variable. Traditionally, iterative algorithms have been used to solve this problem. However, with the rise of AI, these iterations can be transformed into a deep network, allowing for the learning of regularization and data fidelity terms. Each iteration is represented as a network module, incorporating the physical model into the measurement operator within the network. This operator, known as the data consistency layer, maps the parameter maps to the raw data space, ensuring data consistency. Typically, the network is trained in a supervised manner, optimizing the parameter maps by minimizing the discrepancy between the predicted and actual measurements.

A deep model-based magnetic resonance parameter mapping network, referred to as DOPAMINE [132], has been developed for rapid 3D T1 mapping of the brain, utilizing a variable flip angle (VFA) gradient echo sequence. The DOPAMINE framework consists of two primary components: a parameter mapping network and an artifact-removing network. First, the parameter mapping network is used to estimate the initial parameter maps from the undersampled k-space data. Then, the artifact removal network is employed to eliminate the aliasing artifacts in the parameter maps. Notably, an interleaved data consistency layer is embedded within the artifact-removing network to ensure data fidelity, thereby guaranteeing that the reconstructed parameter maps adhere to the physical constraints imposed by the MR signal formation process. Specifically, DOPAMINE represents the regularization term in Equation 20 as

$$\mathcal{R}(\mathbf{X}) = \| \mathbf{X} - \mathcal{D}_{\mathbb{R}}(\mathbf{X}) \|_2^2, \tag{21}$$

where $\mathcal{D}_{\mathbb{R}}(\mathbf{X}): \mathbb{C}^{N\times 1} \mapsto \mathbb{C}^{N\times 1}$ denotes a convolutional neural network denoiser. Then, Equation 21 can be rewritten as follows:

$$\widehat{\mathbf{X}} = \arg\min_{X} \frac{1}{2} \| \mathbf{A}(\mathbf{X}) - \mathbf{B}_t \|_F^2 + \lambda \| \mathbf{X} - \mathcal{D}_{\mathbb{R}}(\mathbf{X}) \|_2^2, \tag{22}$$

where $\mathbf{A}$ is the variable flip angle T1 model. The least squares problem in Equation 22 is typically solved using iterative optimization algorithms based on stochastic gradient descent. When the perturbation is small, the gradient of $\mathcal{D}_{\mathbb{R}}(\mathbf{X})$ can be approximated as zero. The corresponding computation process can be expressed as:

$$\begin{aligned} \mathbf{X}_{k+1} &= \mathbf{X}_k - 2\mu_k \left[\mathbf{J}_{\mathbf{A}}^{\mathbf{H}}(\mathbf{X}_k)\left(\mathbf{A}(\mathbf{X}_k) - \mathbf{B}_t\right) + \lambda_k \left(\mathbf{X}_k - \mathcal{D}_R(\mathbf{X}_k)\right) \right] \\ &= (1 - 2\lambda_k\mu_k)\mathbf{X}_k - 2\lambda_k\mu_k\mathcal{D}_R(\mathbf{X}_k) - 2\mu_k\mathbf{J}_{\mathbf{A}}^{\mathbf{H}}(\mathbf{X}_k)\left(\mathbf{A}(\mathbf{X}_k) - \mathbf{B}_t\right), \end{aligned} \tag{23}$$

where $\mathbf{J_A}$ represents the Jacobian matrix of $\mathbf{A}$, and $\mathbf{J_A^H}$ represents the conjugate transpose of $\mathbf{J_A} \cdot \lambda_k$ and μ_k represent the regularization parameter and step size used by the model at the k-th iteration, respectively, and they are trainable parameters. The initial $\mathbf{X}_1 = (\mathbf{I}_0, \mathbf{T}_1)$ is generated from zero-filling T1-weighted images by the constructed network. In the DOPAMINE framework, the network $\mathcal{D}_{\mathbb{R}}$ is a CNN-based denoiser. Additionally, the physical model is incorporated into the operation of $\mathbf{J_A^H}$ in the model-based data consistency layer, as represented in Equation 23.

Direct Learning-based Reconstruction

Techniques within the direct learning-based reconstruction subcategory seek to complement traditional model-based reconstruction approaches by leveraging deep neural networks to directly estimate quantitative magnetic resonance imaging parameter maps from the acquired undersampled k-space data. Specifically, the neural network, denoted as $\mathcal{H}$, takes the undersampled k-space data $\widehat{\boldsymbol{Z}}$ as input and produces the estimated qMRI parameter maps $\widehat{\boldsymbol{X}}$ as output, which can be mathematically represented as $\widehat{\boldsymbol{X}} = \mathcal{H}(\widehat{\boldsymbol{Z}} \mid \boldsymbol{\theta})$. The optimization of the network parameters $\boldsymbol{\theta}$ is accomplished through a training process akin to Equation 13, where $\boldsymbol{W}_t$ and $\boldsymbol{Z}_t$ represent the reference qMRI parameter maps and undersampled k-space data, respectively, from a training dataset, thereby enabling the network to learn a complex mapping between the undersampled k-space measurements and the desired qMRI parameter maps.

The computational costs of training a deep neural network to directly estimate quantitative magnetic resonance imaging parameter maps from k-space data are high. As a consequence, an alternative strategy has been proposed, wherein neural networks are employed to augment specific components of the traditional direct model-based reconstruction approach [128–132]. For instance, deep learning-based regularization techniques have been developed to refine the estimation of qMRI parameter maps in Equation 24 [132–134]:

$$\widehat{\boldsymbol{X}} = \arg\min_{\boldsymbol{X}} \left\| \boldsymbol{Y} - \varepsilon \mathcal{U}(\boldsymbol{X}) \right\|_2^2, \tag{24}$$

The signal model $\mathcal{U}$ can be adjusted to improve parameter estimation.

Additionally, neural networks have been used to estimate initial parameter maps from undersampled k-space data for direct model-based reconstruction methods [132]. Furthermore, a pretrained neural network has been utilized to predict the derivatives of a direct forward model, thereby reducing the computational time required for direct model-based reconstruction [135]. Additionally, self-supervised learning methods have been used for real-time parameter mapping in transient imaging scenarios [136]. In this work, the Fourier Transform of the parameter maps is first computed from the undersampled k-space data, followed by applying an inverse Fourier Transform to obtain the desired parameter maps, thereby enabling fast and accurate qMRI parameter estimation.

1.3.2.3 Summary

In conclusion, AI-based techniques have emerged as a crucial aspect of fast quantitative magnetic resonance imaging reconstructions. While existing methods have demonstrated promising results, several open questions remain to be addressed in the areas of modeling and theoretical analysis. Specifically, the researchers must further investigate the generalization, uncertainty, and optimization of AI-based qMRI methods to realize their full potential. This includes exploring strategies to improve the robustness of these methods to variations in sequence parameters, physical models, and vendor and site changes, as well as developing more accurate and reliable uncertainty quantification techniques. Additionally, optimizing the design of AI-based qMRI frameworks to achieve better performance and efficiency is essential. By addressing these challenges, the signal processing community can unlock the full potential of AI-based qMRI and enable the development of more accurate, efficient, and reliable imaging techniques.

1.3.3 AI-BASED DIFFUSION MAGNETIC RESONANCE IMAGING

1.3.3.1 Introduction

Diffusion Magnetic Resonance Imaging (dMRI) is a non-invasive imaging technique that enables the investigation of the diffusion process of water molecules in biological tissues. Its significance lies in comprehending the microstructural organization of tissues, particularly in the brain, by providing valuable insights into the direction and magnitude of water diffusion. This information proves invaluable in examining the integrity of white matter tracts, delineating tissue boundaries, and identifying pathologies such as tumors, strokes, and neurodegenerative diseases. dMRI plays a critical role in advancing our knowledge of tissue microstructure and its clinical applications in the realms of neuroimaging and neuroscience research.

Artificial intelligence encompasses developing systems capable of performing tasks that typically necessitate human perception and cognition, including speech, image, and natural language synthesis. Specifically, as a subset of artificial intelligence, deep learning or machine learning trains artificial neural networks with stochastic gradient descent and its variants, making decisions and predictions based on existing data. The evolution of AI algorithms, especially with DL/ML techniques, has been driven by the exponential growth in computing power and resources [137, 138]. Notably, AI-based approaches have made significant strides in the domain of dMRI, encompassing denoising and artifact reduction [130, 139], fiber tractography [140–143], resolution enhancement [144–146], and quantification of microstructural properties [147–150]. These techniques have proven particularly valuable in handling clinical and challenging datasets, leading to advancements in dMRI microstructure parameter imaging, image quality assessment, and image enhancement.

This chapter investigates the application of artificial intelligence in diffusion magnetic resonance imaging (MRI), including "data processing and denoising," "microstructure estimation," and "white matter fiber tractography." Each section thoroughly presents state-of-the-art methodologies and offers detailed explanations using select classic approaches as examples.

1.3.3.2 Approaches

AI-based Data Processing and Denoising for Diffusion MRI

Golkov et al. [151] were the first to introduce the concept of deep learning into dMRI and developed the deep learning-based q-space super-resolution (q-DL) framework, which has had a significant impact on subsequent research in the field. Since then, deep learning has increasingly gained popularity in the field of diffusion magnetic resonance imaging and has become a promising tool for studying WM architecture in living humans, both in healthy conditions and in disease.

Prior to undertaking AI in diffusion MRI research, researchers and clinicians need first to understand its application fields. For instance, dMRI has been successfully used to study patients with acute stroke [92, 152, 153] or brain tumors [154–156], neurodegenerative disorders including multiple sclerosis [157–159], Alzheimer's and mild cognitive impairment [160–164], neuropsychiatric disorders such as schizophrenia [165–168], and so on.

Artifacts in DWI data are primarily related to gradient system hardware, scanning sequences, pulse sequences, and body movement. Therefore, it is important to be familiar with some MRI scanning techniques, the causes of image artifacts, and how to address them [169]. To ensure that the collected DWI data covers the entire brain area, it is typically necessary to acquire multiple scans while varying the diffusion gradient directions or amplitudes. Relatively, DWI data often has lower resolution and signal-to-noise ratio (SNR) and is more susceptible to motion artifacts. Additionally, head motion and eddy current distortions are two major factors causing artifacts during acquisition, affecting the voxel correspondence across all DWI data [169–172].

Quality control and preprocessing procedures are crucial for detecting and correcting artifacts in DWI and excluding those that cannot be corrected, ensuring consistency for reliable downstream analyses. There is no consensus on the ideal workflow for DWI quality control or preprocessing for now. After data preprocessing, the following sections will detail subsequent stages.

Diffusion-weighted images, which rely on the attenuation of MR signals based on the diffusivity of water molecules, often result in noisy images, particularly in acquisitions involving strong diffusion encoding or high spatial resolutions. Image denoising emerges as a viable strategy to enhance the quality of diffusion-weighted images within a shorter scan duration. The goal of image denoising is to recover clean images with a high SNR from noisy measurements, which is a challenging inverse problem. The DeepDTI method described in [130] uses a convolutional neural network to denoise six DWI datasets sampled along optimal diffusion-encoding directions, where the ideal clean data is synthesized from tensors fitted using the dataset. This approach is nearly four times faster than non-denoised images.

Despite the notable performance of deep learning-based denoising techniques, many of them necessitate additional high-quality data for the supervised training of CNNs, making them less straightforward to implement in practical applications than traditional algorithms. The performance of a pre-trained CNN can degrade when employed directly on new datasets acquired using different hardware systems and sequences characterized by distinct image contrasts, spatial resolutions, SNR levels, and other factors. Conversely, developing a tailored CNN optimized for specific application data mandates abundant high-SNR image data as training targets, even for fine-tuning parameters of pre-existing CNNs. Obtaining these high-quality training targets involves typically extensive measurements from prolonged scans, which can be challenging to acquire and are often unavailable for legacy data.

In an effort to overcome these challenges, [139] proposed a novel self-supervised deep learning framework for denoising DTI data, dubbed "SDnDTI," which obviates the need for external high-SNR data during the training process. SDnDTI can generate multiple copies of DWI volumes with consistent image contrast but differing noise observations by applying the diffusion tensor model to diffusion tensor imaging (DTI) data from multiple directions [173]. SDnDTI first uses a deep 3D convolutional neural network to perform preliminary denoising on each copy of the DWI data and then averages the copies of all DWI data as the training target. This approach is similar to classical supervised learning-based denoising methods. Finally, the preliminary denoised images are averaged to obtain images with a higher SNR, effectively removing noise from the images.

AI-based Tissue Microstructure Estimation

Diffusion magnetic resonance imaging (dMRI) leverages its sensitivity to the Brownian motion of water molecules, allowing for observing the brain's microstructure at the cellular level. By modeling the relationship between signals and tissue microstructure, most methods have extracted various biomarkers from dMRI signals, making dMRI an important tool for neuroscience and clinical research. However, several major issues still limit the widespread uptake of these microstructure imaging methods, including long acquisition time, diffusion model fitting susceptible to imaging artifacts, and insufficient specificity in microstructural measures.

Several AI-based methods have been proposed to improve the feasibility of fast and quantitative brain microstructure imaging. The AI-based denoising algorithm referenced in the preceding section typically acquires high-quality DWI through the network before progressing to downstream tasks using the output DWI. However, most AI-based microstructural estimation methods tend to train neural networks to predict the corresponding diffusion metrics from diffusion-weighted images. These works used multilayer perceptrons [151, 174, 175], convolutional neural networks [107, 128, 176], long short-term memory (LSTMs) [147–149],

Graph neural networks (GNNs) [150, 177] and recent Transformer-based network [150, 178].

The q-space deep learning [151] was the first to directly map dMRI signals to microstructural parameters using a limited direction of q-space samples through a multi-layer perceptron (MLP). Then, convolutional neural networks were also utilized to predict high-quality scalar diffusion metrics using a small direction of diffusion data [107, 128, 130, 176]. Beyond the data-driven mapping approaches, model-based neural networks incorporating domain knowledge have been introduced to improve network performance and interpretability. Specifically, the model-based neural network is designed by unfolding the conventional optimization process of a mathematical model to construct deep networks. For example, inspired by accelerated microstructure imaging via convex optimization (AMICO) [179], Ye et al. [147–149] proposed patch-wise dictionary-based DL approaches to estimate parametric diffusion maps of NODDI and the multi-compartment SMT separately. Chen et al. [150, 177] used a subset q-space to estimate the NODDI parameters by explicitly considering the q-space geometric structure with a graph neural network. Zheng et al. [156] introduce a new framework named METSC with the Transformer structure for dMRI model estimation.

MESC-Net consists of two consecutive stages. The first one processes image patches to estimate the spatial-angular sparse representation of diffusion signals. Then, it transforms this sparse representation into tissue microstructure. In contrast to [147], MESC-Net's first stage is designed with inspiration from utilizing historical information adaptively in iterative updates for optimization problem-solving. The objective of the second stage is to create a method for generic microstructure estimation. The network learns the weights in both stages simultaneously from the training data.

Though MESC-Net boasts an enhanced network architecture, the spatial-angular sparse representation of signals and the adaptive integration of previous data may result in a large number of model parameters. This rise in complexity could hinder model training and constrain the estimation accuracy. Additionally, current deep learning methods that directly learn the mapping from diffusion signals to tissue microstructure only provide deterministic predictions. They lack vital information on estimation uncertainty, which is crucial for guiding patient treatment or analysis and benefiting subsequent image processing steps [180–182]. Ye et al. [149] proposed an enhanced deep network model consisting of two functional parts for tissue microstructure estimation alongside a methodology for measuring the network estimates' uncertainty. This method is based on a spatial-angular sparse representation of diffusion signals, with dictionaries that are separable in both the spatial and angular domains [183, 184].

AI-based Identification of White Matter Fiber Tracts

Diffusion magnetic resonance imaging enables the mapping of white matter pathways in the brain via tractography [54]. This technique estimates fiber trajectories by tracking likely tract orientations, allowing the assessment of microstructural properties of fiber pathways [185, 186]. Tractography is valuable for studying neurological development, brain function, and diseases. Yet, generating vast numbers of fibers in whole-brain tractography for a single subject can overwhelm clinicians and researchers. Hence, segmenting white matter tracts to identify anatomically significant fibers is crucial for quantifying and visualizing tracts accurately.

Recently, deep learning-based methods have been used to study white matter tract segmentation [186]. Overall, these methods can be categorized into voxel-based and fiber-based approaches, primarily distinguished by the type of input data used in the models. Voxel-based methods primarily segment fiber tracts based on the "tract presence" volume of the projection, where each voxel encoding can represent the presence and/or direction of fiber tracts, allowing for subsequent segmentation through fiber tracking based on the projected fiber directions [140, 188]. Conversely, fiber-based methods first perform imaging of the fiber tract and then use graph neural networks or convolutional neural networks to segment the acquired fiber tracts into anatomical tracts, as demonstrated in [189], trained on fiber feature descriptors [189–192]. The fiber feature descriptors proposed previously include torsion, curvature, distances to anatomical landmarks [190], as well as spatial coordinates of fiber points [166, 168, 169].

Despite the success of deep learning-based fiber segmentation methods, challenges remain, particularly in achieving consistency in fiber segmentation across dMRI data from different institutions, which may include variations in scanning protocols, healthy populations, patient populations, or different age groups. Consistency in tract segmentation aids in more comprehensive white matter analysis, which is crucial for conducting multicenter and cross-lifespan scientific research on large datasets [62–74, 167]. By predicting a tract presence volume, voxel-based methods offer a normalized and condensed representation of the raw dMRI data, thus exhibiting robustness to variations in data acquisition parameters such as the number of gradient directions, b-values, and other factors [140, 188]. Nevertheless, voxel-based methods may encounter difficulties in handling local anatomical differences from subjects with high anatomical variability. On the other hand, traditional machine learning methods for fiber segmentation (e.g., fiber clustering techniques) can accommodate a large amount of anatomical variability between different subjects. However, these conventional methods often necessitate multiple time-consuming processing steps.

To overcome these challenges, Zhang et al. [187] introduced a fiber-based deep learning method, termed the Deep White Matter Analysis (DeepWMA), tailored for rapid and consistent white matter tract segmentation. DeepWMA stands as the first fiber-based deep learning tract segmentation approach capable of generalizing to dMRI data across various demographics and acquisition methods and multiple tractography methods.

1.3.3.3 Summary

These methods have proven particularly valuable for processing complex clinical datasets, leading to advancements in dMRI microstructural parameter estimation and improving image quality assessment and enhancement. However, it is crucial to acknowledge the potential drawbacks of utilizing these data-driven methods, such as tomographic hallucination and training bias. Therefore, implementing such techniques in clinical dMRI must adhere to best practices to avoid generating erroneous or inconsistent outcomes.

Key AI practices in clinical dMRI include meticulous protocol design and optimization, precise image reconstruction, noise reduction to establish reliable ground truth, and thoughtful data interpretation. Furthermore, incorporating robust validation processes, transparent reporting of limitations, and continuous monitoring of AI algorithms' performance are crucial steps to maintain the integrity and reliability of clinical dMRI results. As technology evolves, interdisciplinary collaboration between scientists, radiologists, and clinicians becomes increasingly imperative for refining AI applications in medical imaging. By proactively addressing these challenges and engaging in ongoing education and training, the healthcare industry can harness the power of AI to revolutionize diagnostic accuracy and patient care in the realm of clinical dMRI.

1.3.4 AI-BASED FUNCTIONAL MAGNETIC RESONANCE IMAGING

1.3.4.1 Introduction

Background on fMRI

Among various imaging modalities, functional magnetic resonance imaging (fMRI) provides researchers with novel insights into observing dynamic brain activity and internal activation states [193]. fMRI is utilized to assess brain activity by detecting low-frequency blood oxygen level-dependent (BOLD) signals [194]. Functional MRI monitors blood flow variations by mapping neuronal activity associated with energy consumption in the brain. This technique indirectly highlights differences in brain activity between patients and healthy individuals, offering new insights into disease pathogenesis [195–197]. A substantial body of literature extensively explains and reviews the fundamental concepts and core principles of fMRI [198–202].

The advantage of fMRI lies in its ability to increase blood flow to regions where neurons are activated. The BOLD technique is one of the most commonly used methods for functional brain mapping [203]. The BOLD signal is quite complex and can reflect changes in local cerebral blood flow, volume, and oxygenation. Therefore, neuronal activity can be indirectly measured based on the magnitude of these signals. Functional MRI has gained popularity in brain imaging because it is non-invasive, does not expose individuals to ionizing radiation, and requires no ingestion of substances [204].

Clinical Application

Task-based fMRI

Also known as stimulus-driven fMRI, this technique infers brain activation in specific regions by measuring the relative changes in BOLD signals compared to baseline during task performance or in response to stimuli.

Presurgical Mapping: Task-based fMRI is extensively used in presurgical planning for patients with brain tumors, epilepsy, and other conditions requiring neurosurgery. By identifying specific brain areas activated during tasks such as language, motor, and sensory functions, surgeons can avoid critical regions, minimizing the risk of postoperative deficits. This approach is particularly useful in mapping eloquent cortices, ensuring better surgical outcomes.

Diagnosis and Management of Neurological Diseases: Task-based fMRI aids in diagnosing and managing neurological diseases like Parkinson's disease, multiple sclerosis, and stroke. It helps understand the functional impact of these diseases on brain activity and assists in tracking disease progression and response to therapy. For instance, in Parkinson's disease, task-based fMRI can reveal alterations in motor network connectivity and functionality.

Cognitive and Behavioral Neuroscience: Task-based fMRI is a valuable cognitive and behavioral neuroscience research tool. It helps study the neural basis of cognitive functions such as memory, attention, decision-making, and emotion. By examining brain activation patterns while performing specific cognitive tasks, researchers can obtain insights into how different brain regions contribute to these functions and how they are affected by various factors, including aging and mental health conditions.

Psychiatric Disorders: Task-based fMRI is used to investigate brain activity patterns in psychiatric disorders such as schizophrenia, major depressive disorder, anxiety disorder, and bipolar disorder. It helps identify dysfunctional brain networks and regions associated with these conditions, aiding their diagnosis and understanding. For example, task-based fMRI can reveal altered activation in the prefrontal cortex during emotion regulation tasks in patients with depression.

Neurodevelopmental Disorders: In the study of neurodevelopmental disorders like autism spectrum disorder (ASD) and attention-deficit/hyperactivity disorder (ADHD), task-based fMRI is employed to examine atypical brain activity patterns during tasks related to social interaction, attention, and executive functions. This application helps understand the neural underpinnings of these disorders and develop targeted interventions.

Resting-State fMRI

Also known as functional connectivity, MRI examines simultaneous activations between spatially distinct regions that occur without a task or stimulus to explore the functional architecture of the brain. Resting-state fMRI provides an important technological tool for understanding the functional organization of healthy brains and various disease states. It has potential clinical applications, including presurgical planning, diagnosis, and prognosis of neurological and psychiatric disorders [205].

Presurgical Localization of Eloquent Cortex: Resting-state fMRI is useful for presurgical planning in patients with brain tumors and epilepsy. It helps identify specific brain RSNs, such as motor and language areas, crucial for surgical planning. This method is advantageous as it can be performed on patients who cannot cooperate with task-based paradigms due to young age, altered mental status, sedation, or other conditions [205].

Diagnosis and Prognosis of Neurological Diseases: Resting-state fMRI assists in the identification of patients with Alzheimer's disease, mild cognitive impairment, and various other forms of dementia. By analyzing the connectivity of the default mode network (DMN) and other RSNs, rs-fMRI can distinguish between different types of dementia and provide diagnostic accuracy. It also shows promise in predicting disease progression and cognitive decline.

Psychiatric Disorders: Resting-state fMRI has been utilized to differentiate patients with psychiatric disorders like autism spectrum disorder, major depressive disorder, schizophrenia, and attention-deficit/hyperactivity disorder. Pattern classification of rs-fMRI data helps identify abnormal functional connectivity associated with these disorders.

Pediatric Applications: Resting-state fMRI is used to study brain development in pediatric populations, including preterm infants and children with neurodevelopmental disorders. It helps in understanding the early formation and maturation of RSNs, providing insights into typical and atypical brain development.

Disorders of Consciousness: Resting-state fMRI assists in diagnosing disorders of consciousness by demonstrating the connectivity of the DMN and its correlation with the level of consciousness impairment. This application is crucial for assessing patients with varying levels of consciousness, including those in comatose states.

Advances and Challenges in fMRI

Compared to neuroimaging methods like MRI and PET, fMRI faces some challenging issues that somewhat impact its applicability. Firstly, the acquisition, cleaning, preprocessing, and analysis of fMRI data are significantly more labor-intensive and complex than MRI and PET data. Secondly, fMRI data are characterized by a low SNR, necessitating highly specialized expertise, and are relatively underrepresented in large-scale databases. Moreover, fMRI often demonstrates lower accuracy than other techniques, such as MRI. Consequently, fMRI methodologies are less popular due to their substantial demands on computational power, extensive resources, and proficiency with related technologies, which are often deemed unjustifiable compared to other techniques, such as cognitive assessments [206].

Therefore, to optimize the process of functional magnetic resonance imaging analysis and obtain the most accurate data interpretations, it may be necessary to consider numerous technical factors, including details of the analytical paradigm, artifacts present in the imaging process, complex protocol definitions, various analysis and processing methods, and the limitations of specific methods. Nevertheless, recent innovations in AI-based technologies have further streamlined the fMRI analysis process. [206].

1.3.4.2 Approaches

Algorithms for Resting-State fMRI

Resting-state functional magnetic resonance imaging (rs-fMRI) is a neuroimaging modality conducted with participants in a quiescent state, devoid of engaging in any particular tasks or being exposed to explicit stimuli. This technique is predominantly utilized to investigate the intrinsic brain activity and the patterns of functional connectivity that emerge during periods of repose. Resting-state fMRI uses a Blood Oxygen Level Dependent (BOLD) contrast mechanism to detect changes in blood flow within the brain. BOLD signals reflect changes in blood oxygen levels associated with neuronal activity, which can reveal spontaneous brain activity in different regions of the brain during rest. Researchers evaluate functional connectivity between brain regions by analyzing the time series data of these spontaneous activities.

Biswal et al. [207] demonstrated that low-frequency spontaneous oscillations exhibit remarkable temporal coherence between distant regions of the primary sensory-motor cortices that are functionally connected, even when no explicit tasks are being performed. This discovery underscores the critical neurological role of activity observed in the resting state. After this pivotal finding, a multitude of studies have reported additional clusters of regions that, while active during various cognitive tasks, including language, motor, attention, auditory, and visual processing, also display synchronized fluctuations in the absence of tasks [208–217]. These regions, characterized by their spontaneous synchronized oscillations, are collectively referred to as resting state networks (RSNs) or intrinsic brain networks. The designation RSN denotes brain networks that are discerned through rs-fMRI and are implicated in shared functional processes.

Unsupervised Learning Methods

Unsupervised learning is crucial in analyzing fMRI (functional magnetic resonance imaging) data, as it can extract valuable information from high-dimensional, complex neuroimaging data and uncover latent patterns and structures of brain activity without relying on pre-labeled data.

In the realm of rs-fMRI, numerous unsupervised learning techniques are dedicated to segmenting the brain into discrete functional subunits, akin to constructing brain atlases. These segmentation algorithms operate based on functional data, which sets them apart from methods reliant on cytoarchitectural structures (e.g., the Brodmann atlas) or macroscopic anatomical landmarks (e.g., the Automatic Anatomical Labeling (AAL) atlas) [218]. Lately, unsupervised learning has been extended to investigate the dynamic functional connectome, yielding promising outcomes [219–223]. Furthermore, unsupervised learning has been employed to discern the latent low-dimensional representation of resting-state functional connectivity (RSFC) to analyze entire subject populations. Machine learning possesses immense potential for delineating neuroanatomical structural boundaries with distinct functionality and identifying clusters of regions within the brain that exhibit functional coupling, which are pivotal objectives in the field of neuroscience.

Clustering algorithms serve to delineate the brain's surface or volume into distinct, non-overlapping functional networks. A pivotal aspect of clustering methodology is selecting an appropriate distance function that quantifies the divergence between voxels or vertices. Within the context of rs-fMRI, this distance metric is derived from either the raw time series data of the voxels or their respective connectivity profiles. While both approaches are predicated on functional homogeneity, variations in the resulting segmentations have been observed when different criteria are employed for optimization [224]. This underscores the significance of carefully choosing the distance measure to ensure meaningful and biologically plausible partitions of the brain's functional architecture.

Independent Component Analysis (ICA) stands as one of the pioneering and most extensively utilized analytical instruments in the domain of rs-fMRI. It has profoundly enhanced our comprehension of the intrinsic networks of the brain. Deployed in the context of rs-fMRI, ICA encapsulates brain activity as a linear amalgamation of assorted spatial patterns or maps, each accompanied by its unique temporal trajectory. These spatial maps may correspond to coherent functional systems or potentially to noise, and they can be discerned automatically by applying diverse criteria. The proficiency of ICA in segregating noise sources renders it an especially appealing technique for analyzing neuroimaging data.

In the nascent stages of rs-fMRI research, a multitude of studies established a notable congruence between ICA-derived spatial maps and the cortical functional networks identified in task-based activation studies [208, 210]. While the conventional ICA model operates under the premise of an absence of noise and posits that the inherent randomness is confined to the sources themselves, a variety of ICA adaptations have been proffered to account for extraneous noise present in the observed signals. Beckmann et al. [208] introduced the Probabilistic ICA (PICA) model to elucidate the connectivity architecture within rs-fMRI data. PICA encapsulates the linear instantaneous mixing process, considering the presence of additional noise and the statistical independence of the sources. De Luca et al. [211] have illustrated that PICA can reliably discern both Resting-State Networks (RSNs) and artifactual patterns, showcasing a high degree of uniformity in resting-state patterns across a diverse array of subjects.

In the absence of a definitive standard for validating ICA patterns or the efficacy of any clustering algorithm, metrics such as reproducibility and reliability are frequently employed for quantitative assessment. Recently, Khoshidi et al. introduced an ICA-based fMRI automatic denoising strategy termed FIX (FMRIB's ICA-based X denoiser). The methodology involves training a classifier with manually annotated markers to identify artifact components based on their distinct spatial and temporal characteristics. These components, indicative of various structured noise sources, can be effectively removed from the data, either by subtraction or regression, to yield purified signals.

Sparse dictionary learning represents an alternative and widely embraced framework for devising succinct representations of observed data. Varoquaux et al. [225] harnessed the dictionary learning approach to segment functional regions from rs-fMRI time series. Their technique accommodates inter-subject variability in spatial maps by allowing individual subject spatial maps to deviate from the population-level atlas. The optimization of a loss function is central to their method, which encompasses a residual term to gauge the approximate discrepancy between the data and its decomposition, a cost term that penalizes significant divergences of individual subject spatial maps from the population-level latent map, and a regularization term designed to foster sparsity.

In the pursuit of enhancing the clarity and spatial coherence of the dominant patterns within each dictionary, a smoothness constraint was additionally implemented. This approach facilitated the creation of distinct partitions. Abraham et al. [226] introduced total variation regularization within the multi-subject dictionary learning framework to counteract the potential for blurred edges that might arise from the imposition of smoothness constraints. Their findings indicated that this technique yielded more organized partitions and demonstrated superior performance in interpreting test data when compared to ICA and clustering, among other competing methodologies. In a similar vein, Lv et al. [227] put forth a strategy aimed at learning a sparse representation of the complete brain fMRI signal for individual subjects. This was achieved by decomposing the time series into a foundational dictionary and corresponding sparse coefficients. In this context, the dictionary encapsulates the prevalent activation patterns of functional networks, while the coefficients correspond to the associated spatial maps. The experimental outcomes revealed that the functional networks extracted exhibited a high degree of spatial overlap, which diverges from the typical ICA output characterized by spatially non-overlapping components.

K-means clustering and mixture models are prevalent techniques for the spatial segmentation of fMRI data [228–231]. The affinity between voxels is often characterized by the correlation of their raw time series [229] or their connectivity profiles [231]. Additionally, Euclidean distance metrics have been utilized to assess the spectral features of time series data [228]. Golland et al. [232] introduced a Gaussian mixture model for the clustering of fMRI signals, wherein each voxel's signal is represented as a composite of N Gaussian densities. Here, N signifies the hypothesized number of functional networks, and the weights indicate the likelihood of association with various networks. This methodology has been applied to large-scale systems across multiple resolutions, uncovering inherent hierarchies in the functional organization of the brain. Yeo et al. [233] leveraged rs-fMRI measurements from approximately 1,000 subjects to deduce the structure of large-scale distributed cortical networks. They employed a mixture model to pinpoint clusters of voxels with analogous cortical-cortical connectivity profiles. The optimal number of clusters was ascertained through stability analysis, culminating in identifying partitions at a coarse resolution of 7 networks and a more granular resolution of 17 networks. The high reproducibility observed across different data samples suggests that these networks can be considered dependable reference maps for functional attributes.

Hierarchical clustering (HC) serves as an intrinsic method for dissecting resting-state functional magnetic resonance imaging data, revealing latent hierarchical patterns. Pioneering implementations of rs-fMRI clustering embraced HC [234, 235], thereby establishing the viability of delineating resting-state networks (RSNs) from rs-fMRI datasets. Contemporary applications have concentrated on demarcating comprehensive brain partitions to facilitate downstream analyses [236–238]. The enforcement of spatial continuity within these partitions is achieved by prioritizing local neighborhoods for potential merging [236]. A distinct advantage of HC is its deterministic nature and the absence of a prerequisite for pre-emptive cluster quantity specification, contrasting with k-means clustering. After forming the dendrogram, it is imperative to identify the optimal cut-point that encapsulates the "natural" clusters. This determination can be guided by the assessment of link inconsistencies [235], inter-subject reliability [234], or established empirical insights [239].

Functional MRI data can be elegantly depicted as a graph, with nodes symbolizing voxels and edges indicating the strength of connections, typically quantified by the correlation coefficient of voxel time series or through connectivity matrices. In order to manage the graph's complexity, thresholds are customarily applied to its edges. The Ncut criterion underpins popular graph partitioning techniques for crafting whole-brain partitions [224, 240]. The derivation of partitions at the population level often unfolds in two phases: initially, individual graphs undergo clustering to delineate regions with functional connectivity, followed by a second phase where these individual cluster graphs are further clustered to reflect the collective coherence of the population-level graph [224, 241]. Spatial continuity is readily ensured by either restricting the connectivity graph to local neighborhoods or by employing shape priors [224, 241]. In a departure from this approach, Shen et al. [240] introduced a unified population clustering method that optimizes individual and population partitions into a single stage, yielding spatially coherent partitions without the need for explicit constraints.

Supervised Learning Methods

Supervised learning is a machine learning paradigm that utilizes labeled data to train models, enabling them to predict target variables for new, unseen input data. In supervised learning, the dataset consists of input-output pairs, where each pair includes an input sample (feature vector) and a corresponding output value (label). The model learns the mapping relationship between these input-output pairs and can make predictions when encountering new inputs. Common algorithms within the supervised learning paradigm encompass a spectrum of techniques, such as linear regression for modeling relationships, logistic regression for classification tasks, support vector machines (SVM) for both linear and nonlinear classification and regression, decision trees for rule-based decision-making, random forests for an ensemble of decision trees, and neural networks for complex pattern recognition and function approximation. These methods are pivotal in training models to predict target variables based on labeled data. Feature extraction is crucial for using supervised learning effectively. In rs-fMRI, various designs are needed to capture relevant neurophenotypes and extract features. Most supervised models extract brain networks or "connectomes" from rs-fMRI time series as input features for learning algorithms.

In some research methodologies, the conventional process of feature extraction is circumvented. Instead, graph-theoretical algorithms are employed where the segmented brain regions are depicted as nodes within a graph, and the weights of the connecting edges denote functional linkages between these regions. This graphical representation of the functional connections, often referred to as the "connectome," facilitates the deduction of a range of topological attributes inherent in brain networks. These include measures such as modularity, clustering coefficients, and identifying small-world characteristics, which are pivotal for understanding the complex architecture of the brain's functional landscape.

In the domain of rs-fMRI analysis, the predominant application of supervised learning techniques is for categorical differentiation, where the algorithms are designed to delineate distinct classes without presupposing any underlying generative mechanisms. The primary objective lies in accurately delineating the demarcation lines that separate the categories of interest. Even when the learning algorithms are tasked with the same class-discriminating function, such as a linear one, they may be founded on a variety of objective functions, leading to the emergence of diverse models.

Machine learning methods have shown promise in studying the developing connectome. In early influential work, Dosenbach et al. [242] demonstrated the feasibility of using RSFC (resting-state functional connectivity) to predict brain maturity, measured by actual age, with research subjects being adolescents and young adults. They developed a functional maturity index based on the predicted brain age using SVM. Subsequent studies have shown that brain maturity can be reasonably predicted even in a diverse population across the entire lifespan [243, 244].

Machine learning (ML) has been extensively used to explore the diagnostic potential of rs-fMRI data for various neurological and psychiatric diseases. ML models, based on functional connectivity biomarkers, have demonstrated promising accuracy in classifying neurodegenerative diseases such as Alzheimer's disease [245–247], its precursor mild cognitive impairment [248–251], Parkinson's disease [252], and amyotrophic lateral sclerosis (ALS) [253]. Notably, brain atrophy patterns in neurological diseases like Alzheimer's disease or multiple sclerosis often manifest long before the onset of behavioral symptoms.

Functional connectivity, a concept in neuroimaging, can be employed to forecast variations among individuals in cognitive processes and behavior, as indicated by reference [254]. rs-fMRI, characterized by its spontaneous activity without the constraints of specific tasks, captures a wide array of cognitive states, thereby serving as a valuable instrument for identifying variations in behavior across various domains. Machine learning (ML) models have demonstrated efficacy in forecasting fluid intelligence [255], sustained attention [256], memory capabilities [257–259], and linguistic proficiency [257], utilizing RSFC (resting-state functional connectivity) as biomarkers in both healthy and diseased populations. The scope of these predictive models has recently broadened to include personality dimensions such as neuroticism, extraversion, agreeableness, and openness [260, 261].

In the realm of rs-fMRI, some research leverages machine learning to anticipate the level of consciousness during scanning. Given the absence of task demands in resting-state studies, participants' states of consciousness can vary, oscillating between wakefulness and drowsiness. Accurately classifying the state of alertness during rs-fMRI is essential for mitigating the influence of consciousness-related biases. SVM classifiers, trained on inter-cortical RSFC, have been validated for their ability to reliably identify periods of sleep during the scanning process [262, 263].

Exploring the influence of genetic factors on the brain's architecture and functionality has long been an aspiration in the field of neuroscience. Ge et al. [280], in a recent investigation, have delved into this area. Furthermore, studies on the genetic and environmental determinants of RSFC have been pursued within a machine-learning framework. Miranda-Dominguez et al. [75] have utilized an SVM classifier to differentiate individual FC characteristics between sibling and twin pairs in contrast to unrelated pairs.

Algorithms Related to Task-based fMRI

Task-based fMRI methods are considered a benchmark for identifying regions of interest (ROI) or voxels based on external stimuli. However, studies reveal the large-scale involvement of brain networks in various brain responses to visual stimuli. Due to high costs and time-consuming issues, determining all these large functional networks in task-based fMRI data becomes challenging. These issues remain to be addressed when working with task-based fMRI datasets. Multivariate Pattern Analysis (MVPA) has been extensively studied in task-based fMRI applications.

In one study, researchers used the General Linear Model (GLM), which supports hypothesis testing for fitting parameters and is easy to support parameter estimation, to decode multivoxel patterns of cognitive states from fMRI data. This approach emphasizes the spatial patterns of activation rather than just the signal intensity, enhancing the understanding of how complex cognitive tasks are represented in distributed brain activity patterns [76]. Kenneth A. Norman explored the use of GLM for multivoxel pattern analysis to decode cognitive states in fMRI data, emphasizing the spatial patterns of activation, which enhances understanding of how complex cognitive tasks are represented in the brain's distributed activity patterns [77]. Toshiharu Nakai introduced a real-time fMRI method using a sliding window GLM analysis to dynamically monitor brain activity, demonstrating the advantage of real-time adjustment of GLM parameters to capture transient brain activity changes during visual tasks [78]. Kay, Rokem, Winawer, Dougherty, and Wandell proposed GLMdenoise, an automated technique to improve the signal-to-noise ratio (SNR) of task-based fMRI data by adding noise regression variables, thereby providing more accurate BOLD response estimation and enhancing the reliability of GLM analysis [79]. Joram Soch discussed the problem of model mismatch in GLM analysis and proposed a cross-validation Bayesian model selection method to improve model accuracy, emphasizing the importance of choosing the correct model to avoid overfitting and improve statistical inference in fMRI research [264]. Safoura Shahin suggested improving the design matrix in sparse Bayesian learning to enhance the detection of brain activity areas, emphasizing the necessity of a flexible design matrix to adapt to different experimental conditions, effectively avoiding overfitting and capturing low signal-to-noise ratio signals [265]. Tom Johnstone investigated the effects of motion correction and the use of motion covariates in multi-subject fMRI analysis, showing how considering motion artifacts in group analysis can significantly improve the accuracy of brain activity detection [266]. Jiansong Xu compared the independent component analysis with traditional GLM methods, showing that ICA can reveal more functional brain activities and supports the combination of ICA with GLM to discover brain activity patterns that GLM may miss [267]. Z. Wang combined GLM with support vector machine (SVM) learning to enhance the analysis of group fMRI data, introducing a method that combines machine learning techniques with GLM, improving the sensitivity and specificity of brain activity detection [268]. Anna Zilverstand utilized window correlation techniques combined with GLM to provide real-time adjustment for task difficulty-based functional connectivity neurofeedback, enhancing the application of GLM in neurofeedback research through dynamic adjustment of real-time brain activity measurements [269].

The Psychophysiological Interaction (PPI) model helps identify voxels where activity is related to a given stimulus seed ROI. This method can identify areas where activity depends on the interaction between the task and the ROI time course. Chris Tailby and colleagues used PPI analysis to capture state-dependent changes in network connectivity. They analyzed fMRI data from 19 healthy controls and 37 patients with temporal lobe epilepsy (TLE) during a semantic word retrieval task, suggesting that a reduction in network flexibility may contribute to cognitive impairment in epilepsy [270]. Lara Lordier and colleagues used the PPI method to compare fMRI data from 35 preterm infants (divided into music intervention and control groups) and 21 full-term newborns under different music conditions, highlighting the positive impact of musical auditory training on brain functional connectivity in preterm infants in the NICU environment [271]. Kristine Boksman and colleagues used a 4.0 Tesla fMRI scanner to compare brain activation and functional connectivity (PPI analysis) in 10 patients with first-episode schizophrenia and 10 healthy volunteers during a lexical fluency task, finding the involvement of the anterior cingulate in the neural circuitry of schizophrenia and emphasizing abnormal brain functional connectivity in the early stages of the disease [272].

Structural Equation Modeling (SEM) is an effective method for examining brain connectivity disorders, and the parameters of this model can be well estimated. Damaraju and colleagues combined Independent Component Analysis and SEM techniques, first separating independent brain networks through ICA and then modeling the structural relationships between these networks using

SEM [273]. Harrison and colleagues used SEM to integrate multi-subject fMRI data, personality trait assessments, and symptom assessments, modeling the path relationships between these variables. Their study emphasized the key role of the prefrontal cortex in emotional regulation and revealed the neural basis of emotional resilience [274]. Jieun Kim and colleagues proposed a unified SEM and Generalized Linear Model method for analyzing multi-subject multivariate fMRI data [275].

In the Dynamic Causal Modeling (DCM) approach, interactions are modeled at the neuronal level using structural equation modeling, which produces a more biologically realistic fitting model. Ronald Sladky and colleagues used DCM to analyze fMRI data, assessing the connectivity between the amygdala and the orbitofrontal cortex and its regulation. Their study provided an in-depth understanding of the dysfunction of the emotional regulation network in patients with social anxiety disorder, highlighting the importance of DCM in revealing causal relationships in neural connections [275]. Bönstrup and colleagues used DCM to analyze multi-subject fMRI data, assessing causal relationships between brain regions [276]. Penny and colleagues combined EEG and fMRI data, using DCM to model dynamic causal relationships between neural networks. Their study demonstrated the potential of multimodal data integration in revealing the dynamics of neural networks, promoting the understanding of the brain's complex functions [277].

Multivariate Pattern Analysis (MVPA) supports the analysis of fMRI response patterns in a large number of voxels, providing higher sensitivity than univariate hypothesis testing. Fangyi Wang and colleagues combined sparse representation techniques with MVPA, selecting and locating brain activation areas corresponding to experimental conditions/tasks. This method aims to identify as many informative variables as possible, providing an effective approach for decoding brain states and simultaneously locating task-specific brain activation areas. Their work demonstrated the potential of sparse representation in processing high-dimensional data [278]. Kay and colleagues used GLMdenoise for MVPA to improve the accuracy of BOLD response estimation. Their study showed the effectiveness of GLMdenoise in enhancing the reliability of fMRI data analysis, providing a powerful tool for future fMRI research [279].

1.3.4.3 Summary

rs-fMRI studies spontaneous brain activity and functional connectivity in resting subjects. It uses Blood Oxygen Level Dependent contrast to detect changes in blood flow, reflecting neuronal activity. This method evaluates functional connectivity by analyzing the time series data of spontaneous activities. Unsupervised learning methods like Independent Component Analysis, sparse dictionary learning, clustering, and graph partitioning play significant roles in rs-fMRI data analysis, extracting connectivity structures and segmenting the brain into functional sub-units. Supervised learning methods use labeled data to train models for predicting new input data, extracting features such as brain networks or "connectomes" for learning algorithms. Techniques like support vector machines predict brain maturity, diagnose diseases, and identify cognitive differences, while genetic basis analysis explores the impact of genetics on functional connectivity.

Task-based fMRI identifies brain regions activated by specific tasks or external stimuli, measuring BOLD signals during task performance to capture brain activity related to specific functions. Methods like the General Linear Model and its variants improve SNR and accuracy in analyzing spatial activation patterns. Psychophysiological Interaction identifies regions where activity depends on the interaction between tasks and ROI time courses, while Structural Equation Modeling models structural relationships between brain networks. Dynamic Causal Modeling analyzes causal relationships between brain regions, and Multivariate Pattern Analysis decodes brain states and locates task-specific activation areas with higher sensitivity. Both rs-fMRI and task-based fMRI provide comprehensive insights into brain function, connectivity, and the impact of various conditions on brain activity.

In conclusion, resting-state and task-based fMRI are essential for studying brain activity and connectivity. Moreover, rs-fMRI uses BOLD contrast to detect spontaneous brain activity, analyzed through unsupervised and supervised learning methods to extract connectivity structures and predict cognitive differences. Task-based fMRI measures BOLD signals during tasks, using models like GLM, PPI, SEM, DCM, and MVPA to analyze task-specific brain activity and functional relationships. Addressing challenges in modeling, optimization, and robustness will enhance the accuracy and efficiency of these techniques, advancing neuroscience research.

REFERENCES

[1] Wright, G.A. 1997. Magnetic resonance imaging. IEEE Signal Process Mag. 14(1): 56–66.

[2] Shanshan Wang, Ruoyou Wu, Sen Jia, Alou Diakite, Cheng Li, Qiegen Liu, et al. 2024. Knowledge driven deep learning for fast MR imaging: Undersampled MR image reconstruction from supervised to unsupervised learning. Magnetic Resonance in Medicine. 92(2): 496–518.

[3] Komal Sharma, Akwinder Kaur and Shruti Gujral. 2014. Brain tumor detection based on machine learning algorithms. International Journal of Computer Applications. 103(1): 7–11.

[4] Niels Hjort, K. Butcher, S.M. Davis, C.S. Kidwell, W.J. Koroshetz, J. Röther, et al. 2005. Magnetic resonance imaging criteria for thrombolysis in acute cerebral infarct. Stroke. 36(2): 388–397.

[5] Nafi Aygun and Thomas J. Masaryk. 2002. Diagnostic imaging for intracerebral hemorrhage. Neurosurgery Clinics. 13(3): 313–334.

[6] Stefan Posse and Walter P Aue. 1990. Susceptibility artifacts in spin-echo and gradient-echo imaging. Journal of Magnetic Resonance (1969). 88(3): 473–492.

[7] Klaas P. Pruessmann, Markus Weiger, Markus B. Scheidegger and Peter Boesiger. 1999. SENSE: sensitivity encoding for fast MRI. Magnetic Resonance in Medicine. 42(5): 952–962.

[8] Mark A. Griswold, P.M. Jakob, R.M. Heidemann, Mathias Nittka, Vladimir Jellus, Jianmin Wang, et al. 2002. Generalized autocalibrating partially parallel acquisitions (GRAPPA). Magnetic Resonance in Medicine. 47(6): 1202–1210.

[9] Michael Lustig, David Donoho and John M. Pauly. 2007. Sparse MRI: The application of compressed sensing for rapid MR imaging. Magnetic Resonance in Medicine. 58(6): 1182–1195.

[10] Yann LeCun, Yoshua Bengio and Geoffrey Hinton. 2015. Deep learning. Nature. 521(7553): 436–444.

[11] Shanshan Wang, Zhenghang Su, Leslie Ying, Xi Peng, Shun Zhu, Feng Liang, et al. 2016. Accelerating magnetic resonance imaging via deep learning. *In*: 2016 IEEE 13th International Symposium on Biomedical Imaging (ISBI). IEEE. 514–517.

[12] Shanshan Wang, Taohui Xiao, Qiegen Liu and Hairong Zheng. 2021. Deep learning for fast MR imaging: A review for learning reconstruction from incomplete k-space data. Biomedical Signal Processing and Control. 68: 102579.

[13] Yutong Chen, Carola-Bibiane Schönlieb, Pietro Liò, Tim Leiner, Pier Luigi Dragotti, Ge Wang, et al. 2022. AI-based reconstruction for fast MRI—A systematic review and meta-analysis. *In*: Proceedings of the IEEE. 110(2): 224–245.

[14] Reinhard Heckel, Mathews Jacob, Akshay Chaudhari, Or Perlman and Efrat Shimron. 2024. Deep learning for accelerated and robust MRI reconstruction: A review. arXiv preprint arXiv:2404.15692.

[15] Jiahao Huang, Yinzhe Wu, F. Wang, Yingying Fang, Yang Nan, Cagan Alkan, et al. 2024. Data and physics driven deep learning models for fast MRI reconstruction: Fundamentals and methodologies. arXiv preprint arXiv: 2401.16564.

[16] Florian Knoll, Kerstin Hammernik, Chi Zhang, Steen Moeller, Thomas Pock, Daniel K. Sodickson, et al. 2020. Deep-learning methods for parallel magnetic resonance imaging reconstruction: A survey of the current approaches, trends, and issues. IEEE Signal Processing Magazine. 37(1): 128–140.

[17] Dong Liang, Jing Cheng, Ziwen Ke and Leslie Ying. 2020. Deep magnetic resonance image reconstruction: Inverse problems meet neural networks. IEEE Signal Processing Magazine. 37(1): 141–151.

[18] Pádraig Cunningham, Matthieu Cord and Sarah Jane Delany. 2008. Supervised learning. *In*: M. Cord, and P. Cunningham (eds). Machine Learning Techniques for Multimedia. Cognitive Technologies. Springer, Berlin, Heidelberg. 21–49.

[19] Olivier Chapelle, Mingmin Chi and Alexander Zien. 2006. A continuation method for semi-supervised SVMs. *In*: Proceedings of the 23rd International Conference on Machine Learning. 185–192.

[20] Semi-Supervised Learning. 2006. Semi-supervised Learning. CSZ2006. html 5. 2.

[21] Kanishka Tyagi, Chinmay Rane, Raghavendra Sriram and Michael Manry. 2022. Unsupervised learning. *In*: R. Pandey, S.K. Khatri, N.K. Singh and P. Verma (eds). Artificial Intelligence and Machine Learning for Edge Computing. Elsevier. 33–52.

[22] Xiao Liu, Fanjin Zhang, Zhenyu Hou, Li Mian, Zhaoyu Wang, Jing Zhang, et al. 2021. Self-supervised learning: Generative or contrastive. IEEE Transactions on Knowledge and Data Engineering. 35(1): 857–876.

[23] Yoseob Han, Jaejun Yoo, Hak Hee Kim, Hee Jung Shin, Kyunghyun Sung and Jong Chul Ye. 2018. Deep learning with domain adaptation for accelerated projection-reconstruction MR. Magnetic Resonance in Medicine. 80(3): 1189–1205.

[24] Kinam Kwon, Dongchan Kim and HyunWook Park. 2017. A parallel MR imaging method using multilayer perceptron. Medical Physics. 44(12): 6209–6224.

[25] Andreas Kofler, Markus Haltmeier, Tobias Schaeffter and Christoph Kolbitsch. 2021. An end-to-end-trainable iterative network architecture for accelerated radial multi-coil 2D cine MR image reconstruction. Medical Physics. 48(5): 2412–2425.

[26] Andreas Kofler, M. Haltmeier, T. Schaeffter, M. Kachelrieß, M. Dewey, C. Wald, et al. 2020. Neural networks-based regularization for large-scale medical image reconstruction. Physics in Medicine and Biology. 65(13): 135003.

[27] Liyue Shen, John Pauly and Lei Xing. 2022. NeRP: Implicit neural representation learning with prior embedding for sparsely sampled image reconstruction. IEEE Transactions on Neural Networks and Learning Systems. 35(1): 770–782.

[28] Bo Zhu, Jeremiah Z. Liu, Stephen F. Cauley, Bruce R. Rosen and Matthew S. Rosen. 2018. Image reconstruction by domain-transform manifold learning. Nature. 555(7697): 487–492.

[29] Taejoon Eo, Hyungseob Shin, Yohan Jun, Taeseong Kim and Dosik Hwang. 2020. Accelerating Cartesian MRI by domain-transform manifold learning in phase-encoding direction. Medical Image Analysis. 63: 101689.

[30] Aniket Pramanik, Hemant Kumar Aggarwal and Mathews Jacob. 2020. Deep generalization of structured low-rank algorithms (Deep-SLR). IEEE Transactions on Medical Imaging. 39(12): 4186–4197.

[31] Tran Minh Quan, Thanh Nguyen-Duc and Won-Ki Jeong. 2018. Compressed sensing MRI reconstruction using a generative adversarial network with a cyclic loss. IEEE Transactions on Medical Imaging. 37(6): 1488–1497.

[32] Cong Quan, Jinjie Zhou, Yuanzheng Zhu, Yang Chen, Shanshan Wang, Dong Liang, et al. 2021. Homotopic gradients of generative density priors for MR image reconstruction. IEEE Transactions on Medical Imaging. 40(12): 3265–3278.

[33] Tianming Du, Honggang Zhang, Yuemeng Li, S. Pickup, M. Rosen, R. Zhou, et al. 2021. Adaptive convolutional neural networks for accelerating magnetic resonance imaging via k-space data interpolation. Medical Image Analysis. 72: 102098.

[34] Jiahao Huang, Yingying Fang, Yinzhe Wu, Huanjun Wu, Zhifan Gao, Yang Li, et al. 2022. Swin transformer for fast MRI. Neurocomputing. 493: 281–304.

[35] Ajil Jalal, Marius Arvinte, Giannis Daras, Eric Price, Alexandros G. Dimakis and Jonathan I. Tamir. 2021. Robust compressed sensing MRI with deep generative priors. Advances in Neural Information Processing Systems. 34: 14938–14954.

[36] Alper Güngör, Salman UH Dar, Şaban Öztürk, Yilmaz Korkmaz, Hasan A. Bedel, Gokberk Elmas, et al. 2023. Adaptive diffusion priors for accelerated MRI reconstruction. Medical Image Analysis. 88: 102872.

[37] Morteza Mardani, E. Gong, J.Y. Cheng, Shreyas S. Vasanawala, Greg Zaharchuk, Lei Xing, et al. 2018. Deep generative adversarial neural networks for compressive sensing MRI. IEEE Transactions on Medical Imaging. 38(1): 167–179.

[38] Dominik Narnhofer, Alexander Effland, Erich Kobler, K. Hammernik, Florian Knoll and Thomas Pock. 2021. Bayesian uncertainty estimation of learned variational MRI reconstruction. IEEE Transactions on Medical Imaging. 41(2): 279–291.

[39] Guanxiong Luo, Na Zhao, Wenhao Jiang, Edward S. Hui and Peng Cao. 2020. MRI reconstruction using deep Bayesian estimation. Magnetic Resonance in Medicine. 84(4): 2246–2261.

[40] Mevan Ekanayake, Kamlesh Pawar, Mehrtash Harandi, Gary Egan and Zhaolin Chen. 2024. McSTRA: A multi-branch cascaded swin transformer for point spread function-guided robust MRI reconstruction. Computers in Biology and Medicine. 168: 107775.

[41] Yong Sun, Xiaohan Liu, Yiming Liu, Ruiqi Jin and Yanwei Pang. 2024. DIRECTION: Deep cascaded reconstruction residual-based feature modulation network for fast MRI reconstruction. Magnetic Resonance Imaging. 111: 157–167.

[42] Kerstin Hammernik, Teresa Klatzer, E. Kobler, M.P. Recht, Daniel K. Sodickson, Thomas Pock, et al. 2018. Learning a variational network for reconstruction of accelerated MRI data. Magnetic Resonance in Medicine. 79(6): 3055–3071.

[43] Hemant K. Aggarwal, Merry P. Mani and Mathews Jacob. 2018. MoDL: Model-based deep learning architecture for inverse problems. IEEE Transactions on Medical Imaging. 38(2): 394–405.

[44] Anish Lahiri, Guanhua Wang, Saiprasad Ravishankar and Jeffrey A. Fessler. 2021. Blind primed supervised (BLIPS) learning for MR image reconstruction. IEEE Transactions on Medical Imaging. 40(11): 3113–3124.

[45] Dianlin Hu, Yikun Zhang, Jianfeng Zhu, Qiegen Liu and Yang Chen. 2022. Trans-Net: Transformer-enhanced residual-error alternative suppres- sion network for MRI reconstruction. IEEE Transactions on Instrumentation and Measurement. 71: 1–13.

[46] Changfeng Wang, Yingjie Huang, Cheng Ci, Hongming Chen, Hong Wu and Yingxin Zhao. 2024. EIDNet: Extragradient-based iterative denoising network for image compressive sensing reconstruction. Expert Systems with Applications. 250: 123829.

[47] Zalan Fabian, Berk Tinaz and Mahdi Soltanolkotabi. 2022. Humus-Net: Hybrid unrolled multi-scale network architecture for accelerated MRI reconstruction. Advances in Neural Information Processing Systems. 35: 25306–25319.

[48] Zheyuan Yi, Jiahao Hu, Yujiao Zhao, Linfang Xiao, Yilong Liu, Alex T.L. Leong, et al. 2023. Fast and Calibrationless low-rank parallel imaging reconstruction through unrolled deep learning estimation of multi-channel spatial support maps. IEEE Transactions on Medical Imaging. 42(6): 1644–1655.

[49] Zi Wang, Chen Qian, Di Guo, Hongwei Sun, Rushuai Li, Bo Zhao, et al. 2023. One-dimensional deep low-rank and sparse network for accelerated MRI. IEEE Transactions on Medical Imaging. 42(1): 79–90.

[50] Jing Cheng, Haifeng Wang, Leslie Ying and Dong Liang. 2019. Model learning: Primal dual networks for fast MR imaging. *In*: Medical Image Computing and Computer Assisted Intervention–MICCAI 2019: 22nd International Conference, Shenzhen, China. Proceedings, Part III 22. Springer. 21–29.

[51] Jinming Duan, Jo Schlemper, Chen Qin, Cheng Ouyang, Wenjia Bai, Carlo Biffi, et al. 2019. VS-Net: Variable splitting network for accelerated parallel MRI reconstruction. *In*: Medical Image Computing and Computer Assisted Intervention–MICCAI 2019: 22nd International Conference, Shenzhen, China. Proceedings, Part IV 22. Springer. 713–722.

[52] Yan Yang, Jian Sun, Huibin Li and Zongben Xu. 2016. Deep ADMM-Net for compressive sensing MRI. Advances in Neural Information Processing Systems. 29.

[53] Yan Yang, Jian Sun, Huibin Li and Zongben Xu. 2020. ADMM-CSNet: A deep learning approach for image compressive sensing. IEEE Transactions on Pattern Analysis and Machine Intelligence. 42(3): 521–538.

[54] Yan Wu, Yajun Ma, Dante Pietro Capaldi, Jing Liu, Wei Zhao, Jiang Du, et al. 2020. Incorporating prior knowledge via volumetric deep residual network to optimize the reconstruction of sparsely sampled MRI. Magnetic Resonance Imaging. 66: 93–103.

[55] Jo Schlemper, Daniel C. Castro, Wenjia Bai, Chen Qin, Ozan Oktay, Jinming Duan, et al. 2018. Bayesian deep learning for accelerated MR image reconstruction. *In*:

Machine Learning for Medical Image Reconstruction: First International Workshop, MLMIR 2018, Held in Conjunction with MICCAI 2018. Granada, Spain. Proceedings 1. Springer. 64–71.

[56] Arjun D. Desai, B.M. Ozturkler, C.M. Sandino, R. Boutin, M. Willis, S. Vasanawala, et al. 2023. Noise2Recon: Enabling SNR-robust MRI reconstruction with semi-supervised and self-supervised learning. Magnetic Resonance in Medicine. 90(5): 2052–2070.

[57] Lisa Lei Morteza Mardani. 2017. Semi-supervised super-resolution GANs for MRI. *In*: 31st Conference on Neural Information Processing Systems (NIPS 2017), Long Beach.

[58] Zhiwei Wang, Yi Lin, Kwang-Ting (Tim) Cheng and Xin Yang. 2020. Semi-supervised mp-MRI data synthesis with StitchLayer and auxiliary distance maximization. Medical Image Analysis. 59: 101565.

[59] Arjun D. Desai, Beliz Gunel, Batu M. Ozturkler, Harris Beg, Shreyas Vasanawala, Brian A. Hargreaves, et al. 2022. VORTEX: Physics-driven data augmentations using consistency training for robust accelerated MRI reconstruction. *In*: Proceedings of The 5th International Conference on Medical Imaging with Deep Learning, PMLR. 172: 325–352..

[60] Mahmut Yurt, Onat Dalmaz, Salman Dar, Muzaffer Ozbey, B. Tınaz, Kader Oguz, et al. 2022. Semi-supervised learning of MRI synthesis without fully-sampled ground truths. IEEE Transactions on Medical Imaging. 41(12): 3895–3906.

[61] Harrison Nguyen, Simon Luo and Fabio Ramos. 2020. Semi-supervised learning approach to generate neuroimaging modalities with adversarial training. *In*: Advances in Knowledge Discovery and Data Mining: 24th Pacific-Asia Conference, PAKDD 2020, Singapore. Proceedings, Part II 24. Springer. 409–421.

[62] Burhaneddin Yaman, Seyed Amir Hossein Hosseini, S. Moeller, Jutta Ellermann, Kâmil Uğurbil and Mehmet Akçakaya. 2020. Self-supervised learning of physics-guided reconstruction neural networks without fully sampled reference data. Magnetic Resonance in Medicine. 84(6): 3172–3191.

[63] Chen Hu, Cheng Li, Haifeng Wang, Qiegen Liu, Hairong Zheng and Shanshan Wang. 2021. Self-supervised learning for MRI reconstruction with a parallel network training framework. *In*: Medical Image Computing and Computer Assisted Intervention–MICCAI 2021: 24th International Conference, Strasbourg, France. Proceedings, Part VI 24. Springer. 382–391..

[64] Mehmet Akçakaya, Steen Moeller, Sebastian Weingärtner and Kâmil Uğurbil. 2019. Scan-specific robust artificial-neural-networks for k-space interpolation (RAKI) reconstruction: Database-free deep learning for fast imaging. Magnetic Resonance in Medicine. 81(1): 439–453.

[65] Burhaneddin Yaman, Seyed Amir Hossein Hosseini, Steen Moeller, Jutta Ellermann, Kâmil Uğurbil, Mehmet Akçakaya. 2021. Ground-truth free multi-mask self-supervised physics-guided deep learning in highly accelerated MRI. In: 2021 IEEE 18th International Symposium on Biomedical Imaging (ISBI). IEEE. 1850–1854.

[66] Burhaneddin Yaman, Hongyi Gu, Seyed Amir Hossein Hosseini, O. Burak Demirel, Steen Moeller, Jutta Ellermann, et al. 2022. Multi-mask self-supervised learning for physics-guided neural networks in highly accelerated magnetic resonance imaging. NMR in Biomedicine. 35(12): e4798.

[67] Bo Zhou, Jo Schlemper, Neel Dey, Seyed Sadegh Mohseni Salehi, Kevin Sheth, Chi Liu, et al. 2022. Dual-domain self-supervised learning for accelerated non-Cartesian MRI reconstruction. Medical Image Analysis. 81: 102538.

[68] Shanshan Wang, Ruoyou Wu, Cheng Li, Juan Zou, Ziyao Zhang, Qiegen Liu, et al. 2023. PARCEL: Physics-based unsupervised contrastive representation learning for multi-coil MR imaging. IEEE/ACM Transactions on Computational Biology and Bioinformatics. 20(5): 2659–2670..

[69] Juan Zou, Cheng Li, Sen Jia, Ruoyou Wu, Tingrui Pei, Hairong Zheng, et al. 2022. SelfCoLearn: Self-supervised collaborative learning for accelerating dynamic MR imaging. Bioengineering. 9: 650.

[70] Tongyao Pang, Yuhui Quan and Hui Ji. 2020. Self-supervised Bayesian deep learning for image recovery with applications to compressive sensing. *In*: Computer Vision–ECCV 2020: 16th European Conference, Glasgow, UK. Proceedings, Part XI 16. Springer. 475–491.

[71] Hemant K. Aggarwal, Aniket Pramanik, Maneesh John and Mathews Jacob. 2023. ENSURE: A general approach for unsupervised training of deep image reconstruction algorithms. IEEE Transactions on Medical Imaging. 42(4): 1133–1144.

[72] Charles Millard and Mark Chiew. 2023. A theoretical framework for self-supervised MR image reconstruction using sub-sampling via variable density Noisier2Noise. IEEE Transactions on Computational Imaging. 9: 707–720.

[73] Yuyang Hu, Weijie Gan, Chunwei Ying, T. Wang, Cihat Eldeniz, Jiaming Liu, et al. 2024. SPICER: Self-supervised learning for MRI with automatic coil sensitivity estimation and reconstruction. Magnetic Resonance in Medicine. 92(3): 1048–1063.

[74] Tobit Klug, Dogukan Atik and Reinhard Heckel. 2024. Analyzing the sample complexity of self-supervised image reconstruction methods. Advances in Neural Information Processing Systems. 36.

[75] Oscar Miranda-Dominguez, Eric Feczko, David S. Grayson, Hasse Walum, J.T. Nigg and Damien A. Fair. 2018. Heritability of the human connectome: A connectotyping study. Network Neuroscience. 02(02): 175–199.

[76] Tom Johnstone, Carien M. van Reekum, Terrence R. Oakes and Richard J. Davidson. 2006. The voice of emotion: An fMRI study of neural responses to angry and happy vocal expressions. Social Cognitive and Affective Neuroscience. 1(3): 242–249.

[77] Kenneth A. Norman, Sean M. Polyn, Greg J. Detre and James V. Haxby. 2006. Beyond mind-reading: Multi-voxel pattern analysis of fMRI data. Trends in Cognitive Sciences. 10(9): 424–430.

[78] Toshiharu Nakai, Epifanio Bagarinao, Kayako Matsuo, Yuko Ohgami and Chikako Kato. 2006. Dynamic monitoring of brain activation under visual stimulation using fMRI—the advantage of real-time fMRI with sliding window GLM analysis. Journal of Neuroscience Methods. 157(1): 158–167.

[79] Kendrick N. Kay, Ariel Rokem, J. Winawer, R.F. Dougherty and Brian A. Wandell. 2013. GLMdenoise: A fast, automated technique for denoising task-based fMRI data. Frontiers in Neuroscience. 7: 247.

[80] Yan Xia, N. Ravikumar, J.P. Greenwood, S. Neubauer, S.E. Petersen and A.F. Frangi. 2021. Super-resolution of cardiac MR cine imaging using conditional GANs and unsupervised transfer learning. Medical Image Analysis. 71: 102037.

[81] Ke Lei, Morteza Mardani, John M. Pauly and Shreyas S. Vasanawala. 2021. Wasserstein GANs for MR imaging: From paired to unpaired training. IEEE Transactions on Medical Imaging. 40(1): 105–115.

[82] Hyungjin Chung and Jong Chul Ye. 2022. Score-based diffusion models for accelerated MRI. Medical Image Analysis. 80: 102479.

[83] Muzaffer Özbey, Onat Dalmaz, Salman U. H. Dar, Hasan A. Bedel, Şaban Öztürk, Alper Güngör, et al. 2023. Unsupervised medical image translation with adversarial diffusion models. IEEE Transactions on Medical Imaging. 42(12): 3524–3539.

[84] Qing Zou, Abdul Haseeb Ahmed, Prashant Nagpal, Sarv Priya, Rolf F. Schulte and Mathews Jacob. 2022. Variational manifold learning from incomplete data: Application to multislice dynamic MRI. IEEE Transactions on Medical Imaging. 41(12): 3552–3561.

[85] Carlo Pierpaoli. 2010. Quantitative brain MRI. Topics in Magnetic Resonance Imaging. 21(2): 63.

[86] Alexander Seiler, Ulrike Nöth, Pavel Hok, Annemarie Reiländer, Michelle Maiworm, Simon Baudrexel, et al. 2021. Multiparametric quantitative MRI in neurological diseases. Frontiers in Neurology. 12: 640239.

[87] Banafshe Shafieizargar, Riwaj Byanju, Jan Sijbers, Stefan Klein, A.J. den Dekker and Dirk H.J. Poot. 2023. Systematic review of reconstruction techniques for accelerated quantitative MRI. Magnetic Resonance in Medicine. 90(3): 1172–1208.

[88] Yanjie Zhu, Jing Cheng, Zhuo-Xu Cui, Qingyong Zhu, Leslie Ying and Dong Liang. 2023. Physics-driven deep learning methods for fast quantitative magnetic resonance imaging: Performance improvements through integration with deep neural networks. IEEE Signal Processing Magazine. 40(2): 116–128.

[89] Yuxin Hu, Y. Xu, Qiyuan Tian, Feiyu Chen, Xinwei Shi, Catherine J. Moran, et al. 2020. RUN-UP: Accelerated multishot diffusion-weighted MRI reconstruction using an unrolled network with U-Net as priors. Magnetic Resonance in Medicine. 85(2): 709–720.

[90] Merry P. Mani, Hemant K. Aggarwal, Sanjay Ghosh and Mathews Jacob. 2020. Model-based deep learning for reconstruction of joint kq under-sampled high resolution diffusion MRI. *In*: 2020 IEEE 17th International Symposium on Biomedical Imaging (ISBI). IEEE. 913–916.

[91] Marcelo V.W. Zibetti, Patricia M. Johnson, Azadeh Sharafi, Kerstin Hammernik, Florian Knoll and Ravinder R. Regatte. 2020. Rapid mono and biexponential 3D-T1ρ mapping of knee cartilage using variational networks. Scientific Reports. 10: 19144.

[92] R Gilberto González. 2012. Clinical MRI of acute ischemic stroke. Journal of Magnetic Resonance Imaging. 36(2): 259–271.

[93] Hemant K. Aggarwal, Merry P. Mani and Mathews Jacob. 2019. MoDL-MUSSELS: model-based deep learning for multishot sensitivity-encoded diffusion MRI. IEEE Transactions on Medical Imaging. 39(4): 1268–1277.

[94] Merry Mani, Baolian Yang, Girish Bathla, Vincent Magnotta and Mathews Jacob. 2021. Multi-band-and in-plane-accelerated diffusion MRI enabled by model-based deep learning in q-space and its extension to learning in the spherical harmonic domain. Magnetic Resonance in Medicine. 87(4): 1799–1815.

[95] Merry Mani, Vincent A. Magnotta and Mathews Jacob. 2021. qModeL: A plug-and-play model-based reconstruction for highly accelerated multi-shot diffusion MRI using learned priors. Magnetic Resonance in Medicine. 86(2): 835–851.

[96] Ketan Fatania, Carolin M. Pirkl, Marion I. Menzel, Peter Hall and Mohammad Golbabaee. 2022. A plug-and-play approach to multiparametric quantitative MRI: Image reconstruction using pre-trained deep denoisers. *In*: 2022 IEEE 19th International Symposium on Biomedical Imaging (ISBI). IEEE. 1–4.

[97] Yang Gao, Martijn Cloos, Feng Liu, Stuart Crozier, G. Bruce Pike and Hongfu Sun. 2021. Accelerating quantitative susceptibility and R2 mapping using incoherent undersampling and deep neural network reconstruction. NeuroImage. 240: 118404.

[98] Sooyeon Ji, J. Jeong, Se-Hong Oh, Yoonho Nam, S.H. Choi, Hyeong-Geol Shin, et al. 2021. Quad-contrast imaging: Simultaneous acquisition of four contrast-weighted images (PD-weighted, T_2-weighted, PD-flair and T_2-flair images) with synthetic T_1-weighted image, T_1 -and T_2-maps. IEEE Transactions on Medical Imaging. 40(12): 3617–3626.

[99] Caohui Duan, He Deng, Sa Xiao, Junshuai Xie, Haidong Li, Xiuchao Zhao, et al. 2022. Accelerate gas diffusion-weighted MRI for lung morphometry with deep learning. European Radiology. 32: 702–713.

[100] Zhiyang Fu, Sagar Mandava, M.B. Keerthivasan, Zhitao Li, Kevin Johnson, Diego R. Martin, et al. 2020. A multi-scale residual network for accelerated radial MR parameter mapping. Magnetic Resonance Imaging. 73: 152–162.

[101] Kuang Gong, Paul Han, Georges El Fakhri, Chao Ma and Quanzheng Li. 2019. Arterial spin labeling MR image denoising and reconstruction using unsupervised deep learning. NMR in Biomedicine. NMR in Biomedicine. 35(4): e4224.

[102] Berkin Bilgic, Itthi Chatnuntawech, Mary Kate Manhard, Q. Tian, Congyu Liao, Siddharth S. Iyer, et al. 2019. Highly accelerated multishot echo planar imaging through synergistic machine learning and joint reconstruction. Magnetic Resonance in Medicine. 82(4): 1343–1358.

[103] Yan Wu, Yajun Ma, Jiang Du and Lei Xing. 2020. Accelerating quantitative MR imaging with the incorporation of B1 compensation using deep learning. Magnetic Resonance Imaging. 72: 78–86.

[104] SShu-Fu Shih, Sevgi Gokce Kafali, Tess Armstrong, Xiaodong Zhong, Kara L. Calkins and Holden H. Wu. 2021. Deep learning-based parameter mapping with uncertainty estimation for fat quantification using accelerated free-breathing radial MRI. *In*: 2021 IEEE 18th International Symposium on Biomedical Imaging (ISBI). IEEE. 433– 437.

[105] Jie Yang, Z. Zhang, Yanchun Zhu and Yaoqin Xie. 2019. An accurate estimation of T2 mapping for fast magnetic resonance imaging. *In*: Proceedings of the Third International Symposium on Image Computing and Digital Medicine. 335–342.

[106] Yong Chen, Zhenghan Fang, Sheng-Che Hung, Wei-Tang Chang, Dinggang Shen and Weili Lin. 2020. High-resolution 3D MR Fingerprinting using parallel imaging and deep learning. NeuroImage. 206: 116329.

[107] Eric K. Gibbons, Kyler K. Hodgson, A.S. Chaudhari, L.G. Richards, J.J. Majersik, Ganesh Adluru, et al. 2019. Simultaneous NODDI and GFA parameter map generation from subsampled q-space imaging using deep learning. Magnetic Resonance in Medicine. 81(4): 2399–2411.

[108] Pingfan Song, Yonina C. Eldar, Gal Mazor and Miguel R.D. Rodrigues. 2019. HYDRA: Hybrid deep magnetic resonance fingerprinting. Medical Physics. 46(11): 4951–4969.

[109] Mohammad Golbabaee, Guido Buonincontri, Carolin M. Pirkl, Marion I. Menzel, Bjoern H. Menze, Mike Davies, et al. 2021. Compressive MRI quantification using convex spatiotemporal priors and deep encoder-decoder networks. Medical Image Analysis. 69: 101945.

[110] Yuze Li, Yajie Wang, Haikun Qi, Zhangxuan Hu, Zhensen Chen, Runyu Yan, et al. 2021. Deep learning–enhanced T1 mapping with spatial-temporal and physical constraint. Magnetic Resonance in Medicine. 86(3): 1647–1661.

[111] Carolin M. Pirk, P.A. Gomez, Ilona Lipp, G. Buonincontri, Miguel Molina-Romero, Anjany Sekuboyina, et al. 2020. Deep learning-based parameter mapping for joint relaxation and diffusion tensor MR Fingerprinting. Medical Imaging with Deep Learning. PMLR. 638-654.

[112] Zhenghan Fang, Yong Chen, Weili Lin and Dinggang Shen. 2017. Quantification of relaxation times in MR fingerprinting using deep learning. In: Proceedings of the International Society for Magnetic Resonance in Medicine. Scientific Meeting and Exhibition. International Society for Magnetic Resonance in Medicine. Scientific Meeting and Exhibition. Vol. 25. NIH Public Access.

[113] Binyu Ouyang, Qizhi Yang, X. Wang, Hongjian He, Lingceng Ma, Qinqin Yang, et al. 2022. Single-shot T2 mapping via multi-echo-train multiple overlapping-echo detachment planar imaging and multitask deep learning. Medical Physics. 49(11): 7095–7107.

[114] Xiaoxia Zhang, Quentin Duchemin, Kangning Liu, Cem Gultekin, S. Flassbeck, C. Fernandez-Granda, et al. 2022. Cramér–Rao bound-informed training of neural networks for quantitative MRI. Magnetic Resonance in Medicine. 88(1): 436–448.

[115] Simin Li, Jian Wu, Lingceng Ma, Shuhui Cai and Congbo Cai. 2022. A simultaneous multi-slice T2 mapping framework based on overlapping-echo detachment planar imaging and deep learning reconstruction. Magnetic Resonance in Medicine. 87(5): 2239–2253.

[116] Carolin M. Pirkl, Laura Nunez-Gonzalez, Florian Kofler, S. Endt, Lioba Grundl, Mohammad Golbabaee, et al. 2021. Accelerated 3D whole-brain T1, T2, and proton density mapping: Feasibility for clinical glioma MR imaging. Neuroradiology. 63: 1831–1851.

[117] Peng Cao, Di Cui, Vince Vardhanabhuti and Edward S. Hui. 2020. Development of fast deep learning quantification for magnetic resonance fingerprinting in vivo. Magnetic Resonance Imaging. 70: 81–90.

[118] Kratika Gupta and Suyash P. Awate. 2019. Random Forests for Simultaneous-Multislice (SMS) Undersampled HARDI Reconstruction and Uncertainty Estimation. *In*: 2019 IEEE International Conference on Image Processing (ICIP). IEEE. 2626– 2630.

[119] Gopal Nataraj, Jon-Fredrik Nielsen, Clayton Scott and Jeffrey A. Fessler. 2018. Dictionary-free MRI PERK: Parameter estimation via regression with kernels. IEEE Transactions on Medical Imaging. 37(9): 2103–2114.

[120] Marco Barbieri, Leonardo Brizi, Enrico Giampieri, F. Solera, David Neil Manners, Gastone Castellani, et al. 2021. A deep learning approach for magnetic resonance fingerprinting: Scaling capabilities and good training practices investigated by simulations. Physica Medica. 89: 80–92.

[121] Refik Soyak, Ebru Navruz, Eda Ozgu Ersoy, Gastao Cruz, Claudia Prieto, Andrew P. King, et al. 2022. Channel attention networks for robust MR fingerprint matching. IEEE Transactions on Biomedical Engineering. 69(4): 1398–1405.

[122] Tilman J.S. Dipl-Ing, Martin Uecker, Susann Boretius and Jens Frahm. 2011. Model-based nonlinear inverse reconstruction for T2 mapping using highly undersampled spin-echo MRI. Journal of Magnetic Resonance Imaging. 34(2): 420–428.

[123] Christopher L. Welsh, Edward W Hsu and Edward VR DiBella. 2011. Strategies for under-sampling and reconstructing MR DTI data. *In*: 2011 IEEE International Symposium on Biomedical Imaging: From Nano to Macro. IEEE. 77–80.

[124] Noam Ben-Eliezer, Daniel K. Sodickson, Timothy Shepherd, Graham C. Wiggins and Kai Tobias Block. 2016. Accelerated and motion-robust *in vivo* T2 mapping from radially undersampled data using Bloch-simulation-based iterative reconstruction. Magnetic Resonance in Medicine. 75(3): 1346–1354.

[125] Marica Pesce, Audrey Repetti and Yves Wiaux. 2019. Fast spatially coherent fiber orientation estimation in diffusion MRI from kq-space sampling. *In*: 2019 IEEE 8th International Workshop on Computational Advances in Multi-Sensor Adaptive Processing (CAMSAP). IEEE. 326–330.

[126] Christopher L. Welsh, Edward V. R. DiBella, Ganesh Adluru and Edward W. Hsu. 2013. Model-based reconstruction of undersampled diffusion tensor k-space data. Magnetic Resonance in Medicine. 70(2): 429–440.

[127] Guillaume Daval-Frérot, A. Massire, Boris Mailhe, Mariappan Nadar, Alexandre Vignaud and Philippe Ciuciu. 2022. Iterative static field map estimation for off-resonance correction in non-Cartesian susceptibility weighted imaging. Magnetic Resonance in Medicine. 88(4): 1592–1607.

[128] Hongyu Li, Zifei Liang, Chaoyi Zhang, Ruiying Liu, Jing Li, Weihong Zhang, et al. 2021. SuperDTI: Ultrafast DTI and fiber tractography with deep learning. Magnetic Resonance in Medicine. 86(6): 3334–3347.

[129] Huan Minh Luu, Dong-Hyun Kim, J.-W. Kim, S.-H. Choi and Sung-Hong Park. 2021. qMTNet: Accelerated quantitative magnetization transfer imaging with artificial neural networks. Magnetic Resonance in Medicine. 85(1): 298–308.

[130] Qiyuan Tian, Berkin Bilgic, Qiuyun Fan, Congyu Liao, Chanon Ngamsombat, Yuxin Hu, et al. 2020. DeepDTI: High-fidelity six-direction diffusion tensor imaging using deep learning. NeuroImage. 219: 117017.

[131] Beomgu Kang, Byungjai Kim, Michael Schär, HyunWook Park and Hye-Young Heo. 2021. Unsupervised learning for magnetization transfer contrast MR fingerprinting: Application to CEST and nuclear Overhauser enhancement imaging. Magnetic Resonance in Medicine. 85(4): 2040–2054.

[132] Yohan Jun, Hyungseob Shin, Taejoon Eo, Taeseong Kim and Dosik Hwang. 2021. Deep model-based magnetic resonance parameter mapping network (DOPAMINE) for fast T1 mapping using variable flip angle method. Medical Image Analysis. 70: 102017.

[133] Fang Liu, Li Feng and Richard Kijowski. 2019. MANTIS: model-augmented neural network with incoherent k-space sampling for efficient MR parameter mapping. Magnetic Resonance in Medicine. 82(1): 174–188.

[134] Fang Liu, Richard Kijowski, Georges El Fakhri and Li Feng. 2021. Magnetic resonance parameter mapping using model-guided self-supervised deep learning. Magnetic Resonance in Medicine. 85(6): 3211–3226.

[135] Hongyan Liu, Oscar van der Heide, Stefano Mandija, Cornelis A. T. van den Berg and Alessandro Sbrizzi. 2022. Acceleration strategies for MR-STAT: Achieving high-resolution reconstructions on a desktop PC within 3 minutes. IEEE Transactions on Medical Imaging. 41(10): 2681–2692.

[136] Yilin Liu, Yong Chen and Pew-Thian Yap. 2021. Real-time mapping of tissue properties for magnetic resonance fingerprinting. Medical Image Computing and

Computer Assisted Intervention–MICCAI 2021: 24th International Conference, Strasbourg, France. Proceedings, Part VI 24. Springer. 161–170.

[137] Christos Davatzikos. 2019. Machine learning in neuroimaging: Progress and challenges. NeuroImage. 197: 652–656.

[138] Ashley N. Nielsen, Deanna M. Barch, Steven E. Petersen, Bradley L. Schlaggar and Deanna J. Greene. 2020. Machine learning with neuroimaging: Evaluating its applications in psychiatry. Biological Psychiatry: Cognitive Neuroscience and Neuroimaging. 5(8): 791–798.

[139] Qiyuan Tian, Ziyu Li, Qiuyun Fan, J.R. Polimeni, Berkin Bilgic, David H. Salat, et al. 2022. SDnDTI: Self-supervised deep learning-based denoising for diffusion tensor MRI. NeuroImage. 253: 119033.

[140] Jakob Wasserthal, Peter Neher and Klaus H. Maier-Hein. 2018. TractSeg-Fast and accurate white matter tract segmentation. NeuroImage. 183: 239–253.

[141] Zhichao Lin, Ting Gong, Kewen Wang, Zhiwei Li, Hongjian He, Qiqi Tong, et al. 2019. Fast learning of fiber orientation distribution function for MR tractography using convolutional neural network. Medical Physics. 46(7): 3101–3116.

[142] Davood Karimi, Lana Vasung, Camilo Jaimes, Fedel Machado-Rivas, Shadab Khan, Simon K. Warfield, et al. 2021. A machine learning-based method for estimating the number and orientations of major fascicles in diffusion-weighted magnetic resonance imaging. Medical Image Analysis. 72: 102129.

[143] Ranjeet Ranjan Jha, S.K. Pathak, Vishwesh Nath, W. Schneider, B.V. Rathish Kumar, Arnav Bhavsar, et al. 2022. VRfRNet: Volumetric ROI fODF reconstruction network for estimation of multi-tissue constrained spherical deconvolution with only single shell dMRI. Magnetic Resonance Imaging. 90: 1 16.

[144] Chuyang Ye, Yu Qin, Chenghao Liu, Yuxing Li, Xiangzhu Zeng and Zhiwen Liu. 2019. Super-resolved q-space deep learning. In: Medical Image Computing and Computer Assisted Intervention–MICCAI 2019: 22nd International Conference, Shenzhen, China. Proceedings, Part III 22. Springer. 582–589.

[145] Yu Qin, Zhiwen Liu, Chenghao Liu, Yuxing Li, X. Zeng and Chuyang Ye. 2021. Super-Resolved q-Space deep learning with uncertainty quantification. Medical Image Analysis. 67: 101885.

[146] Yu Qin, Yuxing Li, Zhizheng Zhuo, Zhiwen Liu, Yaou Liu and Chuyang Ye. 2021. Multimodal super-resolved q-space deep learning. Medical Image Analysis. 71: 102085.

[147] Chuyang Ye. 2017. Tissue microstructure estimation using a deep network inspired by a dictionary-based framework. Medical Image Analysis. 42: 288–299.

[148] Chuyang Ye, Xiuli Li and Jingnan Chen. 2019. A deep network for tissue microstructure estimation using modified LSTM units. Medical Image Analysis. 55: 49–64.

[149] Chuyang Ye, Yuxing Li and Xiangzhu Zeng. 2020. An improved deep network for tissue microstructure estimation with uncertainty quantification. Medical Image Analysis. 61: 101650.

[150] Geng Chen, Haotian Jiang, Jiannan Liu, Jiquan Ma, Hui Cui, Yong Xia, et al. 2022. Hybrid graph transformer for tissue microstructure estimation with undersampled diffusion MRI data. *In*: International Conference on Medical Image Computing and Computer-Assisted Intervention. Springer. 113–122.

[151] Vladimir Golkov, A. Dosovitskiy, J.I. Sperl, M.I. Menzel, M. Czisch, P. Sämann, et al. 2016. Q-space deep learning: Twelve-fold shorter and model-free diffusion MRI scans. IEEE Transactions on Medical Imaging. 35(5): 1344–1351.

[152] Albert Clèrigues, Sergi Valverde, Jose Bernal, Jordi Freixenet, Arnau Oliver and Xavier Lladó. 2020. Acute and sub-acute stroke lesion segmentation from multimodal MRI. Computer Methods and Programs in Biomedicine. 194: 105521.

[153] E.V.R. DiBella, A. Sharma, L. Richards, V. Prabhakaran, J.J. Majersik and S.K. HashemizadehKolowri. 2022. Beyond diffusion tensor MRI methods for improved characterization of the brain after ischemic stroke: A review. American Journal of Neuroradiology. 43(5): 661–669.

[154] Stephan E. Maier, Yanping Sun and Robert V Mulkern. 2010. Diffusion imaging of brain tumors. NMR in Biomedicine. 23(7): 849–864.

[155] T.S. Papageorgiou, D. Chourmouzi, A. Drevelengas, K. Kouskouras and A. Siountas. 2015. Diffusion tensor imaging in brain tumors: A study on gliomas and metastases. Physica Medica. 31(7): 767–773.

[156] Ranliang Hu and Michael J. Hoch. 2021. Application of diffusion weighted imaging and diffusion tensor imaging in the pretreatment and post-treatment of brain tumor. Radiologic Clinics. 59(3): 335–347.

[157] S.D. Roosendaal, J.J.G. Geurts, H. Vrenken, H.E. Hulst, K.S. Cover and J.A. Castelijns. 2009. Regional DTI differences in multiple sclerosis patients. NeuroImage. 44(4): 1397–1403.

[158] Silvia De Santis, Matteo Bastiani, Amgad Droby, Pierre Kolber, Frauke Zipp, Eberhard Pracht, et al. 2019. Characterizing microstructural tissue properties in multiple sclerosis with diffusion MRI at 7 T and 3 T: The impact of the experimental design. Neuroscience. 403: 17–26.

[159] D.A. Lakhani, K.G. Schilling, J. Xu and F. Bagnato. 2020. Advanced multicompartment diffusion MRI models and their application in multiple sclerosis. American Journal of Neuroradiology. 41(5): 751–757.

[160] Talia M. Nir, Neda Jahanshad, J.E. Villalon-Reina, A.W. Toga, Clifford R. Jack, Michael W. Weiner, et al. 2013. Effectiveness of regional DTI measures in distinguishing Alzheimer's disease, MCI, and normal aging. NeuroImage: Clinical. 3: 180–195.

[161] Tijn M. Schouten, Marisa Koini, Frank de Vos, Stephan Seiler, Mark de Rooij, Anita Lechner, et al. 2017. Individual classification of Alzheimer's disease with diffusion magnetic resonance imaging. NeuroImage. 152: 476–481.

[162] Nhat Trung Doan, Andreas Engvig, Karin Persson, Dag Alnæs, Tobias Kaufmann, Jaroslav Rokicki, et al. 2017. Dissociable diffusion MRI patterns of white matter microstructure and connectivity in Alzheimer's disease spectrum. Scientific Reports. 7: 45131.

[163] Judith R. Harrison, Sanchita Bhatia, Zhao Xuan Tan, Anastasia Mirza-Davies, Hannah Benkert, Chantal M.W. Tax, et al. 2020. Imaging Alzheimer's genetic risk using diffusion MRI: A systematic review. NeuroImage: Clinical. 27: 102359.

[164] Xiuwei Fu, Susan Shrestha, Man Sun, Qiaoling Wu, Yuan Luo, Xianchang Zhang, et al. 2020. Microstructural white matter alterations in mild cognitive impairment and alzheimer's disease: Study based on Neurite Orientation Dispersion and Density Imaging (NODDI). Clinical Neuroradiology. 30: 569–579.

[165] Ofer Pasternak, Carl-Fredrik Westin, Brian Dahlben, Sylvain Bouix and Marek Kubicki. 2015. The extent of diffusion MRI markers of neuroinflammation

and white matter deterioration in chronic schizophrenia. Schizophrenia Research. 161(1): 113–118.

[166] Stefani O'Donoghue, Laurena Holleran, Dara M. Cannon and Colm McDonald. 2017. Anatomical dysconnectivity in bipolar disorder compared with schizophrenia: A selective review of structural network analyses using diffusion MRI. Journal of Affective Disorders. 209: 217–228.

[167] Suheyla Cetin-Karayumak, Maria A. Di Biase, Natalia Chunga, Benjamin Reid, Nathaniel Somes, Amanda E. Lyall, et al. 2020. White matter abnormalities across the lifespan of schizophrenia: A harmonized multi-site diffusion MRI study. Molecular Psychiatry. 25: 3208–3219.

[168] Inês Carreira Figueiredo, Faith Borgan, Ofer Pasternak, Federico E. Turkheimer and Oliver D. Howes. 2022. White-matter free-water diffusion MRI in schizophrenia: A systematic review and meta-analysis. Neuropsychopharmacology. 47: 1413–1420.

[169] Denis Le Bihan, Cyril Poupon, Alexis Amadon and Franck Lethimonnier. 2006. Artifacts and pitfalls in diffusion MRI. Journal of Magnetic Resonance Imaging. 24(3): 478–488.

[170] Gustavo Kunde Rohde, A.S. Barnett, P.J. Basser, S. Marenco and C. Pierpaoli. 2004. Comprehensive approach for correction of motion and distortion in diffusion-weighted MRI. Magnetic Resonance in Medicine. 51(1): 103–114.

[171] Siawoosh Mohammadi, Harald E. Möller, Harald Kugel, Dirk K. Müller and Michael Deppe. 2010. Correcting eddy current and motion effects by affine whole-brain registrations: Evaluation of three-dimensional distortions and comparison with slicewise correction. 64(4): 1047–1056.

[172] Jesper L.R. Andersson and Stamatios N. Sotiropoulos. 2016. An integrated approach to correction for off-resonance effects and subject movement in diffusion MR imaging. NeuroImage. 125: 1063–1078.

[173] José M. Soares, Paulo Marques, Victor Alves and Nuno Sousa. 2013. A hitchhiker's guide to diffusion tensor imaging. Frontiers in Neuroscience. 7: 31.

[174] Eric Aliotta, Hamidreza Nourzadeh, Jason Sanders, Donald Muller and D.B. Ennis. 2019. Highly accelerated, model-free diffusion tensor MRI reconstruction using neural networks. Medical Physics. 46(4): 1581–1591.

[175] Eric Aliotta, Hamidreza Nourzadeh and Sohil H. Patel. 2021. Extracting diffusion tensor fractional anisotropy and mean diffusivity from 3-direction DWI scans using deep learning. Magnetic Resonance in Medicine. 85(2): 845–854.

[176] Zhiwei Li, Ting Gong, Zhichao Lin, Hongjian He, Qiqi Tong, Chen Li, et al. 2019. Fast and robust diffusion kurtosis parametric mapping using a three-dimensional convolutional neural network. IEEE Access. 7: 71398–71411.

[177] Geng Chen, Yoonmi Hong, Y. Zhang, Jaeil Kim, Khoi Minh Huynh, Jiquan Ma, et al. 2020. Estimating tissue microstructure with undersampled diffusion data via graph convolutional neural networks. *In*: International Conference on Medical Image Computing and Computer-Assisted Intervention. Springer. 280–290.

[178] Tianshu Zheng, Guohui Yan, Haotian Li, Weihao Zheng, Wen Shi, Yi Zhang, et al. 2023. A microstructure estimation Transformer inspired by sparse representation for diffusion MRI. Medical Image Analysis. 86: 102788.

[179] Alessandro Daducci, E.J. Canales-Rodríguez, H. Zhang, T.B. Dyrby, D.C. Alexander and Jean-Philippe Thiran. 2015. Accelerated microstructure imaging via convex optimization (AMICO) from diffusion MRI data. NeuroImage. 105: 32–44.

[180] Ryutaro Tanno, Aurobrata Ghosh, Francesco Grussu, E. Kaden, Antonio Criminisi and Daniel C. Alexander. 2016. Bayesian image quality transfer. In: Medical Image Computing and Computer-Assisted Intervention–MICCAI 2016: 19th International Conference, Athens, Greece. Proceedings, Part II 19. Springer. 265–273.

[181] Ryutaro Tanno, Daniel E. Worrall, Aurobrata Ghosh, E. Kaden, S.N. Sotiropoulos, Antonio Criminisi, et al. 2017. Bayesian image quality transfer with CNNs: Exploring uncertainty in dMRI super-resolution. *In*: Medical Image Computing and Computer Assisted Intervention- MICCAI 2017: 20th International Conference, Quebec City, QC, Canada. Proceedings, Part I 20. Springer. 611–619.

[182] Ryutaro Tanno, Daniel E. Worrall, Enrico Kaden, A. Ghosh, Francesco Grussu, A. Bizzi, et al. 2021. Uncertainty modelling in deep learning for safer neuroimage enhancement: Demonstration in diffusion MRI. NeuroImage. 225: 117366.

[183] Evan Schwab, René Vidal and Nicolas Charon. 2016. Spatial-angular sparse coding for HARDI. *In*: Medical Image Computing and Computer-Assisted Intervention-MICCAI 2016: 19th International Conference, Athens, Greece. Proceedings, Part III 19. Springer. 475–483.

[184] Evan Daniel Schwab. 2018. Joint Spatial-Angular Sparse Coding, Compressed Sensing, and Dictionary Learning for Diffusion MRI. PhD thesis. Johns Hopkins University.

[185] Peter J. Basser, Sinisa Pajevic, Carlo Pierpaoli, Jeffrey Duda and Akram Aldroubi. 2000. *In vivo* fiber tractography using DT-MRI data. Magnetic Resonance in Medicine. 44(4): 625–632.

[186] Philippe Poulin, Daniel Jörgens, Pierre-Marc Jodoin and Maxime Descoteaux. 2019. Tractography and machine learning: Current state and open challenges. Magnetic Resonance Imaging. 64: 37–48.

[187] Fan Zhang, Suheyla Cetin Karayumak, Nico Hoffmann, Yogesh Rathi, A.J. Golby and Lauren J. O'Donnell. 2020. Deep white matter analysis (DeepWMA): Fast and consistent tractography segmentation. Medical Image Analysis. 65: 101761.

[188] Jakob Wasserthal, P.F. Neher, Dusan Hirjak and K.H. Maier-Hein. 2019. Combined tract segmentation and orientation mapping for bundle-specific tractography. Medical Image Analysis. 58: 101559.

[189] Feihong Liu, Jun Feng, Geng Chen, Ye Wu, Y. Hong, Pew-Thian Yap, et al. 2019. DeepBundle: Fiber bundle parcellation with graph convolution neural networks. *In*: Graph Learning in Medical Imaging: First International Workshop, GLMI 2019, Held in Conjunction with MICCAI 2019, Shenzhen, China. Proceedings 1. Springer. 88–95.

[190] Prince D. Ngattai Lam, Gaetan Belhomme, J. Ferrall, B. Patterson, Martin Styner and Juan C. Prieto. 2018. TRAFIC: Fiber tract classification using deep learning. In: Medical Imaging 2018: Image Processing. Vol. 10574. SPIE. 257–265.

[191] Haotian Xu, M. Dong, Min-Hee Lee, N. O'Hara, E. Asano, Jeong-Won Jeong, et al. 2019. Objective detection of eloquent axonal pathways to minimize post- operative deficits in pediatric epilepsy surgery using diffusion tractography and convolutional neural networks. IEEE Transactions on Medical Imaging. 38(8): 1910–1922.

[192] Vikash Gupta, S.I. Thomopoulos, C.K. Corbin, F. Rashid and Paul M. Thompson. 2018. Fibernet 2.0: An automatic neural network based tool for clustering white matter fibers in the brain. *In*: 2018 IEEE 15th International Symposium on Biomedical Imaging (ISBI 2018). IEEE. 708–711.

[193] Martijn P. Van Den Heuvel and Hilleke E. Hulshoff Pol. 2010. Exploring the brain network: A review on resting-state fMRI functional connectivity. European Neuropsychopharmacology. 20(8): 519–534.

[194] Kenneth K. Kwong. 2012. Record of a single fMRI experiment in May of 1991. NeuroImage. 62(2): 610–612.

[195] David J. Heeger and David Ress. 2002. What does fMRI tell us about neuronal activity? Nature Reviews Neuroscience. 3(2): 142–151.

[196] S.M. Slobounov, M. Gay, K. Zhang, B. Johnson, D. Pennell, W. Sebastianelli, et al. 2011. Alteration of brain functional network at rest and in response to YMCA physical stress test in concussed athletes: RsFMRI study. NeuroImage. 55(4): 1716–1727.

[197] Badari Birur, Nina Vanessa Kraguljac, Richard C. Shelton and Adrienne Carol Lahti. 2017. Brain structure, function, and neurochemistry in schizophrenia and bipolar disorder—A systematic review of the magnetic resonance neuroimaging literature. NPJ Schizophrenia. 3: 15.

[198] Edson Amaro Jr and Gareth J Barker. 2006. Study design in fMRI: Basic principles. Brain and Cognition. 60(3): 220–232.

[199] T. Labbé Atenas, E. Ciampi Díaz, J.P. Cruz Quiroga, S.U. Arancibia and C. Cárcamo Rodríguez. 2018. Functional magnetic resonance imaging: Basic principles and application in the neurosciences. Radiología (English Edition). 60(5): 368–377.

[200] Ophelia Deroy. 2019. Categorising without concepts. Review of Philosophy and Psychology. 10(3): 465–478.

[201] Scott H. Faro and Feroze B. Mohamed. 2006. Functional MRI: Basic Principles and Clinical Applications. Springer Science and Business Media.

[202] Gagan S. Wig, Bradley L. Schlaggar and Steven E. Petersen. 2011. Concepts and principles in the analysis of brain networks. Annals of the New York Academy of Sciences. 1224(1): 126–146.

[203] Seiji Ogawa. 2012. Finding the BOLD effect in brain images. NeuroImage. 62(2): 608–609.

[204] Xiaopeng Song, Yi Zhang and Yijun Liu. 2014. Frequency specificity of regional homogeneity in the resting-state human brain. PLoS One. 9(1): e86818.

[205] Megan H. Lee, Christopher D. Smyser and Joshua S. Shimony. 2013. Resting-state fMRI: A review of methods and clinical applications. American Journal of Neuroradiology. 34(10): 1866–1872.

[206] Samuel L. Warren and Ahmed A. Moustafa. 2023. Functional magnetic resonance imaging, deep learning, and Alzheimer's disease: A systematic review. Journal of Neuroimaging. 33(1): 5–18.

[207] Bharat Biswal, F. Zerrin Yetkin, Victor M. Haughton and James S. Hyde. 1995. Functional connectivity in the motor cortex of resting human brain using echo-planar MRI. Magnetic Resonance in Medicine. 34(4): 537–541.

[208] Christian F. Beckmann, Marilena DeLuca, Joseph T. Devlin and Stephen M. Smith. 2005. Investigations into resting-state connectivity using independent component analysis. Philosophical Transactions of the Royal Society B: Biological Sciences. 360(1457): 1001–1013.

[209] Dietmar Cordes, Victor M. Haughton, Konstantinos Arfanakis, Gary J. Wendt, Patrick A. Turski, Chad H. Moritz, et al. 2000. Mapping functionally related regions of brain with functional connectivity MR imaging. American Journal of Neuroradiology. 21(9): 1636–1644.

[210] J.S. Damoiseaux, S.A.R.B. Rombouts, F. Barkhof, P. Scheltens, C.J. Stam, S.M. Smith, et al. 2006. Consistent resting-state networks across healthy subjects. Proceedings of the National Academy of Sciences. 103(37): 13848–13853.

[211] M. De Luca, C.F. Beckmann, N. De Stefano, P.M. Matthews and S.M. Smith. 2006. fMRI resting state networks define distinct modes of long-distance interactions in the human brain. NeuroImage. 29(4): 1359–1367.

[212] Nico U.F. Dosenbach, Damien A. Fair, Francis M. Miezin, Alexander L. Cohen, Kristin K. Wenger, Ronny A.T. Dosenbach, et al. 2007. Distinct brain networks for adaptive and stable task control in humans. Proceedings of the National Academy of Sciences. 104(26): 11073–11078.

[213] Michael D. Fox, Maurizio Corbetta, Abraham Z. Snyder, Justin L. Vincent and Marcus E. Raichle. 2006. Spontaneous neuronal activity distinguishes human dorsal and ventral attention systems. Proceedings of the National Academy of Sciences. 103(26): 10046–10051.

[214] Michelle Hampson, Bradley S. Peterson, Pawel Skudlarski, James C. Gatenby and John C. Gore. 2002. Detection of functional connectivity using temporal correlations in MR images. Human Brain Mapping. 15(4): 247–262.

[215] Daniel S. Margulies, A.M. Clare Kelly, L.Q. Uddin, B.B. Biswal, F.X. Castellanos and Michael P. Milham. 2007. Mapping the functional connectivity of anterior cingulate cortex. NeuroImage. 37(2): 579–588.

[216] William W. Seeley, Vinod Menon, Alan F. Schatzberg, Jennifer Keller, G.H. Glover, Heather Kenna, et al. 2007. Dissociable intrinsic connectivity networks for salience processing and executive control. Journal of Neuroscience. 27(9): 2349–2356.

[217] Stephen M. Smith, P.T. Fox, K.L. Miller, D.C. Glahn, P.M. Fox, Clare E. Mackay, et al. 2009. Correspondence of the brain's functional architecture during activation and rest. Proceedings of the National Academy of Sciences. 106(31): 13040–13045.

[218] N. Tzourio-Mazoyer, B. Landeau, D. Papathanassiou, F. Crivello, O. Etard, N. Delcroix, et al. 2002. Automated anatomical labeling of activations in SPM using a macroscopic anatomical parcellation of the MNI MRI single-subject brain. NeuroImage. 15(1): 273–289.

[219] Elena A. Allen, Eswar Damaraju, Sergey M. Plis, Erik B. Erhardt, T. Eichele and Vince D. Calhoun. 2014. Tracking whole-brain connectivity dynamics in the resting state. Cerebral Cortex. 24(3): 663–676.

[220] Diego Vidaurre, Stephen M. Smith and Mark W. Woolrich. 2017. Brain network dynamics are hierarchically organized in time. Proceedings of the National Academy of Sciences. 114(48): 12827–12832.

[221] Harini Eavani, T.D. Satterthwaite, Raquel E. Gur, R.C. Gur and Christos Davatzikos. 2013.Unsupervised learning of functional network dynamics in resting state fMRI. In: Information Processing in Medical Imaging: 23rd International Conference, IPMI 2013, Asilomar, CA, USA. Proceedings 23. Springer. 426–437.

[222] Nora Leonardi, J. Richiardi, M. Gschwind, S. Simioni, J.-M. Annoni, M. Schluep, et al. 2013. Principal components of functional connectivity: A new approach to study dynamic brain connectivity during rest. NeuroImage. 83: 937–950.

[223] Nora Leonardi, William R. Shirer, Michael D. Greicius and Dimitri Van De Ville. 2014. Disentangling dynamic networks: Separated and joint expressions of functional connectivity patterns in time. Human Brain Mapping. 35(12): 5984–5995.

[224] R. Cameron Craddock, G.Andrew James, Paul E. Holtzheimer III, Xiaoping P. Hu and Helen S. Mayberg. 2011. A whole brain fMRI atlas generated via spatially constrained spectral clustering. 33(8): 1914–1928.

[225] Gael Varoquaux, Alexandre Gramfort, Fabian Pedregosa, Vincent Michel and Bertrand Thirion. 2011. Multi-subject dictionary learning to segment an atlas of

brain spontaneous activity. In: Information Processing in Medical Imaging: 22nd International Conference, IPMI 2011, Kloster Irsee, Germany. Proceedings 22. Springer. 562–573.

[226] Alexandre Abraham, Elvis Dohmatob, Bertrand Thirion, Dimitris Samaras and Gael Varoquaux. 2013. Extracting brain regions from rest fMRI with total-variation constrained dictionary learning. In: Medical Image Computing and Computer-Assisted Intervention–MICCAI 2013: 16th International Conference, Nagoya, Japan. Proceedings, Part II 16. Springer. 607–615.

[227] Jinglei Lv, Xi Jiang, Xiang Li, Dajiang Zhu, Shu Zhang, Shijie Zhao, et al. 2015. Holistic atlases of functional networks and interactions reveal reciprocal organizational architecture of cortical function. IEEE Transactions on Biomedical Engineering. 62(4): 1120–1131.

[228] Aviv Mezer, Yossi Yovel, Ofer Pasternak, Tali Gorfine and Yaniv Assaf. 2009. Cluster analysis of resting-state fMRI time series. NeuroImage. 45(4): 1117–1125.

[229] Yulia Golland, Polina Golland, Shlomo Bentin and Rafael Malach. 2008. Data-driven clustering reveals a fundamental subdivision of the human cortex into two global systems. Neuropsychologia. 46(2): 540–553.

[230] Megan H. Lee, Carl D. Hacker, Abraham Z. Snyder, Maurizio Corbetta, D. Zhang, E.C. Leuthardt, et al. 2012. Clustering of resting state networks. PLoS One. 7(7): e40370.

[231] Jae-Hun Kim, Jong-Min Lee, Hang Joon Jo, Sook Hui Kim, J.H. Lee, Sung Tae Kim, et al. 2010. Defining functional SMA and pre-SMA subregions in human MFC using resting state fMRI: Functional connectivity-based parcellation method. NeuroImage. 49(3): 2375–2386.

[232] Polina Golland, Yulia Golland and Rafael Malach. 2007. Detection of spatial activation patterns as unsupervised segmentation of fMRI data. *In*: Medical Image Computing and Computer-Assisted Intervention–MICCAI 2007: 10th International Conference, Brisbane, Australia. Proceedings, Part I 10. Springer. 110–118.

[233] B.T. Thomas Yeo, Fenna M. Krienen, Jorge Sepulcre, M.R. Sabuncu, D. Lashkari, M. Hollinshead, et al. 2011. The organization of the human cerebral cortex estimated by intrinsic functional connectivity. Journal of Neurophysiology. 106(3): 1125–1165.

[234] Raymond Salvador, John Suckling, Martin R. Coleman, J.D. Pickard, David Menon and Ed Bullmore. 2005. Neurophysiological architecture of functional magnetic resonance images of human brain. Cerebral Cortex. 15(9): 1332–1342.

[235] Dietmar Cordes, Vic Haughton, John D. Carew, Konstantinos Arfanakis and Ken Maravilla. 2002. Hierarchical clustering to measure connectivity in fMRI resting-state data. Magnetic Resonance Imaging. 20(4): 305–317.

[236] Thomas Blumensath, Saad Jbabdi, Matthew F. Glasser, David C. Van Essen, Kamil Ugurbil, Timothy E.J. Behrens, et al. 2013. Spatially constrained hierarchical parcellation of the brain with resting-state fMRI. NeuroImage. 76: 313–324.

[237] Alexandre Abraham, Michael P. Milham, Adriana Di Martino, R. Cameron Craddock, D. Samaras, Bertrand Thirion, et al. 2017. Deriving reproducible biomarkers from multi-site resting-state data: An Autism-based example. NeuroImage. 147: 736–745.

[238] Bertrand Thirion, G. Varoquaux, E. Dohmatob and J.-B. Poline. 2014. Which fMRI clustering gives good brain parcellations? Frontiers in Neuroscience. 8: 167.

[239] Yanlu Wang and Tie-Qiang Li. 2013. Analysis of whole-brain resting-state fMRI data using hierarchical clustering approach. PLoS One. 8(10): e76315.

[240] X. Shen, F. Tokoglu, X. Papademetris and R.T. Constable. 2013. Groupwise whole-brain parcellation from resting-state fMRI data for network node identification. NeuroImage. 82: 403–415.

[241] N. Honnorat, H. Eavani, T.D. Satterthwaite, R.E. Gur, R.C. Gur and C. Davatzikos. 2015. GraSP: Geodesic graph-based segmentation with shape priors for the functional parcellation of the cortex. NeuroImage. 106: 207–221.

[242] Nico U. F. Dosenbach, Binyam Nardos , Alexander L. Cohen , Damien A. Fair , Jonathan D. Power , Jessica A. Church, et al. 2010. Prediction of individual brain maturity using fMRI. Science. 329(5997): 1358–1361.

[243] Lubin Wang, L. Su, H. Shen and D. Hu. 2012. Decoding lifespan changes of the human brain using resting-state functional connectivity MRI. Plos ONE 7(8): e44530.

[244] Timothy B. Meier, A.S. Desphande, S. Vergun, Veena A. Nair, Jie Song, B.B. Biswal, et al. 2012. Support vector machine classification and characterization of age-related reorganization of functional brain networks. NeuroImage. 60(1): 601–613.

[245] Gang Chen, B. Douglas Ward, Chunming Xie, Wenjun Li, Zhilin Wu, J.L. Jones, et al. 2011. Classification of Alzheimer disease, mild cognitive impairment, and normal cognitive status with large-scale network analysis based on resting-state functional MR imaging. Radiology. 259(1): 213-221.

[246] Ali Khazaee, Ata Ebrahimzadeh and Abbas Babajani-Feremi. 2015. Identifying patients with Alzheimer's disease using resting-state fMRI and graph theory. Clinical Neurophysiology. 126(11): 2132–2141.

[247] Edward Challis, Peter Hurley, Laura Serra, Marco Bozzali, Seb Oliver and Mara Cercignani. 2015. Gaussian process classification of Alzheimer's disease and mild cognitive impairment from resting-state fMRI. NeuroImage. 112: 232–243.

[248] Chong-Yaw Wee, Pew-Thian Yap, Daoqiang Zhang, L. Wang and Dinggang Shen. 2014. Group-constrained sparse fMRI connectivity modeling for mild cognitive impairment identification. Brain Structure and Function. 219: 641–656.

[249] Xiaobo Chen, H. Zhang, Yue Gao, Chong-Yaw Wee, Gang Li and Dinggang Shen. 2016. High-order resting-state functional connectivity network for MCI classification. Human Brain Mapping. 37(9): 3282–3296.

[250] Biao Jie, Daoqiang Zhang, Chong-Yaw Wee and Dinggang Shen. 2014. Topological graph kernel on multiple thresholded functional connectivity networks for mild cognitive impairment classification. Human Brain Mapping. 35(7): 2876–2897.

[251] Chong-Yaw Wee, Sen Yang, Pew-Thian Yap and Dinggang Shen. 2016. Sparse temporally dynamic resting-state functional connectivity networks for early MCI identification. Brain Imaging and Behavior. 10: 342–356.

[252] Dan Long, Jinwei Wang, Min Xuan, Quanquan Gu, Xiaojun Xu, Dexing Kong, et al. 2012. Automatic classification of early Parkinson's disease with multi-modal MR imaging. PLoS One. 7(11): e47714.

[253] Robert C. Welsh, Laura M. Jelsone-Swain and Bradley R. Foerster. 2013. The utility of independent component analysis and machine learning in the identification of the amyotrophic lateral sclerosis diseased brain. Frontiers in Human Neuroscience 7: 251.

[254] Sophia Mueller, Danhong Wang, Michael D. Fox, B.T. Thomas Yeo, Jorge Sepulcre, Mert R. Sabuncu, et al. 2013. Individual variability in functional connectivity architecture of the human brain. Neuron. 77(3): 586–595.

[255] Emily S. Finn, Xilin Shen, Dustin Scheinost, Monica D. Rosenberg, Jessica Huang, M.M. Chun, et al. 2015. Functional connectome fingerprinting: Identifying individuals using patterns of brain connectivity. Nature Neuroscience. 18: 1664–1671.

[256] Monica D. Rosenberg, Emily S. Finn, Dustin Scheinost, X. Papademetris, Xilin Shen, R. Todd Constable, et al. 2015. A neuromarker of sustained attention from whole-brain functional connectivity. Nature Neuroscience. 19: 165–171.

[257] Joshua Sarfaty Siegel, Lenny E. Ramsey, Abraham Z. Snyder, Nicholas V. Metcalf, Ravi V. Chacko, Kilian Weinberger, et al. 2016. Disruptions of network connectivity predict impairment in multiple behavioral domains after stroke. Proceedings of the National Academy of Sciences. 113(30): E4367–E4376.

[258] Djalel-Eddine Meskaldji, M.G. Preti, Thomas A.W. Bolton, M.-L. Montandon, C. Rodriguez, Stephan Morgenthaler, et al. 2016. Prediction of long-term memory scores in MCI based on resting-state fMRI. NeuroImage: Clinical. 12: 785–795.

[259] David C. Jangraw, Javier Gonzalez-Castillo, Daniel A. Handwerker, Merage Ghane, Monica D. Rosenberg, Puja Panwar, et al. 2018. A functional connectivity-based neuromarker of sustained attention generalizes to predict recall in a reading task. NeuroImage. 166: 99–109.

[260] Wei-Ting Hsu, Monica D. Rosenberg, Dustin Scheinost, R. Todd Constable and Marvin M. Chun. 2018. Resting-state functional connectivity predicts neuroticism and extraversion in novel individuals. Social Cognitive and Affective Neuroscience. 13(2): 224–232.

[261] Alessandra D. Nostro, V.I. Müller, D.P. Varikuti, R.N. Pläschke, Felix Hoffstaedter, Robert Langner, et al. 2018. Predicting personality from network-based resting-state functional connectivity. Brain Structure and Function. 223: 2699–2719.

[262] Enzo Tagliazucchi, Frederic von Wegner, Astrid Morzelewski, Sergey Borisov, Kolja Jahnke and Helmut Laufs. 2012. Automatic sleep staging using fMRI functional connectivity data. NeuroImage. 63(1): 63–72.

[263] Enzo Tagliazucchi and Helmut Laufs. 2014. Decoding wakefulness levels from typical fMRI resting-state data reveals reliable drifts between wakefulness and sleep. Neuron. 82(3): 695–708.

[264] Joram Soch, John-Dylan Haynes and Carsten Allefeld. 2016. How to avoid mismodelling in GLM-based fMRI data analysis: Cross-validated Bayesian model selection. NeuroImage. 141: 469–489.

[265] Safoura Shahin, Farzaneh Shayegh, Sepehr Mortaheb and Rassoul Amirfattahi. 2016. Improvement of flexible design matrix in sparse Bayesian learning for multi task fMRI data analysis. *In*: 2016 23rd Iranian Conference on Biomedical Engineering and 2016 1st International Iranian Conference on Biomedical Engineering (ICBME). IEEE. 47–52.

[266] Tom Johnstone, K.S. Ores Walsh, Larry L. Greischar, A.L. Alexander, A.S. Fox, Richard J. Davidson, et al. 2006. Motion correction and the use of motion covariates in multiple-subject fMRI analysis. Human Brain Mapping. 27(10): 779–788.

[267] Jiansong Xu, Marc N. Potenza and Vince D. Calhoun. 2013. Spatial ICA reveals functional activity hidden from traditional fMRI GLM-based analyses. Frontiers in Neuroscience. 7: 154.

[268] Ze Wang, Anna R. Childress, Jiongjiong Wang and J.A. Detre. 2007. Support vector machine learning-based fMRI data group analysis. NeuroImage. 36(4): 1139–1151.

[269] Anna Zilverstand, Bettina Sorger, Jan Zimmermann, A. Kaas and Rainer Goebel. 2014. Windowed correlation: A suitable tool for providing dynamic fMRI-based functional connectivity neurofeedback on task difficulty. PLoS One. 9(1): e85929.

[270] Chris Tailby, Magdalena A. Kowalczyk and Graeme D. Jackson. 2018. Cognitive impairment in epilepsy: The role of reduced network flexibility. Annals of Clinical and Translational Neurology. 5(1): 29–40.

[271] Lara Lordier, Serafeim Loukas, Frédéric Grouiller, A. Vollenweider, Lana Vasung, Djalel-Eddine Meskaldij, et al. 2019. Music processing in preterm and full-term newborns: A psychophysiological interaction (PPI) approach in neonatal fMRI. NeuroImage. 185: 857–864.

[272] Kristine Boksman, Jean Théberge, Peter Williamson, Dick J. Drost, Ashok Malla, Maria Densmore, et al. 2005. A 4.0-T fMRI study of brain connectivity during word fluency in first-episode schizophrenia. Schizophrenia Research. 75(2–3): 247–263.

[273] Prasanna Karunanayaka, Vincent J. Schmithorst, Jennifer Vannest, J.P. Szaflarski, Elena Plante and Scott K. Holland. 2011. A linear structural equation model for covert verb generation based on independent component analysis of fMRI data from children and adolescents. Frontiers in Systems Neuroscience. 5: 29.

[274] Matthew Moore, Steven Culpepper, K. Luan Phan, T.J. Strauman, Florin Dolcos and Sanda Dolcos. 2018. Neurobehavioral mechanisms of resilience against emotional distress: An integrative brain-personality-symptom approach using structural equation modeling. Personality Neuroscience. 1: e8.

[275] Jieun Kim, Wei Zhu, Linda Chang, Peter M. Bentler and Thomas Ernst. 2007. Unified structural equation modeling approach for the analysis of multisubject, multivariate functional MRI data. Human Brain Mapping. 28(2): 85–93.

[276] Ronald Sladky, Anna Höflich, Martin Küblböck, Christoph Kraus, Pia Baldinger, Ewald Moser, et al. 2013. Disrupted effective connectivity between the amygdala and orbitofrontal cortex in social anxiety disorder during emotion discrimination revealed by dynamic causal modeling for fMRI. Cerebral Cortex. 25(4): 895–903.

[277] Will Penny, Jorge Iglesias-Fuster, Yakeel T. Quiroz, Francisco Javier Lopera and Maria A. Bobes. 2018. Dynamic causal modeling of preclinical autosomal-dominant Alzheimer's disease. Journal of Alzheimer's Disease. 65(3): 697–711.

[278] Fangyi Wang, Yuanqing Li and Zhenghui Gu. 2017. An MVPA method based on sparse representation for pattern localization in fMRI data analysis. Neurocomputing. 269: 206–211.

[279] Ian Charest, Nikolaus Kriegeskorte and Kendrick N Kay. 2018. GLMdenoise improves multivariate pattern analysis of fMRI data. NeuroImage. 183: 606–616.

[280] Tian Ge, Avram J. Holmes, Randy L. Buckner, J.W. Smoller and Mert R. Sabuncu. 2017. Heritability analysis with repeat measurements and its application to resting-state functional connectivity. Proceedings of the National Academy of Sciences. 114(21): 5521-5526.

Part 2

MRI-based Brain Disease Prediction

Chapter 2.1

Unveiling the Interdisciplinary Landscape of Brain MRI in Ophthalmology

Mini Han Wang[1,2,3,4] and Yi Pan[5]*

[1]Zhuhai People's Hospital (The Affiliated Hospital of Beijing Institute of Technology, Zhuhai Clinical Medical College of Jinan University), Zhuhai, China

[2]Department of Ophthalmology and Visual Sciences, The Chinese University of Hong Kong, Hong Kong SAR, China

[3]Faculty of Data Science, City University of Macau, Macau, China

[4]Center for Frontier Science Computing, Zhuhai Institute of Advanced Technology Chinese Academy of Sciences, Zhuhai, China

[5]Shenzhen University of Advanced Technology, Shenzhen, China

2.1.1 INTRODUCTION

Brain magnetic resonance imaging (MRI) [1] serves as a crucial diagnostic tool for visualizing and evaluating the structure and function of the brain, aiding in the diagnosis and management of various neurological disorders. Ophthalmology [2] focuses on studying and treating eye diseases [3], encompassing a range of conditions that affect visual health. Research in the intersecting fields of brain MRI and ophthalmology holds significant practical value for the advancement

*For Correspondence: yi.pan@siat.ac.cn

DOI: 10.1201/9781003518754-6

of diagnostic and therapeutic approaches in both domains. On the one hand, the integration of brain MRI and ophthalmic assessment represents a promising approach for utilizing retinal pathology as a biomarker in the identification and monitoring of brain-related diseases, like cognitive impairment and Alzheimer's disease [4]. On the other hand, brain MRI technology provides profound insights into the diagnosis and treatment of ocular diseases. Through MRI technology, physicians can more accurately detect and diagnose neurologic disorders related to the eyes, such as optic neuritis and optic nerve tumors [5]. Furthermore, brain MRI contributes to the exploration of the interaction between the visual system and the brain, facilitating our understanding of how visual information is processed in the brain and laying the groundwork for research in visual cognition and visual injury recovery [6]. Additionally, brain MRI plays a crucial role in the assessment of ophthalmic surgeries, aiding physicians in evaluating surgical outcomes and the restoration of visual function in patients [7], particularly in the early screening and treatment of conditions like retinoblastoma, choroidal melanoma, and retinal lymphoma, as well as in the detection and control of brain metastases from ocular cancers, which is vital for reducing mortality rates associated with eye cancer [8]. Therefore, interdisciplinary research at the intersection of brain MRI and ophthalmology not only advances medical knowledge but also provides more accurate and effective methods for neuro-ophthalmologic clinical diagnosis and treatment.

2.1.2 METHODOLOGIES

The study utilized Citespace (CiteSpace 6.2.R6, 64-bit, released on November 19, 2023) [9, 10] for literature visualization and quantitative analysis. Using the Web of Science Core Collection (WoSCC) database, articles in the field of brain MRI and ophthalmology were retrieved with the search string ("brain" and "MRI" and "Ophthalmolog*") as of March 9, 2024, resulting in 183 articles. These articles covered core topics such as neuro-ophthalmology and the application of MRI in diagnosing ocular diseases. Through quantitative analysis, the research revealed patterns of interrelations among authors, journals, institutions, and countries. By mining the core ideas of clustered authors, the study delved into the current status, perspectives, and future directions of this interdisciplinary field.

2.1.3 RESULTS

The search yielded a total of 183 articles from 89 journals, authored by 861 individuals affiliated with 550 institutions across 104 countries/regions. The study conducted analyses on trends in paper development, authorship, journal distribution, institutional affiliations, geographical representation and keyword distributions, aiming to explore thematic evolution and future research directions.

2.1.3.1 Research Development Trends

The non-redundant literature history development trend of WoSCC related to brain magnetic resonance imaging and ophthalmology is illustrated in Figure 1.1(a). The analysis reveals that the earliest publications in this field date back to 2007, with a continuous growth trend in the total number of publications. It is anticipated that this trend is likely to persist over the next few years.

2.1.3.2 The Distribution and Core Opinions Among Authors

This study examined a cohort of 861 authors, revealing a relatively weak collaboration among them (N = 208, E = 627, Density = 0.0291). As Figure 1.1(b) shows, authors were clustered into seven groups based on their research distribution, and an analysis of their publications and viewpoints yielded several key perspectives Figure 1.1(c). Firstly, the integration of PET-MRI scanning and ophthalmic assessment emerges as a promising avenue for leveraging retinal pathology as a biomarker in both identifying and monitoring cognitive impairment and Alzheimer's disease. Secondly, this study highlighted the role of MRI in diagnosing and managing the metastasis of ocular cancer to cerebral neoplasms. Thirdly, MRI's significance in diagnosing suspected neurological disorders with ocular symptoms is emphasized, such as ocular muscle paralysis. Furthermore, MRI's indispensable role in ocular manifestations of brain anomalies is underscored. Additionally, the essentiality of brain MRI in identifying causative genetic factors contributing to neurological disorders and their associated ocular manifestations is highlighted. Moreover, MRI's contribution as a diagnostic tool in the collaborative management of oncology and ophthalmology is acknowledged. Lastly, the significant importance of employing AI in diagnosing neuroophthalmic diseases based on ophthalmic evidence is recognized. Besides, the study found that, in addition to brain MRI, this field of research encompasses evidence from various ophthalmologic modalities, including optical coherence tomography (OCT), OCT angiography (OCTA), 45-degree visual angle fundus imaging [11], ultra-wide-field fundus imaging [12], fluorescein angiography [13], and ophthalmic MRI.

The integration of PET-MRI scanning and ophthalmic assessment represents a promising approach for utilizing retinal pathology as a biomarker in both the identification and monitoring of cognitive impairment and Alzheimer's disease. Esteemed scholars such as Pellegrini et al. [27] have focused their research on elucidating the correlation between ophthalmic parameters and cognitive function, particularly in the context of Alzheimer's disease. Their studies underscore the potential of MRI and ophthalmic assessments in providing novel insights for early screening, detection, and treatment of cognitive impairment and Alzheimer's disease, with biomarkers derived from ophthalmic evidence emerging as a non-invasive means of detection and a valuable tool for guiding further investigation of the disease. Byun et al. [4] conducted a cross-sectional study at Seoul National University Hospital, aiming to investigate the association between retinal biomarkers and in vivo Alzheimer's disease pathologic abnormalities in cognitively normal older adults, thereby developing a screening tool for detecting preclinical Alzheimer's

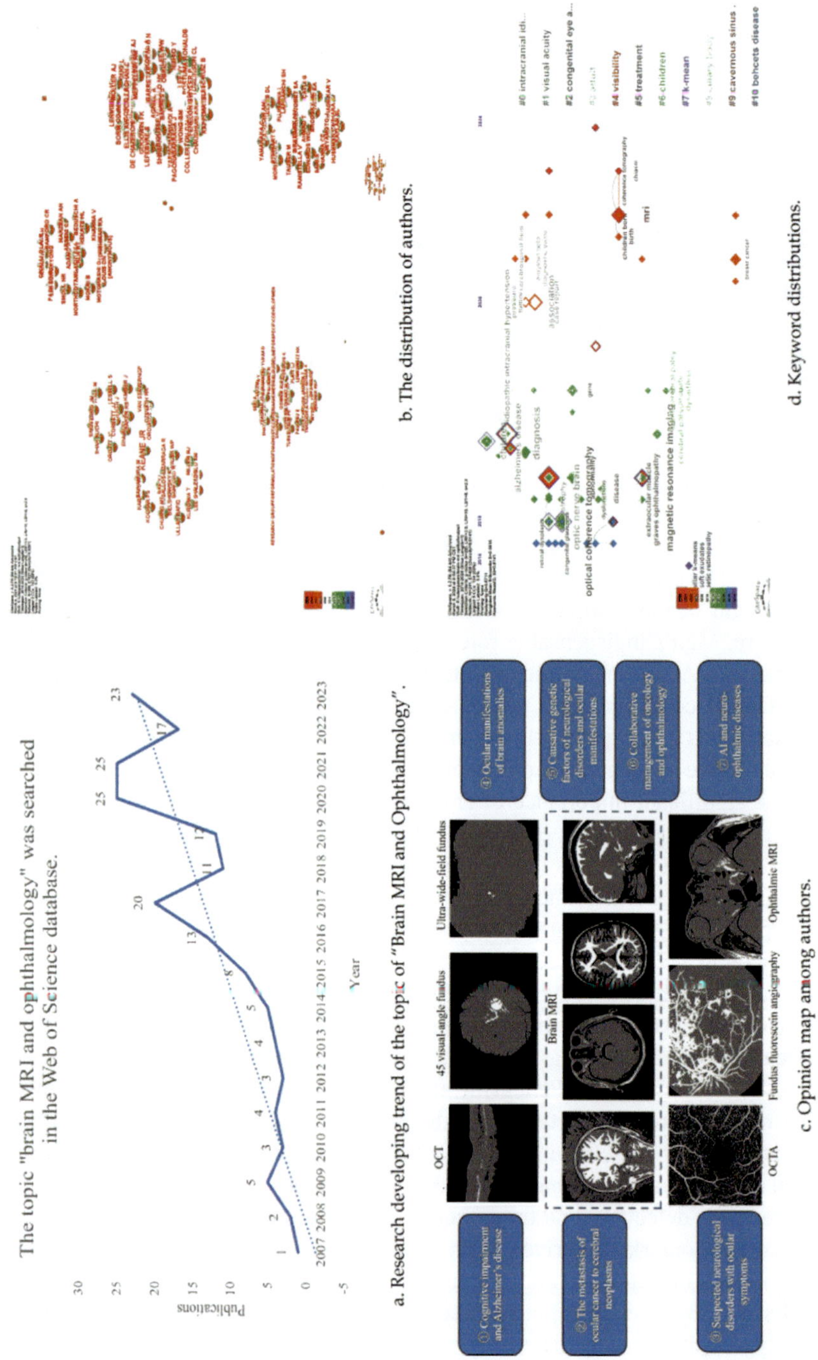

Figure 1.1 Bibliographic study of "Brain MRI and Ophthalmology".

disease. Their findings, based on comprehensive ophthalmic examinations, amyloid-β positron emission tomography, and magnetic resonance imaging in 49 cognitively normal individuals, revealed notable disparities in retinal thickness and function between Aβ+CN and Aβ-CN groups, with the former exhibiting diminished thickness and prolonged implicit time. It suggests the utility of retinal biomarkers as a non-invasive means for early detection of Alzheimer's disease pathologic abnormalities in cognitively normal older adults [4]. Zhang et al. [14] compared measurements of peripapillary retinal nerve fiber layer, retinal nerve fiber layer, and ganglion cell complex thicknesses using spectral domain optical coherence tomography between individuals with early-onset Alzheimer's disease and controls, alongside examining the relationship between these measurements and cognitive function, serum biomarkers for Alzheimer's disease, and cerebral microstructural volume. Their results indicated thinner retinal thicknesses in early-onset Alzheimer's disease patients compared to controls, with observed correlations between retinal thickness and serum biomarker levels, suggesting potential utility in tracking neurodegenerative processes, thereby highlighting the potential of retinal thickness as a marker for assessing neurodegeneration in early-onset Alzheimer's disease [14].

The exploration of brain MRI in diagnosing and managing ocular metastases with cerebral involvement is a pivotal domain of investigation. Ocular metastases, prevalent among ocular malignancies, present diverse clinical scenarios; they share a common therapeutic challenge that necessitates a multidisciplinary approach to selecting systemic and local therapies tailored to individual patient histories. This challenge encompasses achieving tumor control, preserving ocular function, and minimizing iatrogenic harm to surrounding sensitive tissues to safeguard vision and enhance patients' quality of life. Despite systemic molecular therapy for primary tumor management, patients with choroidal metastases often encounter secondary resistance, leading to potential cancer relapse post-initial response. Therefore, a proposition of adjunctive local treatment following systemic therapy is rationalized to sustain treatment response [15]. Scholars such as Fong et al. [16] have been pivotal in researching the diagnosis and treatment of ocular metastases with cerebral involvement, particularly in life-threatening diseases. Thariat et al. [15] demonstrated the utility of brain MRI post-choroidal metastasis discovery, especially in cancers prone to cerebral metastases, allowing for the timely detection of concomitant brain metastases before treatment initiation. Conversely, Fong et al. [16] illustrated a case study showcasing the rapid progression of ocular Vitreoretinal Lymphoma (PVRL), emphasizing the urgency of early diagnosis and intervention. The study advocates for prompt biopsy and close collaboration among pathologists, ophthalmologists, and oncologists to ensure precise and timely diagnosis, as delays may exacerbate intraocular lesion progression and CNS dissemination [16].

Brain MRI plays a crucial role in diagnosing suspected neurological disorders such as ocular muscle paralysis. Scholars such as Bamford R., Bielshowsky A., Chiba A., Fisher M., and Goffette have focused on diagnosing and treating optic nerve diseases and associated ocular manifestations. Their research indicates that neurological disorders often manifest with ocular involvement, and MRI is an essential tool for detecting conditions like internuclear ophthalmoplegia (INO) in individuals with suspected neurological diseases, contributing significantly to the advanced guidance and exploration of neurological disease diagnosis and treatment. Jung et al. [17] evaluated the clinical characteristics and prognosis of patients diagnosed with classical Miller-Fisher syndrome (MFS). Through retrospective analysis, the study investigated clinical and laboratory findings, as well as treatment outcomes in 10 patients diagnosed with MFS. Nine patients had antecedent infectious diseases, with diplopia occurring on average 11 ± 9.7 days after the antecedent infectious systemic illness. The observed triad of symptoms included acute ocular muscle paralysis, ataxia, and areflexia, with additional manifestations such as bilateral eye muscle paralysis, impaired pupil reflexes, limb weakness, speech difficulties, and facial palsy noted in some patients. Brain MRI and cerebrospinal fluid analysis revealed abnormalities in some patients, including optic nerve enhancement and protein-cell separation. Findings show that the consideration of MFS in patients with antecedent infections, along with the presence of acute ocular muscle paralysis, ataxia, and areflexia, as well as the detection of anti-GQ1b antibodies, aids in diagnosis. However, the outcomes in the treatment group did not significantly differ from those in the control group, indicating the need for further research to optimize the management strategies for this disease [17]. Additionally, Y. Ueno and S. Honda (2022) elucidated a case of traumatic medial longitudinal fasciculus (MLF) syndrome diagnosed via brain MRI. The 71-year-old male patient presented with diplopia after a head injury. Clinical examination revealed right medial rectus weakness, mild nystagmus when looking to the left with the left eye, and normal medial rectus function. MRI using susceptibility-weighted imaging (SWI) revealed a low-density area in the right midbrain, suggesting hemorrhage. Based on the patient's history, abnormal eye movement characteristics, and MRI findings, traumatic MLF syndrome was diagnosed. Symptoms improved within 2 weeks, with improvement in eye movements. This case highlights the risk of detecting brainstem hemorrhage using thin-layer MRI combined with SWI and suggests that it may be a precipitating factor for traumatic MLF syndrome [18].

Brain MRI is essential for brain-eye relationship investigations. Scholars such as Passi N., Shaikh A.G., Siavoshi S., Vidmer S., Achrol A.S., Dayani P.N., Hartmann A., and Hernesniemi J.A. have focused on the analysis of the brain-eye relationship, utilizing MRI to provide new insights into the etiology of ocular diseases, especially in patients presenting with sudden blindness or when conventional ophthalmic diagnostic methods fail to detect the underlying cause. Knoors et al. [19] conducted a study on the diagnosis and treatment of Wyburn-Mason syndrome, a rare condition characterized by ipsilateral arteriovenous malformations affecting the eye, brain, and facial skin. Their research highlighted conjunctival vascular dilation as a rare ocular manifestation. They reported a case of a 6-year-old boy presenting with sudden conjunctival vascular lesions in the right eye. Facial examination revealed subtle discoloration and conjunctival vascular structures along the distribution of the right trigeminal nerve. Fundus examination showed retinal vascular dilation and tortuosity. A brain MRI revealed large arteriovenous malformations in the central nuclei and peri-pontine region of the brain, consistent with the diagnosis of Wyburn-Mason syndrome. The sudden appearance of conjunctival vascular anomalies in this case provided a clue for diagnosing Wyburn-Mason syndrome, underscoring the importance of brain MRI in patients with ocular arteriovenous malformations [19]. Florou et al. [20] investigated a case of a 22-year-old Southeast Asian female who experienced unilateral vision loss one week after self-resolving hearing loss. Ophthalmic examination revealed abnormal light perception visual acuity, mild pupillary light reflex abnormalities, normal ocular motility, and a swollen optic disc with indistinct margins in the left eye. Neurological examination did not reveal acute pathological changes, but brain CT-MRI imaging showed a small, nearly subclinical cerebellar tonsillar herniation. After ruling out other causes, such as infection or inflammatory optic neuropathy, neurosurgical intervention was proposed. The patient underwent a successful suboccipital craniectomy and posterior fossa decompression, resulting in the resolution of optic disc swelling and complete visual recovery to 20/20. Chiari malformation is a condition where the posterior fossa volume is reduced, leading to cerebellar tonsillar herniation at least 5 mm below the foramen magnum. Optic disc swelling associated with Chiari malformation is rare. To date, Chiari malformation has been primarily studied in pediatric populations and is often associated with poor visual recovery [20].

The utilization of brain MRI for the detection of brain regions is crucial in identifying causative genetic factors contributing to neurological disorders and their associated ocular manifestations. Scholars such as Achrol A.S., Dayani P.N., Hartmann A., Hernesniemi J.A., Barboni P., Hayashi Shintaro, Kho R.C., and KONTOS have focused on the integration of MRI and ophthalmic diagnostic modalities for the diagnosis and treatment of neuro-ophthalmic diseases, particularly in cases where conventional ophthalmic examinations prove inconclusive, thereby paving the way for innovative diagnostic and therapeutic approaches. Pasqualotto, Bryce (2023) reported a case involving a 19-year-old male who experienced vision loss in the left eye on the first day after a martial arts head kick. A week later, vision loss occurred in the right eye without further trauma. While the initial fundoscopy was unremarkable, the visual field examination revealed temporal depression in the right eye and diffuse depression in the left eye, suggestive of traumatic optic chiasmal injury. A brain MRI demonstrated enlargement of the optic chiasm with internal signal abnormalities but without enhancement. Intravenous corticosteroid injection and hyperbaric oxygen therapy failed to improve vision. Additional investigations for atypical optic neuritis yielded negative results. Luckily, genetic testing for Leber's hereditary optic neuropathy (LHON) revealed positivity for the 11778 mutation. Thus, this case proposed that trauma is a trigger for LHON. The authors highlighted the rare internal signal abnormalities in the optic chiasm within this condition [21]. Almasoudi et al. [22] conducted a study involving two brothers presenting with spastic paraplegia, cognitive impairment, bladder and bowel dysfunction, and gait ataxia. Their unaffected parents had consanguineous relatives. Ophthalmic examination revealed chorioretinal lesions. A brain MRI revealed T2 hyperintensity and T1 hypointensity in the internal capsule, cerebral peduncle, corticospinal tracts, and cerebellar peduncles. Both affected brothers were homozygous for the CYP2U1 c.947A > T p.(Asp316Val) mutation, a known pathogenic variant of SPG56. Two rare autosomal recessive neurological disorders, spastic paraplegia 56 (SPG56) and leukoencephalopathy with spastic paraparesis, were identified in the same family members. However, they also harbored the novel CLCN2 c.607G > T, p.(Gly203Cys) mutation classified as a variant of unknown significance. Testing of other family members revealed another brother also harboring homozygous mutations for both variants, initially thought to be unaffected. Both males carrying CLCN2 mutations were infertile, with one brother showing incomplete spermatogenesis on testicular biopsy. Clinically, he exhibited mild memory impairment and hand tremors, with MRI findings similar to his affected sibling. Considering the neuroimaging and clinical features, including azoospermia, the authors proposed the pathogenicity of CLCN2 c.607G > T [22].

Brain MRI represents a significant advancement in diagnostic methodology for the collaborative management of oncology and ophthalmology. Coordinated care between these specialties is imperative for achieving optimal visual outcomes, with regular follow-up essential for monitoring potential remote ocular toxicity following radiation and/or chemotherapy. Notable scholars such as Aldrees, Sultan, Micieli, and Jonathan A. are actively investigating the diagnostic efficacy of MRI in identifying and managing radiation-induced Optic Neuropathy and Retinopathy. Within 2 months, 27.0% (10/37) and 8.1% (3/37) of eyes demonstrated improvements in best corrected visual acuity (BCVA). After treatment, BCVA restoration was noted in 24.6% (17/69) of eyes, while 13.0% (9/69) exhibited final BCVA improvement. MRI findings revealed optic nerve enhancement in 82.5% (33/40) of eyes, predominantly within the intracranial segment (69.7%), with 36.4% (12/33) showing enhancements concurrent with expansion and T2-high signals [23]. Aldrees et al. [24] report a case of a 68-year-old woman who is with bilateral profound vision loss, occurring over 2 months in the right eye and 1 week in the left eye, following multiple surgeries of radiation therapy for craniopharyngioma. Ophthalmological examination revealed severe visual impairment with bilateral optic disc pallor, suggesting optic nerve damage. Non-contrast MRI demonstrated a reduction of the sellar mass, while gadolinium-enhanced MRI revealed pre-chiasmatic enhancement of both optic nerves, indicative of radiation-induced optic neuropathy. Despite aggressive treatment, including high-dose intravenous corticosteroids, hyperbaric oxygen therapy, and intravenous bevacizumab, the patient's vision deteriorated further to complete blindness in both eyes [24]. Jimene et al. [25] reported a case involving a 72-year-old Hispanic male with extensive stage IV small-cell lung cancer and brain metastasis who developed radiation-induced optic neuropathy and retinopathy subsequent to whole-brain external radiation therapy, chemotherapy, immunotherapy, and thoracic radiation therapy. The report underscores the importance of carefully considering individual fraction sizes administered during radiation therapy, particularly in patients undergoing concurrent chemotherapy and immunotherapy, to mitigate the risk of radiation-induced ocular complications. Recognition of radiation-induced retinopathy and optic neuropathy is crucial, necessitating precise determination of cumulative dosage and fraction size when managing patients previously exposed to radiation. Additionally, an MRI of the brain and orbits can aid in distinguishing radiation-induced optic neuropathy from other forms of optic neuropathy [25].

The application of artificial intelligence (AI) in diagnosing neuro-ophthalmic diseases based on ophthalmic evidence is of significant importance. Scholars such as Alireza Javadzadeh, Ramesh, Hosny, Alzubaidi, and Farabi have been instrumental in exploring the utilization of advanced AI algorithms in ophthalmic and brain MRI settings, offering innovative opportunities for diagnosis and treatment. AI has garnered widespread attention for its immense capability in processing and detecting image markers and making clinical decisions, such as diagnoses, based on imaging data. Retinal vasculature has long been regarded as a promising imaging biomarker for systemic or ocular diseases. Wang et al. [12] indicated that retinal vein occlusion (RVO) entities may be associated with cardiovascular and cerebrovascular events or primary angle-closure glaucoma. Their study investigated the pathogenic differences between branch retinal vein occlusion (BRVO) and central retinal vein occlusion (CRVO) in terms of their correlations with systemic diseases or primary open-angle glaucoma (POAG). This retrospective case-control study included 59 RVO subjects (118 eyes), comprising 25 CRVO and 34 BRVO subjects who underwent routine ophthalmic and brain MRI examinations. Geometric features of retinal and cerebral vasculature diameters and optic nerve sheath width (ONSASW) were measured. Multivariate logistic regression analysis revealed that ONSASW at 3 mm posterior to the globe ($p = 0.044$) and relative retinal vein diameter ($p = 0.031$) were independent risk factors for CRVO-affected eyes compared to BRVO-affected eyes, after adjusting for age, duration of hypertension, BMI, and intraocular pressure. In CRVO-affected eyes, narrower relative retinal artery diameter ($p = 0.041$) and wider relative retinal vein diameter ($p = 0.011$) compared to the contralateral normal eyes were identified as independent risk factors after adjusting for intraocular pressure. The study suggested that BRVO might be more associated with cerebrovascular diseases, while CRVO might be associated with POAG. Geometric differences between retinal and cerebral vasculature could explain the pathological disparities between CRVO and BRVO [12]. Additionally, Alzheimer's disease (AD) is a neurodegenerative disorder primarily affecting brain tissue. Given the shared embryonic origin of the retina and brain, visual defects in AD patients have been well-established in numerous studies. Based on retinal changes in AD patients, many researchers have proposed using AI to predict, diagnose, and prognosticate AD. AD patients undergo changes in retinal thickness and retinal vessel density, sometimes occurring before the onset of clinical symptoms. AI and machine vision can detect and utilize these changes for disease prediction, diagnosis, and prognosis. Past studies have not only developed unique algorithms for this condition but also constructed databases such as the Retinal OCTA Segmentation Dataset (ROSE) [26]. AI-based retinal imaging for AD has achieved high accuracy, sensitivity, and specificity in classification, enabling researchers to identify individuals with a family history of AD based on ocular characteristics.

The continued advancement of AI in medicine holds promise for occupying a significant position in various aspects of managing AD patients, aiding in faster diagnosis of individuals at risk of AD, or assessing the prognosis of AD patients.

2.1.3.3 The Distribution of Journals

The collected literature is from 89 journals. According to the number of papers published, the top 10 journals are the American Journal of Ophthalmology (46 papers, Five-Year Impact Factor: 4.7), Ophthalmology (45 papers, Five-Year Impact Factor: 12.8), Journal of Neuro-ophthalmology (34 papers, Five-Year Impact Factor: 3.2), Neurology (34 papers, Five-Year Impact Factor: 10.3), American Journal of Neuroradiology (25 papers, Five-Year Impact Factor: 4.1), Brain (24 papers, Five-Year Impact Factor: 14.6), Investigative Ophthalmology & Visual Science (23 papers, Five-Year Impact Factor: 4.6), British Journal of Ophthalmology (22 papers, Five-Year Impact Factor: 4.3), Indian Journal of Ophthalmology (20 papers, Five-Year Impact Factor: 2.7). Five-Year Impact Factors were obtained from LetPub on March 17, 2024. These journals are all high-quality journals in the fields of ophthalmology and neurology.

2.1.3.4 The Distribution of Institutions and Countries

Authors of this field of study come from 550 institutions and 104 countries/regions. The result indicates that collaboration (association E) between institutions (N = 202, E = 185, Density = 0.0091) and countries (N = 41, E = 26, Density = 0.0317) is relatively weak. According to the number of published papers, the top 10 institutions are LV Prasad Eye Institute Hyderabad India (4 papers), Ibn Sina University Hospital Center of Rabat (4 papers), University of Toronto (3 papers), Mohammed V University in Rabat (3 papers), Egyptian Knowledge Bank (EKB) (3 papers), Sungkyunkwan University (SKKU) (2 papers), Osaka Medical College (2 papers), University of Birmingham (2 papers), University of Tennessee System (2 papers), and University of Arizona (2 papers). The top 10 countries are the United States (31 papers), India (21 papers), South Korea (14 papers), Japan (11 papers), England (10 papers), Iran (9 papers), Italy (8 papers), Canada (8 papers), Morocco (7 papers), and Saudi Arabia (7 papers), with China ranking 11th (4 papers). It can be seen that the contributing institutions in this study are internationally renowned universities, hospitals, and research centers in the field of medicine. Research in this field in China is still in a relatively nascent stage, with a relatively weak research output.

2.1.3.5 Keyword Distributions

The thematic distribution of this study is illustrated in Figure 1.1(d), where the paper topics are clustered into 10 categories: intracranial, vision, congenital eye, adult, visibility, treatment, children, k-means, ciliary body, sinus, and multiple sclerosis. According to the number of published papers: (1) MRI and OCT are the main medical diagnostic modalities, peaking in 2016 and 2015, respectively; (2) Idiopathic Intracranial Hypertension and Alzheimer's Disease are the primary brain diseases, peaking in 2019 and 2017, respectively; (3) Optic Neuropathy and Ophthalmoplegic Migraine are the main eye diseases, peaking in 2019 and 2015, respectively; (4) Genetics, tumors, treatment, visual pathways, and risk factors are the main research directions in the brain-eye field, peaking in 2018, 2020, 2017, 2021, and 2020, respectively; (5) Fuzzy c-means and Pillar K-means are the main research methods, both peaking in 2014. Thus, the utilization of statistical quantification and advanced AI techniques enables the study of intracranial abnormalities, neurological diseases, common brain diseases, optic nerves, ophthalmoplegia, brain-eye tumor diseases, as well as brain-eye pathway-related diagnosis and treatment, risk factors, genetic factors, and other aspects based on brain MRI and fundus images, serving as the current and future research focus.

2.1.4 DISCUSSION

The findings of this study provide insights into the collaborative networks, emerging topics, and dynamics of knowledge dissemination in the interdisciplinary field intersecting brain MRI and ophthalmology. By employing the Citespace literature quantification method, the research extensively analyzes the interdisciplinary research status of brain MRI in ophthalmology by exploring author patterns, journal distributions, collaborative networks, and keyword distributions. This analysis is a reference for researchers navigating and contributing to this interdisciplinary field. Furthermore, the visualization of co-citation clusters presents the interconnections of concepts and disciplines, facilitating interdisciplinary dialogue and knowledge exchange.

The findings from the literature quantification analysis reveal significant gaps and limited interdisciplinary collaboration in the realm of brain MRI and ophthalmology research. Concurrently, the emergence of AI as a transformative entity in healthcare has brought forth innovative solutions to intricate medical challenges. AI algorithms leveraging deep learning and machine learning technologies have showcased remarkable efficiency and precision in the analysis of medical imaging data. Within the context of brain MRI and ophthalmology, AI stands poised to revolutionize disease diagnosis, monitoring, and treatment. By scrutinizing extensive arrays of brain MRI and ophthalmic images, AI algorithms can discern patterns, anomalies, and disease biomarkers, thereby aiding clinicians in rendering more accurate and timely diagnoses, facilitating early intervention, and devising personalized treatment modalities. Moreover, predictive analytics harnessed through AI can prognosticate disease progression and treatment responses, empowering clinicians to optimize patient care strategies. The symbiotic nexus between AI, brain MRI, and ophthalmology research has fostered the development of innovative applications and tools, encompassing automated image segmentation algorithms for precise delineation of brain structures and ocular tissues, computer-aided diagnostic systems for the detection of neurological and ophthalmic abnormalities, and predictive models for the assessment of disease risks and prognostication. Furthermore, AI-driven research endeavors in brain MRI and ophthalmology engender interdisciplinary collaboration among neurologists, ophthalmologists, radiologists, computer scientists, and engineers, facilitating the exchange of knowledge, ideas, and expertise and propelling advancements in medical imaging technology and clinical practice.

However, AI-driven research in the intersection of brain MRI and ophthalmology faces several challenges, including the need for large-scale and diverse datasets to effectively train and validate AI algorithms, ensuring their robust performance across different patient populations and imaging modalities. Additionally, the interpretability and transparency of AI algorithms remain significant challenges, as clinical practitioners need confidence in understanding how AI systems reach conclusions to trust their diagnostic and therapeutic recommendations. Furthermore, integrating AI technology into clinical workflows presents numerous challenges, including seamless interoperability with existing healthcare systems and addressing data privacy, security, and ethics concerns. Moreover, the dynamic nature of medical imaging technology and the evolving landscape of neurological and ophthalmic diseases require continual refinement and adaptation of AI algorithms to keep pace with advancements in medical science and clinical practice. Lastly, interdisciplinary collaborations among clinical practitioners, data scientists, engineers, and policymakers are essential to address these challenges effectively and fully harness the potential of AI in improving patient care and advancing medical knowledge.

2.1.5 CONCLUSIONS

This study employs the Citespace methodology to conduct a quantitative analysis of the literature, offering a comprehensive assessment of the scholarly landscape within the intersection of brain MRI and ophthalmology. Through querying the WoSCC database, a dataset comprising 183 articles from 89 journals authored by 861 individuals affiliated with 550 institutions across 104 countries/regions was compiled. Examination of the literature revealed the earliest publications in this interdisciplinary domain dating back to 2007. By employing bibliometric analysis, trends in paper evolution, authorship, journal publication, institutional involvement, and geographic distribution were investigated. Additionally, the study undertook core literature extraction among clustered author groups, identifying seven prominent thematic areas, which are brain MRI applications in ocular motility disorders, brain tumors metastasizing to/from the eye, suspected neurogenic diseases inducing ophthalmoplegia, ocular manifestations of brain anomalies, neuro-ophthalmic conditions, brain disorders with associated ocular presentations attributable to genetic factors, and the utilization of AI-based methodologies for the diagnosis and treatment of neuro-ophthalmic ailments. This investigation unveils the collaborative network and emerging trends within the interdisciplinary domain of brain MRI and ophthalmology, underlining the significance of interdisciplinary cooperation and the potential of AI in advancing the diagnosis and treatment of neuro-ophthalmic disorders. The findings deliver valuable insights for researchers and practitioners aiming to deepen their comprehension and contribute to advancing brain MRI and ophthalmology. Furthermore, regarding future research directions, the paper advocates integrating artificial intelligence with brain MRI and ophthalmology research, highlighting its substantial potential to enhance diagnostic precision, ameliorate patient prognoses, and further our understanding of neurological and ophthalmic conditions.

ACKNOWLEDGMENTS

This research was funded by the National Natural Science Foundation of China Natural, grant number U22A2041, 82071915, and 62372047, the Shenzhen Key Laboratory of Intelligent Bioinformatics, grant number ZDSYS20220422103800001, the Shenzhen Science and Technology Program, grant number KQTD20200820113106007, the Guangdong Basic and Applied Basic Research Foundation, grant number 2022A1515220015, and the Zhuhai Technology and Research Foundation, grant number ZH22036201210034PWC, 2220004000131, and 2220004002412. The sub-figures in Figure 1.1(c) are collected from the Kaggle open-source platform and Zhuhai People's Hospital. The document of ethical clearance (No. [2024]-KT-67 and [2023]-54) in this research was obtained from the ethics review board at Zhuhai People's Hospital.

REFERENCES

[1] Ramin Ranjbarzadeh, Annalina Caputo, Erfan Babaee Tirkolaee, S.J. Ghoushchi, and Malika Bendechache. 2023. Brain tumor segmentation of MRI images: A comprehensive review on the application of artificial intelligence tools. Computers in Biology and Medicine. 152: 106405.

[2] Myron Yanoff and Jay S. Duker. 2009. Ophthalmology. Elsevier Health Sciences.

[3] Mini Han Wang, Lumin Xing, Yi Pan, Feng Gu, Junbin Fang, Xiangrong Yu, et al. 2024. AI-based advanced approaches and dry eye disease detection based on multi-source evidence: Cases, applications, issues, and future directions. Big Data Mining and Analytics 7(2): 445–484.

[4] Min Soo Byun, Sung Wook Park, Jun Ho Lee, Dahyun Yi, So Yeon Jeon, Hyo Jung Choi, et al. 2021. Association of retinal changes with Alzheimer disease neuroimaging biomarkers in cognitively normal individuals. JAMA Ophthalmology. 139(5): 548–556.

[5] Kelly A. Townsend, Gadi Wollstein and Joel S. Schuman. 2008. Clinical application of MRI in ophthalmology. NMR in Biomedicine. 21(9): 997–1002.

[6] Linda D'Antona, Hasan Asif, Claudia Craven, James McHugh, Fion Bremner, Laurence D. Watkins, et al. 2021. Brain MRI and ophthalmic biomarkers of intracranial pressure. Neurology. 96(22): e2714–e2723.

[7] Doety Prins, Sandra Hanekamp and Frans W Cornelissen. 2016. Structural brain MRI studies in eye diseases: are they clinically relevant? A review of current findings. Acta Ophthalmologica. 94(2): 113–121.

[8] Thoralf Niendorf, Jan-Willem M. Beenakker, Sönke Langner, Katharina Erb-Eigner, Meritxell Bach Cuadra, Ebba Beller, et al. 2021. Ophthalmic magnetic resonance imaging: where are we (heading to)? Current Eye Research. 46(9): 1251–1270.

[9] Chaomei Chen. 2006. CiteSpace II: Detecting and visualizing emerging trends and transient patterns in scientific literature. Journal of the American Society for Information Science and Technology. 57: 359–377.

[10] Weihong Wang and Chang Lu. 2020. Visualization analysis of big data research based on Citespace. Soft Computing. 24(11): 8173–8186.

[11] Wang Mini Han, Huang Lina, Hou Guanghui, Yang Jie, Xing Lumin, Yuan Qiting, et al. 2024. Deep learning for macular fovea detection based on ultra- widefield fundus images. *In*: Second International Conference on Electrical, Electronics, and Information Engineering (EEIE 2023). 12983: 510–521. SPIE.

[12] Wang Qiyun, Li Ting, Zhang Xinyuan, Zeng Yiyun, Yang Yang, Zhou Yun, et al. 2024. Distinctive Imaging Characteristics of Retinal and Cerebral Vessels between Central and Branch Retinal Vein Occlusion by MRI and AI-Based Image Analyzer. Diagnostics. 14(3): 267.

[13] Wang Mini Han, Zhou Junjie, Huang Chengde, Tang Zhoujie, Yu Xiangrong, Hou Guanghui, et al. 2024. Fusion learning methods for the age-related macular degeneration diagnosis based on multiple sources of ophthalmic digital images. *In*: Second International Conference on Electrical, Electronics, and Information Engineering (EEIE 2023). 12983: 470–492. SPIE.

[14] Zhang Ziyi, Kwapong WR, Cao Li, Feng Zhe, Liu Peng, Wang Ruoyu, et al. 2024. Correlation between serum biomarkers, brain volume, and retinal neuronal loss in early-onset Alzheimer's disease. Neurological Sciences. 45(6): 2615–2623.

[15] Juliette Thariat, Laurys Boudin, Olivier Loria, Anh-Minh Nguyen, Laurent Kodjikian and Thibaud Mathis. 2022. How to manage a patient with ocular metastases? Biomedicines 10(12): 3044.

[16] Joseph W. Fong, Riley N. Sanders, David L. Baker, S. Pina-Oviedo and S. Uwaydat. 2022. Rapidly progressive bilateral vitreoretinal lymphoma. Cureus. 14(11): e31639. https://doi.org/10.7759/cureus.31639.

[17] Jae Woo Jung, Jong Heon Lee and Jae Ho Jung. 2017. The Characteristics and Prognosis of Miller Fisher Syndrome. Journal of the Korean Ophthalmological Society. 58(2): 197–202.

[18] Yosuke Ueno and Shigeru Honda. 2022. A case of traumatic medial longitudinal fasciculus syndrome whose causal lesion was detected by thin-section MRI with susceptibility- weighted imaging. Case Reports in Ophthalmology. 13(2): 368–373.

[19] Knoors Louise, Buyse Gunnar, Lagae Lieven, Demaerel Philippe, Kesteloot Frank, Casteels Ingele, et al. 2018. Conjunctival vascular malformation as a rare presenting sign of Wyburn–Mason syndrome. Journal of Pediatric Neurology. 16(04): 239–242.

[20] Florou Chrysoula, Andreanos Konstantinos, Georgakoulias Nikos, Espinosa Edroulfo, Papakonstantinou Evangelia, Georgalas Ilias, et al. 2020. Acute visual loss secondary to Arnold Chiari type I malformation completely resolving after decompressive posterior fossa surgery. International Medical Case Reports Journal. 657–661.

[21] Bryce Pasqualotto. 2023. Mitochondrial form and function in patient-derived fibroblasts harbouring the G11778A mutation of Leber's hereditary optic neuropathy. (Thesis) Ph.D., Summit Research Repository.

[22] Wejdan Almasoudi, Christer Nilsson, Ulrika Kjellström, Kevin Sandeman and Andreas Puschmann. 2023. Co-occurrence of CLCN2-related leukoencephalopathy and SPG56. Clinical Parkinsonism and Related Disorders. 8: 100189.

[23] Wang Yongping, Fu Junxia, Zhou Huanfen, Li Hongen, Xu Quangang, Wei Shihui, et al. 2023. Clinical characteristics of radiation-induced optic neuropathy: A single-center retrospective study. Advances in Ophthalmology Practice and Research. 3(3): 141–146.

[24] Sultan Aldrees and Jonathan A. Micieli. 2020. Catastrophic vision loss from radiation- induced optic neuropathy. BMJ Case Reports CP. 13(2): e233706.

[25] Brittney Jimenez, Angelina Tran, Lisa Huang and Bhagya Segu. 2023. A Case of Radiation-Induced Optic Neuropathy and Retinopathy after Radiation Therapy, Chemotherapy, and Immunotherapy for Brain Metastasis. Canadian Journal of Optometry. 85(1): 73–82.

[26] Hamidreza Ashayeri, Ali Jafarizadeh, Milad Yousefi, Fereshteh Farhadi and Alireza Javadzadeh. 2024. Retinal imaging and Alzheimer's disease: A future powered by Artificial Intelligence. Graefe's Archive for Clinical and Experimental Ophthalmology. 1–13.

[27] Francesco Pellegrini, Andrew G. Lee and Pietro Zucchetta. 2017. Homonymous hemianopsia due to posterior cortical atrophy. Neuroophthalmology. 41(3): 154–158.

Chapter **2.2**

Brain Disease Diagnosis Through AI-MRI Integration

Baiying Lei
National-Regional Key Technology Engineering Laboratory for Medical Ultrasound,
Guangdong Key Laboratory for Biomedical Measurements and Ultrasound Imaging,
School of Biomedical Engineering,
Shenzhen University Medical School, Shenzhen University,
Shenzhen 518060, China

2.2.1 INTRODUCTION

Brain disorders are conditions that affect the function of the brain and central nervous system, potentially caused by various factors, including genetics, infection, metabolic disorders, environmental factors, lifestyle, and aging [1]. As a result, the definition and classification of brain diseases are quite broad, encompassing neurodegenerative diseases, mental disorders, developmental and genetic diseases, and more. It is reported that neurological disorders within brain diseases are the leading cause of the global burden of disease, with a 59% increase in the number of cases worldwide since 1990. Additionally, research predicts that by 2050, the global burden of brain diseases will increase significantly [2]. Despite progress in our understanding of the brain and its diseases, there is a lack of precise biological markers, and issues such as data sharing and standardization still face considerable challenges in diagnosing and treating brain diseases. Therefore, research on the diagnosis of brain diseases is of great importance and urgency.

*For Correspondence: Email: leiby@szu.edu.cn

DOI: 10.1201/9781003518754-7

Magnetic Resonance Imaging (MRI) is a non-invasive medical imaging technique that uses a strong magnetic field and radio waves to obtain images of the internal structures of the human body. MRI and its advanced technologies, such as Diffusion Tensor Imaging (DTI), can detect early changes in brain diseases, have extremely high contrast resolution for different parts of the brain tissue (such as gray matter, white matter, cerebrospinal fluid, etc.), and can provide more information about the characteristics of brain tissue and pathological processes, making them indispensable tools in the field of brain disease diagnosis. However, the early diagnosis of brain diseases needs to rely on the subjective experience of doctors, and there is a lack of objective diagnostic methods suitable for clinical practice. The development of Artificial Intelligence (AI) technology has improved the accuracy of brain disease diagnosis. Moreover, studies have shown that over the past decade, the number of studies on AI models as auxiliary diagnostic tools for brain diseases has increased exponentially [3]. The above indicates that brain disease diagnosis through AI-integrated MRI has become a significant focus in medical imaging. In recent years, brain disease diagnosis through AI-integrated MRI has been primarily focused on deep learning. These methods have significantly improved the diagnostic performance of brain diseases by characterizing the deeper linear and nonlinear complex interactions between regions of interest. These primary methods include convolutional neural networks (CNN) [4–7], recurrent neural networks (RNN) [8–11], and transformers [12, 13], which have helped doctors make many complex diagnoses in the medical field. However, these studies have a common limitation: dependence on single modality brain imaging data. This dependence may result in an inability to provide a comprehensive set of brain features, such as only providing anatomical structural information [14–16] or functional information [17–19], which affects the integrity and accuracy of brain information extraction, ultimately affecting the model's performance and generalization ability.

To overcome this limitation, researchers have adopted the method of multimodal data fusion to provide a more comprehensive perspective for diagnosing brain diseases and improving the diagnostic effect of brain diseases [20, 21]. Many studies have successfully used multi-modal brain images to diagnose brain diseases [22–26] and used the canonical correlation analysis (CCA) method to perform a linear fusion of gray matter features extracted from sMRI with the time-varying FC state profiles based on functional MRI (fMRI) features.

Moreover [27], considering that the different types of data exhibit nonlinear links that provide rich information, an RNN-based method was used to fuse fMRI and structural MRI (sMRI) data. Considering [28] that traditional autoencoders always mix shared information and complementary information from different modalities into a single latent variable, where the information from one modality may act as the noise obstructing the reconstruction of the other, a disentangled multimodal adversarial autoencoder (DMM-AAE) model was used to fuse sMRI and fMRI data based on the blood oxygenation level-dependent (BOLD) signal (BOLD-fMRI). Although these methods have made significant progress in diagnosing brain diseases, they only use simple fusion techniques and do not consider the heterogeneity, asynchrony, information redundancy and complementarity, and imbalance of data fusion between different brain imaging data modes.

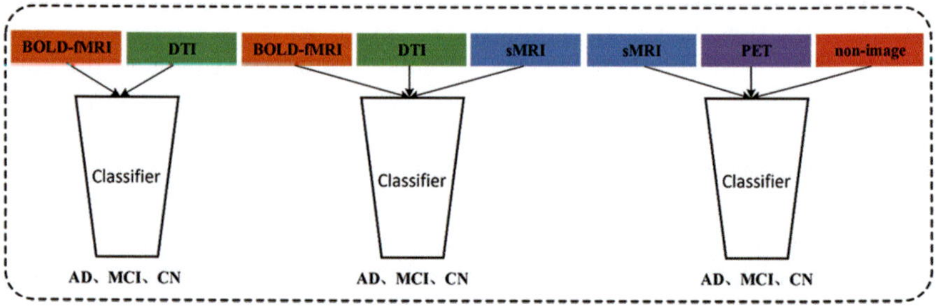

Figure 2.1 Classification of AI-integrated MRI multimodal data fusion models.

Inspired by the above observations, we have proposed a series of AI-integrated MRI multimodal data fusion models to achieve more effective integration of multimodal features for diagnosing brain disease. As shown in Figure 2.1, these models are as follows:

1. Fusion models for BOLD-fMRI and DTI data. We considered that BOLD-fMRI primarily provides information on brain functional activity, such as activating brain regions under specific tasks or stimuli. DTI, on the other hand, mainly includes detailed information on the structure of the brain's white matter, including the pathways and organizational structure of nerve fibers. These two data types have their respective advantages and limitations in neuroscience research and clinical diagnosis. By combining these two technologies, researchers can gain a more comprehensive understanding of the brain's function and structure. However, the fusion of these two types of data has many shortcomings. We have introduced the cross-modal transformer generative adversarial network (CT-GAN) [29] and the brain structure-function fusing-representation learning (BSFL) model [30] to address the complexity of linear and nonlinear correlations in this data and the reliance of existing fusion models on empirical methods, combining structural and functional connectivity for brain disease analysis.
2. Fusion models for BOLD-fMRI, DTI, and sMRI data. We considered that sMRI provides macroscopic structural information about the brain, including the volume, shape, and location of gray and white matter. There is a significant difference between the functional brain information provided by BOLD-fMRI and the microscopic structural information about white matter fiber bundles provided by DTI, and there is a complementary relationship between the information. By combining these three technologies, researchers can better understand the brain's function and structure. At the same time, to address the differences in the regions of interest across different modalities and the various higher-order correlations, we have introduced the stacked sparse nonnegative autoencoder (SSNAE) [31] and the prior-guided adversarial learning

with hypergraph (PALH) model [32]—fusion models of MRI data with other imaging modalities' data or non-image modalities' data. In the fusion of various MRI modalities, we found that adding other image and non-image information, such as positron emission tomography (PET), age, gender, etc., can improve the detection accuracy of brain diseases to some extent. To address the difficulty in finding interpretability between different modality image data and the difficulty in unifying the dimensions of non-image information and image information fusion, we have introduced the multimodal diagnosis network based on multi-fusion and disease-induced learning (MDL-Net) [33] and the multi-scale enhanced graph convolutional network (MSE-GCN) model [34].

2.2.2 FUSION MODELS FOR BOLD-FMRI AND DTI DATA

BOLD-fMRI measures changes in blood oxygen levels, reflecting brain functional activity, while DTI measures the anisotropic diffusion of water molecules, reflecting the structure of white matter fibers. These two imaging techniques are based on different biological processes, so when integrating them, it is necessary to consider how to integrate functional and structural information effectively. The design challenge of the BOLD-fMRI and DTI data fusion model lies in the unknown and complex correlations between the two data types, and the over-reliance on domain experience by existing models. Inspired by the above observations, we have proposed two models for fusing BOLD-fMRI and DTI data.

2.2.2.1 CT-GAN

This section introduces the CT-GAN model to effectively fuse the functional and structural information contained in BOLD-fMRI and DTI. The CT-GAN can learn topological features and generate multimodal connectivity from multimodal imaging data in an efficient end-to-end manner. Moreover, the swapping bi-attention mechanism is designed to gradually align common features and effectively enhance the complementary features between modalities. By analyzing the generated connectivity features, the proposed model can identify Alzheimer's disease (AD)-related brain connections. Evaluations of the public Alzheimer's disease neuroimaging initiative (ADNI) dataset show that the proposed CT-GAN can dramatically improve prediction performance and detect AD-related brain regions effectively. The proposed model also provides new insights into detecting AD-related abnormal neural circuits.

Method

Given bimodal images (i.e., BOLD-fMRI and DTI), the proposed model can learn a non-linear learning network that transforms imaging space into topological connectivity space. To obtain multimodal connectivity, we designed the CT-GAN with four components: (1) the cross-modal transformer generator (G) that is used for inference and generates multimodal connectivity; (2) the dual-channel separator (DS) that decomposes the multimodal connectivity into structural connectivity (SC) and functional connectivity (FC); (3) the structural-functional consistency (SFC) discriminator, which contains two sub-discriminators (i.e., $\mathbf{D}_s$ and $\mathbf{D}_f$). Each discriminates whether an SC or FC comes from the proposed generator or the software toolboxes; (4) the predictor that assigns AD stages based on the generated multimodal connectivity.

Cross-Modal Transformer Generator

1. **Embedding Extractor:** To embed regions of interest-based (ROIs) features into the transformer-based network, a routine convolutional neural network is adopted to extract ROI-based features from brain imaging. We design two extractors, including a structural embedding (SE) extractor and a functional embedding (FE) extractor. The embedding S is computed by successive convolutional filters on the DTI.
2. **Swapping Bi-Attention Mechanism:** To mine the complementary information between BOLD-fMRI and DTI, we devise the swapping bi-attention mechanism (SBM) to align functional features with microstructural information. It can facilitate the synergistic exchange of information between bimodal images.
3. **Feed Forward Mapping:** After the bi-attention mechanism, the cross-modal bi-attention features $F^{Att}$and S^{Att} represent the mixed functional feature sequence and mixed structural feature sequence, respectively. We apply linear mapping to them for effective information adjustment.
4. **Connectivity Computation:** After the L layers of the transformer, we obtained the updated mixed structural and functional features S' and F'. These mixed features contain common and unique information for both modalities, where we utilize the PCC to define multimodal connectivity. We first project one modal feature onto the other modal feature, then compute the relationship of paired ROIs with the following formula:

$$MC = S'F'F'^T S'^T \tag{1}$$

where, MC means the final multimodal connectivity (MC) with the size $N \times N$. In the experiment, we follow the fourth method of FC definition to recompute the multimodal connectivity for AD analysis. The elements in the MC matrix below the threshold are represented by 0, and those above the threshold remain unchanged.

Dual-Channel Separator

The MC contains both structural and functional connectivity information. To stabilize the learning process, we design the dual-channel separator to recover the SC and FC from the MC. The dual-channel separator projects the MC back to two modality-specific connectivities. Considering the topological properties of the human brain, we adopt the cross-weighting scheme to extract global connectivity information for better detachment between structural and functional connectivity. It consists of two branches, which share the first layer and have different weighting parameters in the second and third layers, respectively. The filter is a cross-shape parameter with step size 1. The input and the output for each layer have the same size, except for different channels. Finally, the third layer outputs the reconstructed SC and FC.

Structural-Functional Consistency Discriminator

To make the reconstructed SC and FC have the same distribution as the empirical SC and FC, the SFC discriminator is designed to distinguish empirical SC and FC from the reconstructed SC and FC and provide feedback loss on the generator. It not only makes the dual-channel separator robust but also improves the generator's learning abilities. The SFC discriminator contains two sub-discriminators (i.e., $\boldsymbol{D_s}$ and $\boldsymbol{D_f}$). Both discriminators share the same network structure. For the sake of narration, we take D_s as an example to describe the computing process in detail. The input SC is passed through two branches, including local convolution (top) and global convolution (bottom). The top branch contains four 3×3 convolution operations, one average pooling operation, and one flattened layer. The bottom branch contains two kinds of convolution filters (1×90 and 90×1) and one flattened layer. The final output is a value ranging from 0 to 1, which indicates whether the input is a reconstructed or empirical SC.

Loss Function

To effectively fuse the functional and structural information contained in BOLD-fMRI and DTI, the proposed CT-GAN model is optimized using a hybrid loss function that incorporates three types of objective losses: adversarial loss, classification loss, and pair-wise connectivity reconstruction loss. These three loss functions can ensure the quality of multimodal connectivity generation.

Experiments

To demonstrate the generation effect of the proposed model. Different connectivity characteristics can be seen in the local area; the MC at the AD stage has the sparsest connectivity features. We conducted three binary classification tasks (i.e., normal control (NC) vs. early mild cognitive impairment (EMCI), EMCI vs. late mild cognitive impairment (LMCI), and LMCI vs. AD) for a quantitative analysis of the proposed model's classification, as shown in Table 2.1. Under different classification tasks, our model achieves superior results to others in terms of different classifiers. Both classifiers have similar classification performances.

Additionally, we can find that the decreased connections are greater than the increased connections at the stages of EMCI and AD, while the phenomenon is reversed at the LMCI stage.

2.2.2.2 BSFL

This section introduces the BSFL model to effectively learn fused representation from DTI and BOLD-fMRI for mild cognitive impairment (MCI) analysis. Specifically, the decomposition-fusion framework is developed to decompose

Table 2.1 Performance comparison for different models and classifiers across different classification tasks

Models	**Classifiers**	**NC vs. EMCI**				**EMCI vs. LMCI**				**LMCI vs. AD**			
		ACC	**SEN**	**SPE**	**AUC**	**ACC**	**SEN**	**SPE**	**AUC**	**ACC**	**SEN**	**SPE**	**AUC**
	GCN	87.20	91.25	83.33	89.35	89.26	87.80	90.00	90.70	92.31	92.06	92.68	93.46
MMEGCN	GBDM	87.80	85.00	90.48	90.95	88.43	87.80	88.75	89.45	93.27	93.65	92.68	94.39
	Ours	**89.63**	90.00	89.29	**93.44**	**93.39**	**92.68**	**93.75**	**94.51**	**94.23**	93.65	**95.12**	**95.20**
	Brainnetcnn	88.41	87.50	89.29	90.71	88.43	90.24	87.50	88.17	91.35	90.48	92.68	89.47
MMEGCN	GBDM	88.41	90.00	86.90	90.31	91.74	90.24	92.50	89.42	93.27	92.06	95.12	91.99
	Ours	**90.24**	90.00	**90.48**	**93.26**	**92.56**	90.24	**93.75**	**93.93**	**95.19**	**95.24**	95.12	**94.27**

the feature space into the union of the uniform and the unique spaces for each modality and then adaptively fuse the decomposed features to learn MCI-related representation. Moreover, a knowledge-aware transformer module is designed to capture local and global connectivity features throughout the brain. Also, a uniform-unique contrastive loss is further devised to make the decomposition more effective and enhance the complementarity of structural and functional features. The extensive experiments demonstrate that the proposed model performs better than other competitive methods in predicting and analyzing MCI. More importantly, the proposed model could be a potential tool for reconstructing unified brain networks and predicting abnormal connections during the degenerative processes in MCI.

Method

After some preprocessing steps, given the BOLD-fMRI and DTI, the introduced model learns a complicated non-linear mapping network to transform the bimodal images into brain networks for detecting abnormal brain connections at different stages of MCI. The proposed model consists of four parts: (1) knowledge-aware transformer, (2) decomposed variational graph autoencoders, (3) representation-fusing generator, and (4) dual discriminator. The last three parts are defined as the decomposition-fusion framework. First, the transformer-based network extracts structural features from DTI by incorporating location and volume information of predefined ROIs. Then, the feature space is decomposed into unique and uniform spaces for each modality by the decomposed variational graph autoencoders. Finally, the decomposed representations are fused to generate unified brain networks by the representation-fusing generator and the dual discriminator. The proposed model is featured by incorporating the following objective functions: the Kullback-Leibler (KL) loss, the reconstruction loss, the adversarial loss, the classification loss, and the uniform-unique contrastive loss. These loss functions aim to ensure decomposition thoroughness and enhance structural-functional fusion.

Knowledge-Aware Transformer

In this section, the transformer-based network is adopted to extract structural features for each predefined ROI from DTI. The knowledge-aware transformer (KAT) consists of a stem module, a prior knowledge normalization (PKN) module, and a transformer block. A stem is a common form of convolution with defined kernels and strides. Prior knowledge means the spatial location and morphology information of the predefined ROIs. The standard anatomical template can provide the central location (i.e., x, y, and z) and volume (i.e., v) information for each ROI. The PKN module normalizes the location and volume information into the range [–1, 1]. Both outputs of the stem and PKN are sent to the transformer block to learn spatial and morphological features for each ROI. One stage of the transformer block consists of prior multi-head self-attention (PMS) and feed-forward network (FFN).

Decomposed Variational Graph Autoencoders

After the structural features $X_s \in \mathbf{R}^{N\times d}$ and the functional features $X_f \in \mathbf{R}^{N\times d}$ extracted from the empirical method have been mined separately, decomposing the bimodal features can significantly improve the common and complementary information fusion for representation learning. Given features extracted from two modalities, this section can learn decomposed representations among modalities. There are two parts: two encoders and two decoders. The graph convolutional network (GCN) is a two-layer network with 128 and 64 neurons. Each layer is followed by the rectified linear unit (ReLU) activation function. The brain connectivity central attention (BCCA) block is added to capture the global correlation between two ROIs iteratively. The dual graph convolutional network (DGCN) block is added to generate a pair of latent variables. It consists of two separate GCNs with one h-neuron layer and can output one pair of latent variables representing common and complementary information. In a structural decoder, a network is the reverse operation of the structural encoder, followed by an inner product operation and a sigmoid activation function. Similarly, the functional decoder is the inverse network structure of the functional encoder.

Representation-Fusing Generator

Since the latent representations have been decomposed into unique and uniform components, it is easy to find the best weighting parameters between different components in the fusion process. The Multi-Layer Perceptron (MLP) based generator is designed to fuse the decomposed representations to generate unified brain networks Ap. The generator can adaptively adjust the weight between decomposed representations, fully reflecting the common and complementary information among modalities.

Dual Discriminator

The conventional discriminator is used to keep the output (i.e., A_p) consistent with the real sample (i.e., A_b) distribution, where the real sample is computed using the graph-based deep model (GBDM) [...]. The label-aware discriminator can classify if the input matrix is normal control or patients. It comprises one convolution layer, three residual attention blocks (RAB), and a fully-connected layer.

Hybrid Loss Function

In this section, the KAT, encoders, decoders, generator, and discriminators are combined into the BSFL model to learn MCI-related representations and jointly trained with the KL Loss, reconstruction loss, adversarial loss, classification loss, and uniform-unique contrastive loss.

Experiments

The introduced model aims to generate unified brain networks for disease analysis. This section analyzes the generated brain networks in terms of prediction tasks. To compare the performance of our method with other related methods, three binary prediction tasks are conducted using a cross-validation strategy to calculate the mean values of evaluation indicators, i.e., accuracy (ACC), sensitive (SEN), specificity (SPE), and area under the curve (AUC). Three different classifiers are adopted to evaluate the prediction performance of the generated brain networks. The quantitative prediction results are displayed in Table 2.2. The results show

Table 2.2 Mean prediction results of the generated brain networks by different classifiers (%)

Classifiers	Brain Networks Generated By	SMC vs. NC				EM CI vs. NC				LMCI vs. NC			
		ACC	SEN	SPE	AUC	ACC	SEN	SPE	AUC	ACC	SEN	SPE	AUC
SVM	Empirical	76.8	85.3	68.2	77.8	78.0	73.1	82.9	75.0	82.2	82.8	81.7	83.2
	GBDM	77.4	85.3	69.5	78.8	79.8	73.1	86.5	79.9	85.4	84.2	85.5	84.5
	Ours	**79.8**	**89.0**	70.7	87.0	**84.1**	74.3	**93.9**	**95.0**	**87.9**	**88.1**	**87.8**	**95.3**
DNN	Empirical	78.0	81.7	71.9	77.5	81.7	85.3	78.0	86.8	84.1	78.9	89.0	82.5
	GBDM	78.6	81.7	75.6	78.4	83.5	86.5	80.4	88.1	86.0	82.8	89.0	86.2
	Ours	**82.9**	**84.1**	81.7	86.9	**89.0**	**87.8**	**90.2**	**96.0**	**91.7**	**88.1**	**95.1**	**94.7**
GCN	Empirical	79.2	87.8	70.7	78.7	84.7	89.0	80.4	86.9	88.6	85.5	91.4	88.1
	GBDM	81.7	89.0	74.3	81.8	86.5	89.0	84.1	89.7	91.1	86.8	95.1	89.6
	Ours	**85.9**	**96.3**	**75.6**	**93.8**	**90.8**	**93.9**	**87.8**	**97.8**	**94.3**	**93.4**	**95.1**	**98.1**

that our method achieves the best prediction performance among the three methods. This may indicate that the proposed model can fully use the common and complementary information from the structural-functional data and thus make the fusion more effective.

2.2.3 FUSION MODELS FOR BOLD-FMRI, DTI, AND SMRI DATA

BOLD-fMRI reflects changes in blood oxygen levels in the brain under resting or active states, and DTI provides microscopic structural information of white matter; the fusion of these two types of data lacks a focus on the macroscopic information of the brain. However, sMRI can provide detailed anatomical information about the brain, which helps in more precise spatial normalization and localization in the integrated analysis of BOLD-fMRI and DTI. The fusion of sMRI with BOLD-fMRI and DTI faces challenges, such as discrepancies in the location of ROIs and differences in higher-order correlations between the modalities. Inspired by the above observations, we propose two data fusion models.

2.2.3.1 SSNAE

In this section, we introduce a network combining feature selection method with feature learning to obtain the most discriminative feature representation for longitudinal early diagnosis and clinical score prediction. Specifically, we first preprocess the multi-modal neuroimaging data at multiple time points to extract original longitudinal multi-modal features. Then, the feature selection method is performed to preliminary reduce the feature dimensions. Finally, the SSNAE is employed to obtain more discriminative longitudinal multi-modal features to improve the accuracy of early diagnosis and clinical score prediction at multiple time points. To verify our proposed network, diverse and extensive experiments are performed on the Parkinson's Progression Markers Initiative dataset, which aims to identify biological markers of Parkinson's disease (PD) risk, onset, and progression. The results demonstrate that our proposed method is more efficient and achieves promising performance on longitudinal early diagnosis and clinical score prediction compared to state-of-the-art methods.

Method

We first segment and extract three sets of features (WM, GM, and MD) from the longitudinal multi-modal data of PD at each time point. Next, we use the joint learning from multiple modalities and relations (JLMMR) method to complete the initial dimension reduction in features and screen out the key features. Then, SSNAE is used for feature learning and obtaining longitudinal discriminative information. Finally, the longitudinal discriminative features are processed by support vector classification (SVC) and support vector regression (SVR) for classification and regression tasks.

Joint Learning from Multiple Modalities and Relations

We define a joint classification and regression model by a least square regression function as follows:

$$F(\mathbf{W}) = \mathbf{Y} - \widehat{\mathbf{Y}}_F^2 = \mathbf{Y} - \mathbf{W}^{\mathrm{T}}\mathbf{X}_F^2, \tag{2}$$

where **X** and **Y** represent the training data and the response matrix, respectively. $\widehat{\mathbf{Y}}$ is the predicted response matrix, and **W** is the weight coefficient matrix. Our goal is to make the predicted matrix $\widehat{\mathbf{Y}}$ as similar as possible to the response matrix **Y**. To this end, we measure the similarity between **Y** and $\widehat{\mathbf{Y}}$ by examining the relationships between their corresponding column or rows. Secondly, we define two regularization terms for exploring the relationship between the response variables. Finally, we perform a $\ell_{2,1}$ norm on the weight matrix to select the informative features for classification and regression. Combining the regression function and all regularization terms, we can define the final objective function of JLMMR as follows:

$$\min_{\mathbf{W}} F(\mathbf{W}) + R_1(\mathbf{W}) + R_2(\mathbf{W}) + R_3(\mathbf{W}) + \lambda_4 \mathbf{W}_{2,1}, \tag{3}$$

where λ_4 denotes the penalty factor of $\ell_{2,1}$-norm.

The Stacked Sparse Nonnegative Autoencoder

Sparse learning has been proven to learn more effective data descriptions between fully distributed and single-form descriptions. To ignore most of the useless information and capture a matrix with sparse data but containing key information, a sparse constraint term can be considered. In order to alleviate the overfitting problem, a weight decay term can be added. To improve the performance of the autoencoder in the reconstruction of input data, it needs to separate the data into sparse parts in the encoding layer and then add them together in the decoding layer. In order to achieve this goal, a nonnegative constraint term is imposed on the connecting weights U. To boost nonnegativity in U, the weight decay term can be replaced by a quadratic function. Then, we can formulate the following loss function for sparse nonnegative autoencoder (SNAE) as below:

$$J_{SAE}(\theta,\theta') = \frac{1}{n}\sum_{k=1}^{n}\left[L\left(\overline{\mathbf{X}}_k, g_{\theta'}(f_\theta(\overline{\mathbf{X}}_k))\right)\right] + \alpha\sum_{m=1}^{h} D(\rho \,\|\, \rho'_m) + \frac{\beta}{2}\sum_{l=1}^{2}\sum_{i=1}^{s_l}\sum_{j=1}^{s_l+1} f(u_{ij}^{(l)}) \tag{4}$$

$$f\left(u_{ij}^{(l)}\right) = \begin{cases} u_{ij}^2, & u_{ij} < 0 \\ 0, & u_{ij} \geq 0 \end{cases} \tag{5}$$

where α is the penalty factor of the sparse constraint. The second term of Eq. 4 is a sparse constraint, where $D(\rho \,\|\, \rho'_m) = \rho \log \frac{\rho'_m}{\rho} + (1-\rho)\log\frac{1-\rho'_m}{1-\rho}$ is the KL divergence. ρ represents the pre-defined desired activation, and

$\rho' = \frac{1}{n}\sum_{k=1}^{n}\left[f_\theta\left(\bar{\mathbf{X}}_k\right)\right]$ denotes the average activation of the hidden node. β is the penalty factor to control the weight decay, s_l and s_{l+1} represent the sizes of adjacency layers.

Finally, we iteratively update the encoding and decoding weight matrix **U** and bias vector ***b*** to minimize the difference between input and output. After optimization, the information in the hidden layer is regarded as the input of the next SNAE to form a stacked SNAE. The features of the hidden layer of the last SNAE are the most discriminative features for building classification and regression models.

Experiments

To compare the performance of our method with other related methods, we first compare our JLMMR method with other comparative feature selection methods. Next, the related common deep learning networks are used to compare with our SSNAE method for feature learning. Tables 2.3, 2.4, and 2.5 summarize the classification results for NC vs. PD from the baseline to the 24 months. In all data, our joint model of JLMMR and SSNAE achieves impressive accuracy. Compared with deep belief networks (DBN) and CNN, the performance of both SSNAE and stacked sparse autoencoder (SSAE) is better. For feature selection, we can observe that the experimental results of JLMMR are almost better than multi-modal sparse learning (MMSL) and joint embedding and sparse regression (JESR).

Table 2.3 Classification performance of baseline

Time	Feature Selection	Feature Learning	NC vs. PD			
			ACC	SEN	SPE	F1-score
	MMSL	DBN	75.98±1.08	40.48±2.02	91.57±2.0	48.17±2.0
	JESR		76.40±1.22	44.76±2.22	92.86±3.2	51.42±1.8
	M3T		75.50±1.42	35.71±2.62	94.43±5.3	41.84±1.7
	JLMMR		74.85±1.32	42.60±2.30	90.48±1.8	47.38±2.1
Baseline	MMSL	SSAE	78.98±1.52	39.29±2.89	96.43±2.0	49.74±2.0
	JESR		78.45±1.02	51.67±1.62	90.05±3.0	57.02±1.5
	M3T		71.07±1.47	47.86±4.32	90.05±1.02	49.99±2.6
	JLMMR		79.02±1.28	42.14±2.44	95.00±1.6	52.41±1.3
	MMSL	CNN	72.09±1.02	46.33±4.12	83.65±1.0	53.44±1.28
	JESR		71.57±1.28	55.24±1.42	79.00±4.52	54.70±1.3
	M3T		71.60±1.82	56.90±4.99	82.29±4.08	51.16±1.5
	JLMMR		74.14±1.62	55.64±4.82	89.60±4.72	53.09±1.2
	MMSL	SSNAE	79.04±1.92	39.05±4.23	**96.43±2.0**	49.16±2.1
	JESR		78.50±1.84	42.38±4.92	94.38±3.6	51.82±4.0
	M3T		75.64±1.49	**60.00±4.20**	82.38±4.12	**59.50±1.5**
	JLMMR		**79.95±1.92**	45.71±2.82	95.00±2.6	55.55±2.08

Then, we can conclude that the generalization of our JLMMR method is superior to the above two.

Table 2.4 Classification performance of 12 m

Time	Feature Selection	Feature Learning	NC vs. PD			
			ACC	SEN	SPE	F1-score
	MMSL	DBN	73.54±1.52	24.55±2.92	95.06±2.8	34.02±2.3
	JESR		72.76±1.08	22.36±2.82	**99.20±1.4**	35.29±2.5
	M3T		72.12±1.02	26.00±2.62	89.49±6.2	36.84±2.3
	JLMMR		74.81±1.20	25.68±2.30	96.54±4.2	36.15±2.8
	MMSL	SSAE	78.54±1.62	36.91±2.02	96.80±2.8	49.28±2.2
12m	JESR		75.10±1.22	34.91±2.00	92.73±4.8	43.24±2.0
	M3T		73.72±1.82	36.38±2.02	90.90±6.2	44.00±2.2
	JLMMR		79.04±1.32	51.45±1.90	91.13±3.6	58.23±2.8
	MMSL	CNN	71.92±1.78	53.82±4.92	79.86±8.2	53.09±4.2
	JESR		71.82±1.48	40.91±1.36	85.39±4.72	46.85±4.2
	M3T		71.53±1.92	51.67±1.52	80.38±4.18	53.10±4.1
	JLMMR		71.55±1.92	43.33±1.70	86.48±4.08	47.41±1.8
	MMSL	SSNAE	**80.71±1.02**	46.36±4.82	95.79±2.8	58.42±4.2
	JESR		76.26±1.62	42.36±4.62	91.13±4.3	51.44±1.9
	M3T		79.22±1.78	**57.33±1.62**	82.34±1.12	**63.56±4.2**
	JLMMR		78.13±1.72	37.45±1.82	96.00±2.6	47.29±1.8

Table 2.5 Classification performance of 24 m

Time	Feature Selection	Feature Learning	NC vs. PD			
			ACC	SEN	SPE	F1-score
	MMSL	DBN	93.41±1.02	30.00±2.02	99.00±1.2	10.00±4.29
	JESR		92.14±1.22	40.00±3.02	**100.00±0**	**73.33±4.20**
	M3T		94.37±1.42	60.00±4.12	97.00±3.4	56.67±4.72
	JLMMR		91.67±1.32	60.00±2.50	**100.00±0**	50.00±2.32
24m	MMSL	SSAE	97.23±1.84	60.00±2.92	**100.00±0**	66.67±1.82
	JESR		96.18±1.22	60.00±1.90	98.89±1.6	60.00±1.12
	M3T		96.28±1.72	60.00±2.02	**100.00±0**	60.00±2.12
	JLMMR		97.09±1.12	50.00±2.22	**100.00±0**	53.33±1.92
	MMSL	CNN	94.29±1.43	30.00±2.02	**100.00±0**	41.26±4.35
	JESR		93.41±1.45	20.00±4.40	**100.00±0**	30.28±4.72
	M3T		93.41±1.22	10.00±4.22	99.00±2.8	10.00±4.22
	JLMMR		95.22±1.28	40.00±4.20	99.00±4.3	40.00±4.72
	MMSL	SSNAE	97.34±1.92	70.00±4.12	99.00±1.2	62.00±1.52
	JESR		96.32±1.32	60.00±2.00	99.00±1.2	63.33±4.12
	M3T		97.09±1.11	60.00±3.02	**100.00±0**	63.33±4.16
	JLMMR		**97.99±1.62**	60.00±1.72	**100.00±0**	60.00±1.82

2.2.3.2 PALH

In this section, the PALH model is introduced to predict abnormal brain connections using triple-modality medical images. Concretely, a prior distribution from anatomical knowledge is estimated to guide multimodal representation learning using an adversarial strategy. Also, the pairwise collaborative discriminator structure is further utilized to narrow the difference in representation distribution. Moreover, the hypergraph perceptual network is developed to effectively fuse the learned representations while establishing high-order relations within and between multimodal images. Experimental results demonstrate that the proposed model outperforms other related methods in analyzing and predicting AD progression. More importantly, the identified abnormal connections are partly consistent with previous neuroscience discoveries. The introduced model can evaluate the characteristics of abnormal brain connections at different stages of AD, which is helpful for cognitive disease study and early treatment.

Method

Assuming subjects have the three modal images (i.e., BOLD-fMRI, DTI, and MRI), our goal is to learn a complex nonlinear mapping network to fuse multimodal images for predicting abnormal brain connections at different stages of AD. Our method consists of three components: (1) prior distribution estimation, (2) adversarial representation learning, and (3) the hypergraph perceptual network (HPN).

First, a kernel density estimation (KDE) method is introduced to estimate the prior distribution from graph data regarding subject labels. Second, the estimated distribution is incorporated into a bidirectional adversarial learning network for multimodal representation learning. It should be stressed that the designed pairwise collaborative discriminator (PCD) is used to constrain the representations in a joint embedding space. Then, a hypergraph-based network is developed to fuse the learned representations to produce united connectivity (UC)-based features. Finally, our network is trained with the following objective functions: (1) adversarial loss, (2) reconstruction loss, (3) classification loss, and (4) sparse regularization loss. The goal of loss functions is to improve the representation learning ability and the effect of multimodal image fusion.

Prior Distribution Estimation

The standard normal $\mathbf{N(0, 1)}$ distribution is inadequate for accurately representing the distribution of graph data. Introducing an appropriate distribution, denoted as $\boldsymbol{P_Z(Z)}$, becomes crucial in enhancing the representation learning capability of the adversarial network. In this scenario, there is no additional prior information apart from the provided graph data, denoted as $\boldsymbol{X}$ and $\boldsymbol{A}$. It remains plausible to derive a prior distribution from the available graph data. The intrinsic heterogeneity between $\boldsymbol{A}$ (edge data) and $\boldsymbol{X}$ (node data) poses challenges in directly estimating $\boldsymbol{P_Z(Z|X, A)}$. Nonetheless, these elements do exhibit structural consistency. Leveraging a cross-domain prototype approach bridges effectively the gap between the node domain ($\boldsymbol{X}$) and the edge domain ($\boldsymbol{A}$). Consequently, the conditional distribution $\boldsymbol{P_Z(Z|X, A)}$ can be substituted with $\boldsymbol{P_Z(Z|X_{U_0}, A_{U_0})}$, where U_0 denotes the index set of prototypes containing m_0 ROIs. Then, the determinantal point process (DPP)-based prototype learning method is adopted to select a diversified prototype subset U_1 containing m_1 ROIs.

According to the prototype index set U_0 with $|U_0| = m_0$, the corresponding node features are selected from X to form the features matrix X_{U_0}. Then, the feature dimension is reduced by principal component analysis (PCA) to get Z_{U_0}. A nonparametric estimation method (i.e., KDE) is introduced to estimate the prior distribution. Assuming $z_i \in Z_{U_0}$ is a latent representation of each node with the size $1 \times q$, $P_Z(Z|X_{U_0}, A_{U_0})$ is defined as:

$$\mathbf{P_Z}\left(\mathbf{Z}\,|\,\mathbf{X}_{\mathbf{U}_0},\mathbf{A}_{\mathbf{U}_0}\right)=\frac{1}{\mathbf{m}}\sum_{i=1}^{\mathbf{m}_0}\mathbf{K}_b\left(\mathbf{Z}-\mathbf{z}_i\right)=\frac{1}{\mathbf{m}_0 b}\sum_{i=1}^{\mathbf{m}_0}\mathbf{K}\left(\frac{\mathbf{Z}-\mathbf{z}_i}{b}\right), \tag{6}$$

Here, $K(\cdot)$ represents a multidimensional Gaussian kernel function, while b represents the bandwidth governing the level of smoothness in the estimated prior distribution. Finally, the approximation of the prior distribution $P_Z(Z)$ is derived using the following expression:

$$P_z(Z) \rightarrow P_z(Z|X, A) \rightarrow P_z(Z|X_{U_0}, A_{U_0}) \tag{7}$$

Adversarial Representation Learning

The multi-modal data is limited, so it is challenging to learn discriminative latent representations for disease prediction. In order to solve this problem, a bidirectional adversarial mechanism is introduced to incorporate the estimated distribution to augment samples, which can enhance the ability of multimodal representation learning. Specifically, we design a PCD for learning latent representations and keeping their unimodal features by applying reconstruction and classification modules. This part has three phases: (1) the adversarial phase, (2) the reconstruction phase, and (3) the classification phase.

Hypergraph Perceptual Network

Compared with the conventional graph characterized by pairwise relationships between paired nodes, hypergraph is more appropriate for capturing high-order relations among multiple brain regions. Hence, a hypergraph-based network combined with MLP and convolution is utilized to fuse the learned representations (i.e., $\hat{Z}$ and $\hat{V}$). The obtained UC matrix is sent to the classifier C_2 for task learning.

Hybrid Loss Function

Success in effectively fusing multimodal images requires joint representation learning. The outputs of generator G1 and encoder S should have the same distribution despite the heterogeneity of the input data. Besides, the learned fused representation must be discriminative concerning class labels, and the output UC matrix of HPN is believed to be sparse. An extensive object function is designed to optimize the network to achieve this goal in the proposed model. There are four types of loss functions: (1) adversarial loss, (2) reconstruction loss, (3) classification loss, and (4) sparse regularization loss.

Experiments

The experimental prediction results of all models are displayed in Table 2.6. It can be seen that the introduced model using BOLD-fMRI and DTI and MRI achieves the highest-mean accuracy on the prediction of AD versus NC, LMCI versus NC, and EMCI versus NC, respectively. It can be concluded that our model performs better than other methods in terms of unimodality, bimodality, or triple-modality medical images. In order to analyze the prediction results, BOLD-fMRI and DTI-based methods are selected to compare the learned latent features—the projection of learned latent features on a 2-D plane using t-SNE tools. The features obtained by our model give the best discriminative map among the three methods. Furthermore, the results of triple-modality imaging-based methods are superior to those of bimodality imaging-based methods.

2.2.4 FUSION MODELS OF MRI DATA WITH OTHER IMAGING MODALITIES' DATA OR NON-IMAGE MODALITIES' DATA

MRI demonstrates excellent performance in soft tissue contrast, offering high-resolution anatomical images; PET is more sensitive in displaying biochemical processes and functional activities, such as metabolic rates and receptor distributions. Non-image information can help researchers gain a deeper understanding of the pathophysiological mechanisms of diseases. The fusion of MRI data with PET or non-image information can offer more comprehensive patient information, aiding in improving diagnostic accuracy. Inspired by the above perspectives, we have proposed data fusion models for both MRI and PET, as well as fusion models for MRI with non-image information.

2.2.4.1 MDL-Net

In this section, we introduce the MDL-Net model to enhance early AD diagnosis by efficiently fusing multimodal data. Specifically, MDL-Net proposes a multi-fusion joint learning (MJL) module, which effectively fuses multimodal features and enhances the feature representation from global, local, and latent learning perspectives. MJL consists of three modules: global-aware learning (GAL), local-aware learning (LAL), and outer latent-space learning (LSL) modules. GAL, via a self-adaptive Transformer (SAT), learns the global relationships among the modalities. LAL constructs local-aware convolution to learn the local associations. The LSL module introduces latent information through outer product operation to enhance feature representation further. MDL-Net integrates the disease-induced region-aware learning (DRL) module via gradient weight to enhance interpretability, which iteratively learns weight matrices to identify AD-related brain regions. We conduct extensive experiments on public datasets, and the results confirm the superiority of our proposed method.

Table 2.6 Mean prediction performance of the proposed and other related methods (%)

Modality	Method	AD vs. NC				LMCI vs. NC				EMCI vs. NC			
		ACC	SEN	SPE	AUC	ACC	SEN	SPE	AUC	ACC	SEN	SPE	AUC
fMRI	N2NE	79.57	70.31	87.17	87.68	74.02	72.36	75.64	80.75	72.50	68.29	75.64	79.57
	Ours	**80.98**	**76.56**	84.61	**88.92**	74.68	**76.32**	73.08	**82.79**	73.12	**78.04**	71.79	**81.31**
	MPCA	80.28	70.31	88.46	85.37	75.98	73.68	78.20	80.58	74.37	79.27	69.23	83.22
fMRI and DTI	DCNN	84.51	87.50	82.06	89.40	79.87	77.63	82.06	84.30	76.25	76.83	75.64	82.68
	Ours	**88.73**	**84.37**	**92.31**	**97.48**	**84.42**	**84.21**	**84.62**	**94.02**	**82.50**	**82.93**	**82.05**	**91.65**
fMRI and DTI	SPMRM	94.37	95.31	93.59	97.02	90.91	96.05	85.90	89.05	83.75	90.24	76.93	87.74
and MRI	Ours	**96.47**	**98.43**	**94.87**	**99.59**	**92.70**	**96.05**	**88.46**	**94.83**	**87.50**	**92.68**	**82.05**	**92.72**

Method

The proposed framework can be summarized as follows: (1) 3DResNet18-based backbone network to extract multimodal features. (2) Multi-fusion joint learning to fuse multimodal features. (3) DRL module to identify salient brain regions.

Multimodal Feature Extraction

Let X_p, X_g, $X_w \in \mathbf{R}^{d \times h \times w \times c}$ denote PET, gray matter (GM), extracted from sMRI, and white matter (WM) extracted from sMRI modality brain image features, respectively, where d, h, w, and c represent the depth, height, width, and channel, respectively. We extract multimodal features using 3DResNet18 as the backbone network. To facilitate the dimensional transformation of the feature fusion process, we first dimensionally transformed the input features using an upsampling layer. Then, we set the number of channels of the used 3DResNet to [16] and performed multimodal feature extraction using a dimensionality reduction layer (layer0) and four residual layers. Finally, we obtain the multimodal features $H_p^m, H_g^m, H_w^m \in \mathbf{R}^{d_m \times h_m \times w_m \times c_m}$ (m denotes different layers).

Multi-Fusion Joint Learning

Due to the little relationship between the specific intramodal representations of the two modalities, it is almost impossible for simple fusion methods to learn the complementary information between the multimodal features efficiently. In order to address this limitation, the MJL module is designed to improve the learnability of multimodal fusion features, which consists of three modules: SAT, LSL, and LAL. SAT leverages the benefits of multi-head self-attention (MHSA) and window attention (WA), enabling adaptive global learning within multimodal features. LAL utilizes local-aware learning block to learn local connections between scales. Moreover, LSL utilizes outer products to introduce latent learnable information between modal features and enhance inter-modal feature representation. Subsequently, we obtain $F_s \in \mathbf{R}^{c_4}$, $F_o \in \mathbf{R}^{c_4}$, and $F_l \in \mathbf{R}^{c_4}$ from SAT, LSL, and LAL, and the three fusion features are dimensionally unified and summed to obtain the final fusion feature $F_c \in \mathbf{R}^{c_4}$. For detailed explanations of the SAT, LSL, and LAL modules.

Disease-Induced Region-Aware Learning

As AD is a stage-specific disorder that evolves over time, it is crucial to analyze salient brain regions at different stages. Motivated by Scouter, DRL is proposed to identify salient brain regions effectively. Briefly, the key aspect of DRL is that we first set iteration times t and initialize a brain region ROI weight matrix $\omega_i \in \mathbf{R}^{1 \times 90}$ (i = 1, 2, …, t, here i = 1), and our goal is to learn continuously and update ω_1 within t as a way to assign the corresponding importance to different brain regions.

Experiments

To demonstrate the superiority of our method, we evaluate the proposed method on the ADNI and Australian Imaging Biomarkers and Lifestyle (AIBL)

Table 2.7 Performance comparison of different methods of three classification tasks in ADNI and AIBL datasets

Dataset	Method	AD vs. NC				MCI vs. NC				AD vs. MCI			
		ACC	SEN	SPE	AUC	ACC	SEN	SPE	AUC	ACC	SEN	SPE	AUC
ADNI	ResNet	85.36±7.47	84.09±7.19	85.60±11.10	90.87±6.24	63.78±4.98	40.41±9.21	77.10±21.39	62.51±7.05	72.98±3.84	48.59±10.63	50.80±19.02	76.91±3.84
	ID3	80.88±6.32	91.05±8.42	69.54±8.91	87.48±3.71	60.76±4.46	42.11±6.94	73.39±24.06	62.03±5.20	72.72±3.55	89.18±7.18	42.34±15.81	78.18±3.58
	MFNet	95.54±8.06	95.79±3.43	95.16±4.22	98.19±1.76	70.47±2.82	44.05±0.58	74.41±10.05	73.52±6.73	64.28±4.48	88.63±7.86	75.74±5.19	90.23±4.47
	SSFTT	86.33±4.24	92.87±5.20	78.49±11.30	91.71±4.03	67.55±9.19	40.49±7.34	76.73±14.95	71.20±4.91	77.62±3.97	90.72±10.26	53.66±9.69	82.95±5.70
	Yang et al.	94.56±3.77	95.18±4.98	83.91±4.53	96.95±2.70	70.83±2.66	46.00±9.11	78.24±11.87	73.31±3.60	85.17±4.29	88.07±8.24	79.29±7.98	89.96±4.71
	Ours	**96.37±2.82**	**97.40±3.50**	**95.84±3.66**	**98.54±1.81**	**74.61±3.85**	**73.01±10.97**	**73.02±11.06**	**76.05±4.39**	**85.29±4.48**	**95.09±4.81**	**72.00±11.13**	**88.16±5.51**
AIBL	ResNet	88.03±5.36	87.84±7.04	88.42±13.28	89.42±8.38	74.98±6.84	40.95±12.02	56.71±21.30	81.30±4.01	75.95±5.40	86.13±12.30	57.17±18.66	76.24±7.66
	ID3	91.36±7.48	96.44±3.88	75.11±25.10	92.42±10.46	65.35±10.19	65.12±22.15	59.35±20.32	70.48±10.39	67.67±9.63	76.28±16.36	57.96±24.26	68.27±13.96
	MFNet	95.46±8.49	97.49±5.99	88.56±11.04	96.92±3.57	80.14±7.68	62.41±22.47	84.18±10.27	79.62±8.22	86.46±4.25	71.28±19.07	81.46±4.92	86.49±9.92
	SSFTT	89.67±3.77	89.42±4.72	70.09±4.26	92.05±4.32	71.57±14.39	40.84±8.48	64.41±5.30	87.66±4.85	74.81±9.10	72.25±4.67	80.15±4.71	59.05±8.17
	Yang et al.	98.58±4.49	95.54±5.72	87.09±12.87	95.60±7.00	71.32±8.96	89.94±9.64	62.12±23.18	82.21±9.86	52.79±7.87	75.76±14.30	60.56±14.18	96.80±20.41

datasets and compare it with different 3D classification methods under the same experimental conditions. We conducted experiments on the ADNI and AIBL datasets, respectively, the results of which are presented in Table 2.7. MDL-Net outperforms other 3D methods in almost all metrics, improving the ACC (0.83%/2.78%/0.12%), and SEN (1.61%/13%/2.37%) for the three tasks in the ADNI dataset, respectively. This suggests the essential role of the attention mechanism in enhancing model performance. Moreover, we apply a two-sample t-test between the proposed method and other comparison methods. The p-values of all evaluation metrics are less than 0.05 or 0.001, providing strong evidence for the significant superiority of our method over the others. The results in the AIBL dataset also demonstrate the superiority of our method. The above results demonstrate the effectiveness of our 3D method.

2.2.4.2 MSE-GCN

In this section, we introduce the MSE-GCN model in this paper, which fuses the functional and structural information from the resting-state functional magnetic resonance imaging and diffusion tensor imaging, respectively. Then, both functional and structural information in connectivity networks are integrated via the local weighted clustering coefficients (LWCC), which are concatenated as the feature vectors to represent the vertices of the population graph. Simultaneously, the subject's gender and age information is combined with the multimodal neuroimaging feature to build a sparse graph. Then, we design multiple parallel GCN layers with different inputs by random walk embedding, which can identify the intrinsic MCI graph information from the embedding in GCN. Finally, we concatenate the output of all the GCN layers in the full connection layer for detection. The proposed method is capable of simultaneously representing the individual features and information associations among subjects from potential patients. The experimental results on the public ADNI dataset demonstrate that our proposed method achieves impressive EMCI identification performance compared with all competing methods.

Method

Specifically, we first use a non-overlapping slide window to divide resting state fMRI (R-fMRI) into several subseries and obtain dynamic FCs by calculating the Pearson correlation (PC) coefficient of the pair-subseries. Simultaneously, the connection of white matter fiber bundles between each pair of brain regions is regarded as a structural network. Then, we extract the LWCC of both FC and SC and concatenate it as a feature vector to represent the vertices of the population graph. The edges of the graph represent the similarity between subjects and incorporate the non-image information. Finally, MSE-GCN is used for MCI detection.

LWCC Extraction and Data Fusion

Most existing research gets the upper half matrix of FC or SC of the subject as the feature vector. However, such an operation will bring a high feature dimension and destroy the original structure of the network. To address this problem, for a connectivity matrix $\boldsymbol{W}^{ij} \in \mathbf{R}^{r \times r}$, we first extract the LWCC $\boldsymbol{F} = \{\boldsymbol{f}_i, \mid (\boldsymbol{i} = 1, 2,\ldots,\boldsymbol{r})\}$ from both FC and SC to compose a feature vector. If one subject has $\boldsymbol{\lambda}$ FCs and one SC, we can get $\boldsymbol{\lambda} + \mathbf{1}$ feature vector $\boldsymbol{F}$. Then, we concatenate the LWCC extracted from one subject as a feature vector $\boldsymbol{S}_N = \{\boldsymbol{f}_1, f_2,\ldots, \boldsymbol{f}_{((\lambda+1)r)}\}$, where $\boldsymbol{N}$ is subject's number. Compared with traditional methods, our method not only reduces the feature dimension but also quantifies the clustering of each node in the weighted network.

Graph Construction

In this section, we construct a sparse graph to combine information on the image data (including **BOLD-fMRI** and **DTI**) and demographic information (e.g., gender and age). Incorporating both information in our model can reveal the similarity between each subject's features and help predict labels. Supposing the proposed undirected graph is defined as $\boldsymbol{G}(\boldsymbol{V}, \boldsymbol{E}, \boldsymbol{A})$, where $\boldsymbol{V}$ is the feature vector set extracted from subjects. Edges $\boldsymbol{E}$ models the similarity between the corresponding subjects and incorporates the phenotypic information. The adjacency matrix $\boldsymbol{A}$ describes the vertex connectivity and can be obtained by calculating the similarity matrix $\boldsymbol{S}$ of the sample point distance metric.

Spectral Convolution

GCN effectively implements convolution operations on non-Euclidean spatial data. The convolution operation of graph data can be regarded as the multiplication of both the filter and the signal into the Fourier domain.

Multi-Scale GCN

Recent studies show that traditional GCNs may lead to suboptimal detection accuracy due to the limitation of the receptive field. To address this problem, we use random walk embedding techniques on graphs to obtain node representations. Random walk is a special form of Markov chain, representing the probability of the information from a vertex going to another vertex of the graph. This probability matrix is statistically known as a co-occurrence matrix Y. Therefore, random walk essentially transforms the vertices of a graph into a continuous vector space. In one case, the GCN can simulate the principle of a random walk. Therefore, our MSE-GCN model can combine information from various graph scales. Using the p power of the normalized adjacency matrix A as input can explore the higher-order similarity of features, which is beneficial to the understanding of diseases. Motivated by this, we further design p parallel GCN layers. Finally, we concatenate the output of all the GCN layers into the full connection layer for MCI detection.

Experiments

In this section, three kinds of binary detection tasks are performed, i.e., (1) LMCI vs. NC; (2) EMCI vs. NC; (3) LMCI vs. EMCI. We use a leave-one-out (LOO) cross-validation strategy in all methods. For all the GCN-based

Table 2.8 Detection performance of different methods in three tasks (%)

Method	EMCI vs. NC				LMCI vs. NC				LMCI vs. EMCI			
	ACC	SEN	SPE	F1-score	ACC	SEN	SPE	F1-score	ACC	SEN	SPE	F1-score
SVM(B)	63.19	67.53	58.12	66.24	69.16	62.50	73.13	60.24	68.38	47.50	79.22	50.69
SVM(D)	63.19	75.32	49.25	68.43	75.70	69.05	72.65	69.05	72.65	67.50	75.32	62.79
SVM(F)	68.75	61.19	75.32	64.57	78.50	67.50	85.07	70.13	76.07	72.50	77.92	67.44
GCN(B)	60.42	77.92	40.30	67.80	70.09	83.58	47.50	77.78	57.26	66.23	40.00	67.11
GCN(D)	68.50	59.35	77.61	58.46	71.03	85.07	47.05	78.62	64.10	76.92	56.41	59.82
GCN(F)	71.53	67.53	76.12	71.72	73.83	85.57	52.50	80.56	75.84	84.42	57.50	81.76
MS-GCN(B)	75.69	76.12	75.32	74.45	78.63	75.02	79.22	71.58	80.34	85.71	70.00	85.16
MS-GCN(D)	70.14	65.67	74.03	67.18	74.77	74.63	75.00	78.74	79.49	87.01	65.00	84.81
MS-GCN(F)	81.25	72.73	91.04	80.58	85.05	89.55	77.50	88.24	88.11	72.50	88.61	85.31
Ours(B)	77.08	85.71	67.16	80.00	86.92	89.55	82.50	90.55	91.15	94.81	82.50	92.31
Ours(D)	81.94	89.61	73.13	84.15	89.72	92.54	85.00	91.85	90.60	94.81	82.50	92.99
Ours(F)	**85.42**	**86.57**	**84.42**	**84.67**	**93.46**	**94.03**	**92.50**	**94.74**	**92.31**	**93.51**	**90.00**	**94.12**

competing methods, we use the same model parameters: 20% dropout rate, 10^{-5} weight of the regularization term, 0.002 learning rate, and 200 epochs. We tested our models at different scales and selected the best scale p from the average cross-validation results. Table 2.8 shows the detection performance of our method and other competing methods. It is found that GCN has the advantages in analyzing EMCI compared with traditional machine learning methods. In addition, experiments show that increasing the receptive field of GCN is beneficial for EMCI detection. Moreover, the experiments also demonstrate that the EMCI detection is significantly improved after random walk graph embedding. Our analysis suggests that a random walk graph embedding may efficiently extract the brain's high-order information. Our proposed method has the best average accuracy of 84.72%, 89.72%, and 92.31% in EMCI vs. NC, LMCI vs. EMCI, and LMCI vs. NC, respectively. The fused data achieves better detection results than the single modality in the detection tasks of LMCI vs. NC and LMCI vs. EMCI.

2.2.5 CONCLUSION

This chapter explores the evolution and application of multimodal fusion models for brain disease diagnosis through AI-MRI integration. We introduce innovative strategies to overcome the shortcomings of unimodal data models in providing comprehensive brain features and the existing multimodal fusion models' inability to fully consider the heterogeneity, complementarity, and redundancy of information across various brain imaging modalities. Initially, to address the complex differences in correlations across imaging modalities, differences in regions of interest, difficulties in finding interpretability between data, difficulties in unifying the dimensions of information fusion, and over-reliance on empirical methods in existing fusion models, we start with the fusion of BOLD-fMRI with DTI data, the fusion of BOLD-fMRI, DTI, and sMRI data, and the fusion of MRI data with other imaging modality data or non-imaging modality data fusion in three aspects to summarize and introduce our past work in the field of multimodal fusion models for the brain diseases diagnosis through AI-MRI integration. Subsequently, our experimental validations reveal that our model yields favorable outcomes in the fusion of data from disparate imaging modalities. Integrating multimodal data enhances brain characterization and substantially elevates the precision of brain disease diagnosis. These findings offer fresh insights and methodologies for forthcoming brain disease diagnosis and research, underscoring the transformative potential of AI in medical image analysis.

REFERENCES

[1] Juliane S. Freitas, A. Kupsco, G. Diamante, Andreia A. Felicio, Eduardo A. Almeida and Daniel Schlenk. 2016. Influence of temperature on the thyroidogenic effects of Diuron and its metabolite 3,4-DCA in tadpoles of the American bullfrog (Lithobates catesbeianus). Environmental Science and Technology. 50(23): 13095–13104.

[2] C. Patterson. 2018. World Alzheimer Report 2018. *In*: The State of the Art of Dementia Research: New Frontiers.

[3] Geert Litjens, Thijs Kooi, Babak Ehteshami Bejnordi, Arnaud A. Adiyoso Setio, Francesco Ciompi, Mohsen Ghafoorian, et al. 2017. A survey on deep learning in medical image analysis. Medical Image Analysis. 42: 60–88.

[4] Asma Naseer, Tahreem Yasir, Arifah Azhar, Tanzeela Shakeel, and Kashif Zafar. 2021. Computer-aided brain tumor diagnosis: performance evaluation of deep learner CNN using augmented brain MRI. International Journal of Biomedical Imaging. 2021(1): 5513500.

[5] Duaa AlSaeed and Samar Fouad Omar. 2022. Brain MRI analysis for Alzheimer's disease diagnosis using CNN-based feature extraction and machine learning. Sensors. 22(8): 2911.

[6] Chiyu Feng, Ahmed Elazab, Peng Yang, Tianfu Wang, Feng Zhou, Huoyou Hu, et al. 2019. Deep learning framework for Alzheimer's disease diagnosis via 3D-CNN and FSBi-LSTM. IEEE Access. 7: 63605–63618.

[7] Katia Maria Poloni, Ricardo José Ferrari and Alzheimer's Disease Neuroimaging Initiative. 2022. A deep ensemble hippocampal CNN model for brain age estimation applied to Alzheimer's diagnosis. Expert Systems with Applications. 195: 116622.

[8] Protima Khan, Md. Fazlul Kader, S.M. Riazul Islam, Aisha B. Rahman, Md. Shahriar Kamal, Masbah Uddin Toha, et al. 2021. Machine learning and deep learning approaches for brain disease diagnosis: principles and recent advances. IEEE Access. 9: 37622–37655.

[9] Sidratul Montaha, Sami Azam, A.K.M. Rakibul Haque Rafid, Md. Zahid Hasan, Asif Karim and Ashraful Islam. 2022. Time-distributed-CNN-LSTM: A hybrid approach combining CNN and LSTM to classify brain tumor on 3D MRI scans performing ablation study. IEEE Access. 10: 60039–60059.

[10] A. Shoeibi, M. Khodatars, M. Jafari, N. Ghassemi, P. Moridian, R. Alizadehsani, et al. 2023. Diagnosis of brain diseases in fusion of neuroimaging modalities using deep learning: A review. Information Fusion. 93: 85–117.

[11] Ritu Priya Singh, Sandeep Kumar, Fateh Singh Rana, Saloni Singh, Akarsh Anand, Dikshit Kukreja, et al. 2024. Exploring Neural Network Approaches for Alzheimer's Disease Detection: An Analysis of RNN and CNN Performance. *In*: 2024 International Conference on Communication, Computer Sciences and Engineering (IC3SE). IEEE. 1028–1033.

[12] Andronicus A. Akinyelu, Fulvio Zaccagna, James T. Grist, Mauro Castelli and Leonardo Rundo. 2022. Brain tumor diagnosis using machine learning, convolutional neural networks, capsule neural networks and vision transformers, applied to MRI: A survey. Journal of Imaging. 8(8): 205.

[13] Xuegang Song, Kaixiang Shu, Peng Yang, C. Zhao, Feng Zhou, Alejandro F. Frangi, et al. 2024. Knowledge-aware Multisite Adaptive Graph Transformer for Brain Disorder Diagnosis. IEEE Transactions on Medical Imaging. 44(6): 2370–2383.

[14] Yanteng Zhang, Qizhi Teng, Yuyang Liu, Yan Liu and Xiohai He. 2022. Diagnosis of Alzheimer's disease based on regional attention with sMRI gray matter slices. Journal of Neuroscience Methods. 365: 109376.

[15] Selene Tomassini, N. Falcionelli, P. Sernani, H. Müller and Aldo Franco Dragoni. 2021. An end-to-end 3D ConvLSTM-based framework for early diagnosis of Alzheimer's disease from full-resolution whole-brain sMRI scans. *In*: 2021 IEEE 34th International Symposium on Computer-Based Medical Systems (CBMS). IEEE. 74–78.

[16] Jinwang Feng, Shao-Wu Zhang, Luonan Chen, Chunman Zuo and Alzheimer's Disease Neuroimaging Initiative. 2022. Detection of Alzheimer's disease using features of brain region-of- interest-based individual network constructed with the sMRI image. Computerized Medical Imaging and Graphics. 98: 102057.

[17] Megan H. Lee, Christopher D. Smyser and Joshua S. Shimony. 2013. Resting-state fMRI: A review of methods and clinical applications. American Journal of Neuroradiology. 34(10): 1866–1872.

[18] Paul M. Matthews, Garry D. Honey and Edward T. Bullmore. 2006. Applications of fMRI in translational medicine and clinical practice. Nature Reviews Neuroscience. 7(9): 732–744.

[19] Paul M. Matthews and Adam Hampshire. 2016. Clinical concepts emerging from fMRI functional connectomics. Neuron. 91(3): 511–528.

[20] K.B. Walhovd, A.M. Fjell, J. Brewer, L.K. McEvoy, C. Fennema-Notestine, D.J. Hagler, et al. 2010. Combining MR imaging, positron-emission tomography, and CSF biomarkers in the diagnosis and prognosis of Alzheimer disease. American Journal of Neuroradiology. 31(2): 347–354.

[21] Anders M. Fjell, Kristine B. Walhovd, C. Fennema-Notestine, Linda K. McEvoy, Donald J. Hagler, Dominic Holland, et al. 2010. CSF biomarkers in prediction of cerebral and clinical change in mild cognitive impairment and Alzheimer's disease. Journal of Neuroscience. 30(6): 2088–2101.

[22] Manhua Liu, Danni Cheng, Kundong Wang, Yaping Wang and Alzheimer's Disease Neuroimaging Initiative. 2018. Multi-modality cascaded convolutional neural networks for Alzheimer's disease diagnosis. Neuroinformatics. 16: 295–308.

[23] Zhi Chen, Yongguo Liu, Yun Zhang, Qiaoqin Li and Alzheimer's Disease Neuroimaging Initiative. 2023. Orthogonal latent space learning with feature weighting and graph learning for multimodal Alzheimer's disease diagnosis. Medical Image Analysis. 84: 102698.

[24] Shangran Qiu, Matthew I. Miller, Prajakta S. Joshi, Joyce C. Lee, Chonghua Xue, Yunruo Ni, et al. 2022. Multimodal deep learning for Alzheimer's disease dementia assessment. Nature Communications. 13(1): 3404.

[25] Tong Tong, Katherine Gray, Qinquan Gao, Liang Chen, Daniel Rueckert and Alzheimer's Disease Neuroimaging Initiative. 2017. Multi-modal classification of Alzheimer's disease using nonlinear graph fusion. Pattern Recognition. 63: 171–181.

[26] Anees Abrol, Zening Fu, Yuhui Du and Vince D. Calhoun. 2019. Multimodal data fusion of deep learning and dynamic functional connectivity features to predict Alzheimer's disease progression. *In*: 2019 41st Annual International Conference of the IEEE Engineering in Medicine and Biology Society (EMBC). IEEE. 4409–4413.

[27] Vince D. Calhoun and Jing Sui. 2016. Multimodal fusion of brain imaging data: a key to finding the missing link(s) in complex mental illness. Biological Psychiatry: Cognitive Neuroscience and Neuroimaging. 1(3): 230–244.

[28] Dan Hu, Han Zhang, Zhengwang Wu, Fan Wang, Li Wang, J. Keith Smith, et al. 2020. Disentangled-multimodal adversarial autoencoder: Application to infant age prediction with incomplete multimodal neuroimages. IEEE Transactions on Medical Imaging. 39(12): 4137–4149.

[29] Qiankun Zuo, Yanyan Shen, Ning Zhong, CL Philip Chen, Baiying Lei and Shuqiang Wang. 2023. Alzheimer's disease prediction via brain structural-functional deep fusing network. IEEE Transactions on Neural Systems and Rehabilitation Engineering. 31: 4601–4612.

[30] Qiankun Zuo, Ning Zhong, Yi Pan, Huisi Wu, Baiying Lei and Shuqiang Wang. 2023. Brain structure-function fusing representation learning using adversarial decomposed-VAE for analyzing MCI. IEEE Transactions on Neural Systems and Rehabilitation Engineering. 31: 4017–4028.

[31] Haijun Lei, Yukang Lei, Zihao Chen, Shiqi Li, Zhongwei Huang, Feng Zhou, et al. 2023. Early diagnosis and clinical score prediction of Parkinson's disease based on longitudinal neuroimaging data. Neural Computing and Applications. 35(22): 16429–16455.

[32] Qiankun Zuo, Huisi Wu, CL Philip Chen, Baiying Lei and Shuqiang Wang. 2024. Prior-guided adversarial learning with hypergraph for predicting abnormal connections in Alzheimer's disease. IEEE Transactions on Cybernetics. 54(6): 3652–3665.

[33] Zifeng Qiu, Peng Yang, Chunlun Xiao, Shuqiang Wang, Xiaohua Xiao, Jing Qin, et al. 2024. 3D Multimodal Fusion Network with Disease-induced Joint Learning for Early Alzheimer's Disease Diagnosis. IEEE Transactions on Medical Imaging. 43(9): 3161–3175.

[34] Shuangzhi Yu, Shuqiang Wang, Xiaohua Xiao, Jiuwen Cao, Guanghui Yue, Dongdong Liu, et al. 2020. Multi-scale enhanced graph convolutional network for early mild cognitive impairment detection. *In*: Medical Image Computing and Computer Assisted Intervention–MICCAI 2020: 23rd International Conference, Lima, Peru. Proceedings, Part VII 23. Springer. 228–237.

Chapter 2.3

Advancements in Intelligent Auxiliary Diagnosis for Glioma using Multimodal MRI Images

Jianhong Cheng* and Rui Feng
Institute of Guizhou Aerospace Measuring and Testing Technology, Guiyang 550009, China

2.3.1 INTRODUCTION

Brain glioma, the most common primary intracranial tumor, is caused by the malignant transformation of glial cells in the brain and accounts for 80% of adult malignant brain tumors [1], characterized by high incidence, high recurrence, and high mortality rates. According to the 2020 global cancer burden data released by the International Agency for Research on Cancer (IARC) [2], China ranks first globally in prevalence, incidence, and mortality rates of central nervous system tumors. Thus, brain glioma has become a significant threat to the health and safety of the Chinese population. As early as 2016, the World Health Organization (WHO) first incorporated both histopathological and molecular features into the classification of tumor subtypes in its classification of central nervous system (CNS) tumors [3]. In 2021, the WHO updated the classification and grading standards for tumors again [4]. For instance, in adult diffuse gliomas, an important molecular marker is the mutation of isocitrate dehydrogenase (IDH). The diagnosis is oligodendroglioma, when an IDH mutation is accompanied by 1p19q co-deletion. If there is an IDH mutation without 1p19q co-deletion, the diagnosis is astrocytoma,

*For Correspondence: jianhong_cheng@csu.edu.cn

DOI: 10.1201/9781003518754-8

and IDH wild-type diffuse gliomas with histological features of necrosis or microvascular proliferation can be diagnosed as glioblastoma.

The symptoms, treatment decisions, and prognosis of brain gliomas must be comprehensively evaluated based on clinical characteristics such as patient age, tumor type, lesion location, and overall health status [3, 4]. Imaging-based diagnosis can provide neurosurgeons with information on tumor size, extent, adjacency to critical structures, and morphological characteristics, which significantly aids in the diagnosis and treatment of brain gliomas. Magnetic resonance imaging (MRI), as an important kind of medical image, can show the signal intensity and mass effect of glioma hemorrhage, necrosis, and edema, as well as the extent of the lesion invasion. Clinically, routine MRI imaging for diagnosing brain gliomas includes four modalities: Fluid-Attenuated Inversion Recovery (FLAIR), T1-weighted imaging (T1), T1-weighted contrast-enhanced imaging (T1ce), and T2-weighted imaging (T2). However, due to the unclear boundaries of gliomas, blurred surrounding edema areas, and varying degrees of blood-brain barrier disruption caused by tumors, neurosurgeons face significant challenges in imaging-based diagnosis and differentiation.

Radiology is extracting high-throughput information from images for deep mining and analysis to realize non-invasive biological prediction of potential tumors [5, 6]. In the diagnosis and treatment process based on radiology, neurosurgeons need to manually mark gross tumor volume and important endangered organs on conventional MRI images. Manual delineation of tumor areas requires careful consideration of multimodal MRI images (FLAIR, T1, T1ce, T2), each of which may have hundreds of slices, and the delineation process is highly dependent on the medical knowledge and clinical experience of neurosurgeons. Therefore, manual annotation is not only tedious and time-consuming but also highly subjective, which is likely to lead to deviation in results [7]. In addition, diagnosing glioma requires obtaining samples by resection or biopsy and carrying out histological and molecular pathological examination to determine the pathological grade and molecular subtype. There is no doubt that this detection method is invasive for patients, may also lead to the risk of tumor implantation and metastasis in obtaining tissue samples [8, 9], and is expensive at the same time. Therefore, an efficient and accurate automatic recognition and segmentation method for glioma is urgently needed.

AI technology empowers medical image processing, which can not only relieve doctors from the time-consuming and laborious manual labeling work but also assist doctors in non-invasive and accurate grading diagnosis of glioma [10]. Grading glioma is an important part of determining the treatment plan and prognosis prediction. WHO classifies gliomas into four grades at the tissue level, namely grade I to grade IV gliomas. According to the malignant degree of glioma cells, grade II and III gliomas are classified as low-grade gliomas (LGG), and grade IV gliomas are defined as high-grade glioma (HGG) in the WHO tumor grading standards in 2016. LGG tumor cells grow slowly and are less invasive, and some patients can be cured by surgery with a good prognosis. However, HGG tumor cells grow rapidly and are aggressive, and most patients can't be cured at present, so the prognosis is poor. At present, histopathological analysis is a common method in diagnosing glioma. It is also the baseline method in the diagnosis of glioma. However, this is a time-consuming and invasive technology, and there may be sampling inaccuracy and subjective differences between testers [11]. How to accurately grade glioma patients earlier and adopt more targeted treatment schemes is the key to realizing personalized diagnosis and treatment and improving the overall survival of glioma.

Accurate molecular typing of glioma is directly related to the prognosis of patients. Currently, the diagnostic guidelines for gliomas have reported important pathological molecular markers that affect the survival time of patients with gliomas, such as IDH and 1p19q. However, invasive histopathological biopsy is needed to detect the subtype status of these genes, and there may be subjective differences in the detection results. Preoperative MRI images contain the global information of tumors, which can better describe the heterogeneity of tumors than local pathological sections. Therefore, it is of great significance to establish a non-invasive prediction model by using preoperative multimodal MRI image data and necessary clinical survival data for studying the survival analysis of glioma. Clinical studies have shown that the fusion of phenotypic features in MRI images can improve the survival and prognosis of glioma [12, 13]. It is a new idea to study the survival analysis of glioma by modeling with deep learning method, establishing end-to-end mapping between image and survival, and automatically mining the potential characteristics related to survival from MRI images. However, research on the clinical system of assistant diagnosis of glioma still faces some challenges at present. Firstly, the accuracy of the automatic segmentation of glioma lesions needs to be improved, and the generalization ability of the segmentation model is insufficient [14]. Secondly, the imaging biomarkers related to pathological grading [15], important gene typing [16–20], and survival prognosis of glioma are not very clear.

Therefore, under the tide of the deep integration of medical images and artificial intelligence, the research on automatic segmentation algorithm of glioma lesions based on multimodal MRI images, pathological grading, genotyping, and survival prediction of glioma can promote the sustainable improvement of the research and development of auxiliary diagnosis technology and diagnosis system for glioma in China, which has far-reaching strategic significance for rapid diagnosis and accurate treatment of glioma. By aiming at the difficulty or complexity of accurate preoperative diagnosis of gliomas, this chapter reviews four aspects: automatic segmentation of glioma, grading diagnosis of glioma, genotyping of glioma, and survival analysis of glioma.

2.3.2 BRAIN GLIOMA DATASET AND PREPROCESSING

2.3.2.1 Dataset

The Brain Tumor Segmentation Challenge (BraTS) is among the most important challenges in all Medical Image Computing and Computer Aided Intervention (MICCAI) seminars. It was held as early as 2012, and the organizer provided multimodal MRI image data of patients with high and low levels of glioma, as well as tumor segmentation labels for corresponding patients in the training set.

BraTS datasets before 2016 were scarce, and the segmentation criteria were not uniform. Since 2017, medical scientists have uploaded and shared MRI images, clinical information, and genetic data of nearly 500 patients with glioma in the Cancer Image Archive Database (TCIA) and Cancer Genome Map Database (TCGA), the data sample size of BraTS 2017 Challenge has been expanded. In recent years, the BraTS Challenge has provided more mission types. For instance, BraTS2024 also provides other types of tasks, such as tumor grading and brain tumor survival prediction, in addition to brain tumor segmentation. Therefore, the data set of glioma in this study mainly comes from the BraTS Challenge, TCIA image archive, and TCGA gene archive. Table 3.1 summarizes the datasets published in the BraTS Challenge from 2017 to 2020.

Table 3.1 AUC values of all methods on two datasets

Dataset	Dataset Modalities	Number of Sample		
		Training Set	Validation Set	Total Number
BraTS2017	FLAIR, T1, T1ce, T2	285	46	331
BraTS2018	FLAIR, T1, T1ce, T2	285	66	351
BraTS2019	FLAIR, T1, T1ce, T2	337	125	462
BraTS2020	FLAIR, T1, T1ce, T2	369	125	494

Each sample includes four multimodal MRI images, namely FLAIR, T1, T1ce, and T2. According to the BraTS criteria, tumor regions are clinically stratified into three subregions: the Whole Tumor (WT), Tumor Core (TC), and Enhancing Tumor (ET). The histopathological features of these subregions can be differentiated through intensity variations across multimodal imaging. In typical high-grade glioma cases, distinct phenotypic characteristics are manifested across imaging modalities. Generally, FLAIR and T2 modalities can exhibit marked hyperintensity at edema boundaries, with T2 additionally showing characteristic hyperintensity in the tumor core. T1 demonstrates hypointensity in non-enhancing regions (including necrotic tissue), while T1ce reveals pronounced hyperintensity in enhancing tumor areas while maintaining hypointensity in non-enhancing regions.

Based on the annotation standards of the BraTS, histopathological components within each subregion correspond to the following label values: the non-enhancing tumor/necrotic regions (label 1), the edema regions (label 2), the enhancing tumor regions (label 4), and the background and normal brain tissue (label 0).

This multimodal imaging synergy provides multidimensional biomarkers for preoperative glioma evaluation: FLAIR and T2 modalities enhance sensitivity to edema boundaries, aiding WT delineation. T1ce highlights enhancement effects for precise ET identification. TC characterization (encompassing ET and necrotic areas) relies on integrating T1 hypointensity with T2/FLAIR morphological features. Table 3.2 systematically summarizes the pathological components and imaging characteristics of each subregion.

Table 3.2 AUC values of all methods on two datasets

Name of Subregion	Contained Area	Labels	Annotation
WT	Edema area, enhanced area, non-enhanced area	1,2,4	The tumor structures of all subareas are obvious on FLAIR and T2
TC	Non-enhanced area, enhanced area	1,4	The region of WT, except edema, is more obvious on T1ce
ET	Enhanced area	4	The enhanced part of brain glioma is obvious on T1ce
Background	Normal area	0	Normal tissue except for the lesion area

2.3.2.2 Data Preprocessing

Multimodal MRI images are scanned by instruments. Different medical institutions, scanning equipment, scanning protocols, image collectors, and even scanned patients will cause large heterogeneity problems in multimodal MRI images. In order to alleviate this problem, preprocessing is necessary for the collected image data. The preprocessing process mainly includes format conversion, LPS coordinates, relocation, registration, skull removal, N4 bias field correction, etc. Multimodal MRI images are initially presented in DICOM format, and the image resolution and scanning thickness differ among patients. First, the DICOM format of each modality image is converted into NIFTI format through the dcm2nii software package [21], and the patient information can be anonymized during the conversion process. In order to standardize the image window, the multimodal MRI images of all patients will be located in the left-posterior-superior (LPS) coordinate system using the coordinate relocation function in FSL. Then, the modal images used are registered to the standard T1 modal atlas in the SRI24 atlas [22] by using the FSL tool or **NiftyReg** matching tool to realize the unification of all brain image tissues into the standard space and the resolution of all images is $240 \times 240 \times 155$, and the granularity is $1 \times 1 \times 1$ mm^3. Finally, the skull was removed by FSL or BET brain extraction tools, and all images were corrected by N4 bias field by ANTs tools. Through the above-standardized data preprocessing process, the differences of image data collected by different institutions and different equipment can be alleviated.

2.3.3 AUTOMATIC SEGMENTATION OF GLIOMA

Brain glioma segmentation can help clinicians extract important semantic features of tumor patients so as to make diagnoses and radiotherapy plans. At the same time, glioma segmentation is an essential pretreatment step in many studies, such as grading diagnosis, gene and molecular prediction, prognosis prediction, and biomarker prediction. The glioma information contained in multimodal and multi-dimensional medical MRI image data can provide guidance, observation, and intervention for patients' treatment plans. However, it is a challenging task to accurately segment glioma from multimodal MRI images, which covers professional categories including imaging, oncology, data science, computer science, etc. The particularity of glioma also makes it difficult to segment automatically. For example, the size, shape, and position of glioma in MRI images are varied, and the tumor boundary is blurred. In addition, the gray distribution of MRI images of the same modality collected by different equipment and hospitals is quite different. Glioma may be deformed by glioma squeezing the surrounding normal tissues. The edema area caused by the tumor will also change the gray characteristics of the surrounding areas of the tumor. When faced with these difficulties and challenges, it is extremely difficult and time-consuming for even senior oncologists to segment tumors manually. Therefore, it is of great clinical significance and practical value to design a stable, accurate, and robust automatic glioma segmentation algorithm.

In recent years, the automatic segmentation technology of glioma has been widely favored by researchers at home and abroad, and glioma segmentation algorithms based on different principles have been proposed. From the perspective of technical development, the existing glioma segmentation algorithms can be classified into two categories: machine learning-based image segmentation and deep learning-based image segmentation.

2.3.3.1 Machine Learning-based Glioma Segmentation

MRI segmentation methods based on machine learning mainly include the threshold method [23–25], region growing method [26, 27], random field method [28, 29], edge detection method [30], and graph theory method.

Threshold-based Segmentation Method

Threshold segmentation-based method is the most extensive method in traditional image segmentation methods. Because of its simple design and strong interactivity, this method is one of the earliest algorithms widely used in the field of image processing. The threshold segmentation-based method sets single or multiple thresholds empirically and extracts pixels within the threshold range from medical images as segmentation target areas. Whether the appropriate threshold can be selected is the key to the success of the threshold segmentation method. The parameter optimization strategy based on the image gray histogram can further improve the segmentation accuracy of the image [23]. Hidetomo et al. used a threshold method based on iterative optimization to extract soft tissue from MRI images of the head [24]. Some scholars calculate the volume of each region and then estimate the threshold of each part with prior knowledge so as to segment gray matter, white matter, and cerebrospinal fluid on MRI images [31]. In addition, Gaussian distribution was also applied to determine the threshold of brain tumors in MRI [32]. Nevertheless, the segmentation results obtained by the threshold method are still rough. This is because the imaging process of medical images is often accompanied by noise, which has a great influence on the performance of threshold segmentation. Therefore, the threshold-based method is often used in the pre-processing or post-processing stage of medical images, such as removing the skull and isolating voxels.

Region Growth-based Segmentation Method

Region growing method is a serial region segmentation technique and a typical region segmentation method. The basic idea is to set one or more seed points in the region to be segmented, then merge similar pixels around the seed points into the region where the seed pixels are located based on a certain rule determined in advance until no other pixels meet the set conditions [26, 27]. The challenge lies in the selection of seed points and the determination of growth criteria and growth stop conditions. The selection of seed points needs an automatic detection method or manual intervention method to determine the most suitable pixel points according to the characteristics of specific problems. The regional growth criteria and growth stop conditions also need to be set according to the characteristics and objectives of specific problems, and the quality of the setting will directly affect the segmentation results. It is as easy to realize and operate as the threshold method. However, it is time-consuming to search for pixels. Therefore, the region growth-based method usually needs to be combined with other algorithms. For example, Thomas et al. combined region growth-based and fuzzy clustering methods to segment brain tumors in T1 and T2 weighted imaging [33]. In addition, the region-growing method is also used as a post-processing technology to ensure the connectivity of brain tumor segmentation results [34].

Random Field-based Segmentation Method

The random field-based segmentation method is an image segmentation algorithm based on the statistical model, a random variable with a certain probability of the pixel gray value in the image. The spatial relationship among image pixels considered in this algorithm can correct the gray-scale nonuniformity and local volume effect in medical images. A more commonly used method is the inference mechanism based on the prior probability of bay leaf. The Conditional Random Field (CRF) [28] and the Markov Random Field (MRF) [29] are two representative random field segmentation methods. Nie et al. use the Markov random field to perform brain tumor segmentation on multi-channel MRI images [35]. In general, the segmentation models based on random fields perform well in a complex background, but the high complexity of the algorithm and the length of the time limit the promotion and application in medical image processing. Therefore, it is often used in the post-processing stage for structured prediction.

Edge Detection-based Segmentation Method

The edge detection algorithm is inspired by the high sensitivity of the human visual system to the boundary information of objects. A series of studies show that there is a high correlation between simple closed contour and object representation, and then many operators are proposed for edge detection, such as the Sobel operator, Canny operator, Prewitt operator, Roberts operator, and Laplacian operator. Through these operators, irrelevant data information in the image can be filtered, and important structural attributes of the image are retained. A Canny operator is widely used, and its core idea is to find the maximum value of the local gradient and suppress the smaller value to realize boundary detection. Zhao et al. segmented lung parenchyma from CT images with an edge detection algorithm and mathematical morphology technology [30]. Although edge detection can detect the focus quickly, it is ineffective for the foreground focus with a closed contour. Especially in the segmentation of three-dimensional medical images, the pixel boundary between the focus area and normal tissue is blurred, which increases its detection difficulty.

Graph Theory-based Segmentation Method

Graph theory-based segmentation method is a research hotspot in the field of image segmentation. This method first builds a graph model composed of nodes, edges, and weights. The specific implementation regards each pixel in the image as a node, and every two adjacent pixels form an edge, and the weight of the edge depends on the boundary smoothing energy term. Through the graph model, the problem of segmentation can be transformed into the problem of label weight distribution of nodes by connection characteristics, which can be realized by minimizing the graph cutting energy function. Njeh et al. proposed a graph-cut distribution matching algorithm for multimodal MRI glioma segmentation [36]. In order to improve the segmentation performance, Pedoia et al. combined graph-cutting technology and a competitive expectation maximization (CEM) algorithm to improve the segmentation performance of tumors [37]. Although the methods based on graph theory are widely used in medical images, there are still some challenges. With the expansion of medical image resolution, data dimension, and modal number, the number of nodes and edges in the graph model increases sharply, and the computational complexity also increases, which brings great challenges to the requirements of hardware equipment.

2.3.3.2 Deep Learning-based Glioma Segmentation

Reliable segmentation of glioma is important for accurate diagnosis and treatment planning [38]. Manual segmentation of neurosurgeons is a very time-consuming, boring, and subjective task, so practical automatic segmentation methods are needed. However, because the size, shape, and position of glioma in MRI images are highly variable, and the heterogeneity between tumors and within tumors is extremely strong, automatic and accurate segmentation of glioma has always been a challenging task [39].

In order to promote the development of automatic brain glioma segmentation methods, the MICCAI launched the Multimodal BraTS in 2012 [41]. The BraTS database contains a large number of multimodal MRI images, which can be publicly obtained and used to develop and test the latest brain tumor segmentation algorithm. The representative and advanced methods are the DeepMedic network proposed by Kamnitsas et al. in BraTS 2016, a dual-channel 3D convolution network combined with 11 residual connections [42]. This network increases the receptive field of neurons while maintaining low computational overhead and improves the segmentation performance of the model by using the residual mechanism. Olaf et al. also first proposed using a U-Net network for medical image segmentation [40]. U-Net network is a CNN structure, which consists of a path for context contraction and a symmetric expansion path for accurate positioning in images. Subsequently, Casamitjana et al. applied 3D U-Net to the BraTS 2016 Challenge and achieved an excellent segmentation effect on the whole tumor and tumor core [43]. Fidon et al. proposed a ScaleNet network architecture, which consists of two parts: SN-BackEnd and FrontEnd [44]. SN-BackEnd is an end-to-end multimodal feature extraction processing method that performs a convolution operation on each mode of brain tumor itself and between modes, respectively, and effectively complements the information. It plays a key role in the accuracy of brain tumor segmentation. Because 3D images will bring a lot of calculation overhead, which further limits the resolution and the number of features of images in the network, resulting in the limited complexity of the model and greatly reducing the representation ability of the model. Based on this, Wang et al. propose a new brain tumor segmentation method [45]. In order to extract global features and reduce computational overhead as much as possible, the multi-class brain tumor segmentation problem is decomposed into three binary segmentation problems: Whole Tumor, Tumor Core, and Enhancing Tumor region according to the hierarchical structure of sub-regions. In addition, Isensee et al. also proposed an improved version of the U-Net network [46], which introduced a residual mechanism and dropout layer into the context module to make the network have better segmentation performance and then successively proposed networks such as No New-Net [47] to be used in the subsequent brain tumor segmentation challenge.

2.3.4 GRADING DIAGNOSIS OF GLIOMA

Grading diagnosis of glioma is a key link to improving treatment plans, detection, and clinical experiments, and an important factor related to prognosis prediction. WHO classifies gliomas into I-IV grades [48], and its grading standard still requires pathological examination or biopsy, which is an invasive and expensive detection method, and there may be inaccurate sampling and knowledge differences among observers. Therefore, as a critical development requirement in precision medicine, personalized medicine needs to accurately identify the grade and other genetic characteristics of glioma so that clinicians can adopt more targeted treatment programs and improve the prognosis of patients. Nowadays, MRI imaging technology has become the most potential non-invasive diagnostic tool, and significant progress has been reached.

2.3.4.1 Machine Learning-based Grading Diagnosis of Glioma

The appearance of radiology provides a new idea for non-invasive grading diagnosis of glioma. The automatic grading model is constructed by conventional MRI images and traditional machine learning methods; that is, the grading method of glioma based on traditional imaging methods is widely used. This method usually includes manual definition and segmentation of the region of interest (ROI), feature extraction, feature selection, classification modeling, and performance evaluation [49, 50]. It aims at mining important image markers related to glioma grading through a machine learning algorithm, which has strong interpretability and is favored by professional scholars.

Zacharaki et al. developed a computer-aided diagnosis grading system, which extracted the features of radiology from T1ce mode and then used the SVM-RFE feature selection method and SVM classifier to distinguish the types of brain tumors [51]. Vamvakas et al. also used the SVM-RFE algorithm to determine 12 image features related to glioma classification and achieved good classification performance on a small data set [52]. Cho et al. found that two kinds of spherical displacement (compactness) in the tumor region are significant for glioma grading and designed a grading model that achieves a prediction performance of AUC of 0.94 [53]. Based on the same data set, Reza et al. fused pathological image features based on MRI image omics features and established a classification model through the SVM classifier, achieving a classification performance of AUC of 0.97 [54]. In order to alleviate the tedious work of manually segmenting tumors, Zhao et al. adopted a slice pooling mechanism to compress MRI so as to reduce the workload of doctors in segmenting tumor areas and established an image group model for grading [55]. Chen et al. first proposed a two-stage computer-aided model, which automatically segmented glioma on FLAIR mode and then automatically graded glioma [56]. Zhuge et al. also used the U-Net model to automatically segment multimodal MRI and then input the segmentation results into a convolutional neural network for classification [57].

Although the existing research has made great achievements in distinguishing HGG from LGG, extracting more valuable image features to improve prediction accuracy is still a challenge. Recently, a multi-center study showed that the larger the residual volume of unenhanced tumor after operation, the worse its prognosis [58]. With the increasing awareness of the prognostic importance of non-enhanced tumor areas in malignant gliomas (GBM), some experts suggest that the scope of surgical resection should be extended to non-enhanced tumors, not just enhanced tumor areas [59, 60]. These studies indirectly provide the possibility of improving the accuracy by using non-enhanced tumors to grade gliomas.

2.3.4.2 Deep Learning-based Grading Diagnosis of Glioma

Although the above research methods have achieved good classification performance, the research process is complicated and highly dependent on the experts' prior knowledge. The rise of deep learning provides a new idea for automatic diagnosis of glioma grading. Therefore, the automatic grading diagnosis method of glioma based on deep learning has been developed rapidly. Unlike traditional imaging methods, deep learning-based methods directly take a series of MRI images as input and use the advanced artificial neural network model to extract features and models automatically. Xiao et al. used the pre-trained model VGG-16 as the depth feature extractor and combined it with the traditional imaging features to construct a glioma grading model [62]. Yang et al. combined two pre-training models, AlexNet and GoogLeNet, to achieve better prediction performance in glioma grading [61]. Similarly, Zhang and Ding et al. also combined deep learning features and imaging features to grade glioma [57, 68]. Cheng et al. leveraged a multimodal disentangled variational autoencoder (MMD-VAE) to disentangle features of MRI images into common and distinctive representations to obtain the shared and complementary data among modalities and designed a cross-modality reconstruction loss and common-distinctive loss to ensure the effectiveness of the disentangled representations [69]. In order to meet the clinical needs of tumor segmentation and grading, Naser et al. jointly developed a glioma segmentation network and grading model for automatic segmentation and grading diagnosis of glioma [63]. These methods of glioma classification based on transfer learning all take two-dimensional images as input, and it is necessary to select one or more slice images to represent the whole sample for classification research. One drawback of such methods is that they can not fully characterize the three-dimensional structural information of tumors and may not fully explore the spatial heterogeneity of glioma grading. To avoid this problem, researchers designed an artificial neural classification network. At first, the deep learning segmentation model was used to segment tumors automatically; then, the segmented results were used as the input of the classification network for classification research [57, 64, 66]. Table 3.3 summarizes the data modes, data samples, and grading performance of the above-mentioned glioma grading methods.

2.3.5 GENOTYPING OF GLIOMA

In 2016, WHO added molecular features during the tumor classification of the central nervous system for the first time, among which the most important ones are the IDH gene and chromosome 1p19q deletion [3]. Clinical studies have found that patients with glioma with IDH mutation have a longer survival time. The prognosis of glioma with combined deletion of 1p19q in IDH mutation is better than that without combined deletion of 1p19q, and it is more sensitive to adjuvant chemotherapy with methylbenzyl hydrazine, lomustine, and vincristine [70, 71]. Therefore, in clinical practice, non-invasive and accurate identification of IDH gene mutation and combined deletion of 1p19q in glioma will be helpful for clinical diagnosis and treatment, and the clinical value and significance of preoperative MRI images are particularly important. A large number of studies show that there are some relationships between tumor morphological characteristics extracted

Table 3.3 Summary of grading methods of glioma

Manuscript	Dataset Modality	Method	Grading Performance
[51]	T1ce 102 (0.51)	Use SVM-RFE for feature selection, then use the SVM classifier for classification.	AUC: 0.899 ACC: 0.865
[53]	FLAIR/T1ce/T1/T2 285 (0.74)	Use mRMR for feature selection, then use RF for classification.	AUC: 0.940 ACC: 0.920
[61]	T1ce 100 (0.65)	With rectangular ROI as input, using the GoogleNet model for fine tuning.	AUC: 0.968 ACC: 0.945
[52]	Advanced MRI 40 (0.50)	Use SVM-RFE for feature selection, then use SVM classifier for classification.	AUC: 0.950 ACC: 0.935
[54]	FLAIR/T1ce/T1/T2 285 (0.74)	Combining MRI image features and pathological image features, then use SVM to classify tumors.	AUC: 0.970 ACC: 0.860
[62]	T1ce 285 (0.74)	Combining the image omics features and VGG16 depth features, the traditional classifier was used for classification.	AUC: 0.940 ACC: 0.890
[63]	FLAIR/T1ce/T1 108 (0.54)	The U-Net model was used for tumor segmentation, and the segmentation results were then input into VGG16 for grading.	AUC: 0.970 ACC: 0.950
[64]	FLAIR/T1ce/T1/T2 628 (0.54)	Using the U-Net model to extract tumor regions and then the CNN network to grade.	AUC: 0.940 ACC: 0.900
[65]	DTI 108 (0.60)	Combining the features of radiology and deep learning and using the SVM classifier for classification.	AUC: 0.930 ACC: 0.940
[57]	FLAIR/T1ce/T1/T2 285 (0.74)	Using the U-Net model for tumor segmentation and then 3DConvNet to grade.	— ACC: 0.975
[55]	FLAIR/T1ce/T1/T2 400	Compressing MRI images by slice pooling mechanism, then establishing an image classification model.	AUC: 0.860 —
[56]	FLAIR 137 (0.57)	Extracting local features by directional gradient histogram, then using SVM for classification.	AUC: 0.806 ACC: 0.763
[66]	FLAIR/T1ce 285 (0.74)	Extracting multimodal knowledge and grading using deep learning multimodal interaction module.	AUC: 0.952 ACC: 0.943
[67]	T2 322 (0.51)	Using the rectangular ROI image as input, and then using the pre-training model Resnet18 for classification.	— ACC: 0.958

from MRI images and gene subtypes. Therefore, it is of great clinical significance to predict the micro-genotype state using macro-imaging technology.

In recent years, image genomics has become a rapidly developing research field, combining image genomics with genomics to provide more accurate diagnostic information. As early as 2017, Patel et al. found that the T2-FLAIR mismatch signal can be used as an imaging biological marker of IDH mutation and 1p19q non-joint deletion molecular subtype in low-grade gliomas, with high specificity [72]. Subsequently, Broen et al. confirmed this discovery again [73]. In 38 cases of glioma, the T2-FLAIR mismatch signal has 100% specificity for IDH mutation. Aliotta et al. considered adding an ADC threshold feature to combine with the T2-FLAIR mismatch signal to maintain high specificity and improve sensitivity [74]. There are also reports that there are false positives in this finding, especially in children with glioma [75]. Such methods of judging the semantic information of T2-FLAIR mismatch signal by artificial naked eyes are subjective. To further capture the potential imaging features, Lu et al. extracted high-throughput image features from multimodal MRI images and then used the SVM classifier to predict IDH gene mutation [76]. Van et al. extracted 87 imaging features from T1 and T2 image modes and combined them with the gender and age characteristics of patients [77]. Then, the machine learning method SVM classifier was used to predict the mutation state of 1p19q, which achieved an AUC of 0.72. Other scholars use not only conventional multimodal MRI images but also imaging characteristics such as ADC or DWI to establish machine learning models for genotyping [78, 79]. The genotyping method based on traditional radiology needs to manually label ROI region and extract prior features, which is easily influenced by human subjective factors.

In order to avoid these problems, researchers are committed to automatic genotyping from the original MRI images by using deep learning methods. For example, Chang et al. used a residual convolution neural network to predict the IDH mutation state of glioma through preoperative MRI data [70]. The network was experimentally verified on a multi-center data set, achieving an AUC of 0.95 and an accuracy of 89.1%. Choi et al. established the LSTM network to predict IDH genotyping by combining conventional multimodal MRI images and DCS-MRI sequence information, achieving an AUC of 0.95. Tang et al. [80] also used advanced DWI image data to extract B0, FA, and MD sequences from DWI and combined them with T1ce images to construct a multi-genotyping depth network model, which can simultaneously predict IDH, MGMT, 1p19q, and TERT. The performance of these models depends on advanced DWI and ADC modal images. In addition, Gao et al. tried directly using the tumor histogram information of advanced modality images such as DTI, DKI, NODDI, and MAP to identify tumor genotyping [81].

Cheng et al. proposed a multi-task learning (MTL) network. It devised a hybrid CNN-Transformer encoder to capture the correlation and heterogeneity of data and used a multi-task learning loss designed to balance the two tasks by combining the segmentation and classification loss functions with uncertain weights [82]. Some scholars consider the correlation between tumor segmentation

Table 3.4 Summary of genotyping methods for glioma

Manuscript	Dataset Modality	Method	Performance
[72]	T2/FLAIR	T2-FLAIR mismatch signal differentiates IDH mutation and 1p19q non-deletion type in low-grade glioma.	SEN: 0.760 SPE: 1.000
[73]	FLAIR/T1/T1ce/T2	Identification of IDH mutant 1p19q non-deletion glioma by T2-FLAIR mismatch signal.	SEN: 0.510 SPE: 1.000
[76]	FLAIR/T1/T1ce/T2	Extract image features using traditional image genomics methods and perform IDH genotyping and 1p19q deletion status prediction by SVM classifier.	AUC: 0.889 ACC: 0.800
[70]	FLAIR/T1/T1ce/T2	Extract the key sections of preoperative multimodal MRI, use the Resnet34 model to classify IDH, and improve the classification performance by combining age characteristics.	AUC: 0.950 ACC: 0.891
[83]	MPRAGE	Using a cascade deep neural network for the brain stem glioma segmentation, then predicting the mutation of the H3 K27M gene.	AUC: 0.952 ACC: 0.965
[78]	T1ce/T2/ADC	Extract histogram and statistical characteristics of tumor by image genomics method, and carry out IDH classification by logistic regression model.	AUC: 0.980 ACC: 0.905
[86]	FLAIR/T1/T1ce/T2/ADC	Use the LSTM network for IDH genotyping prediction combined with conventional multimodal MRI images with DSC-MRI sequence information.	AUC: 0.950 ACC: 0.917
[74]	FLAIR/T1/T1ce/T2/ADC	Carry out IDH classification by combining ADC threshold and T2-FLAIR mismatch features and add ADC features to improve sensitivity.	SEN: 0.590 SPE: 0.910
[79]	FLAIR/T1/T1ce/T2/ADC	Establish a logistic regression model to classify IDH using the minimum and average value of ADC, morphological characteristics, and age.	AUC: 0.860
[80]	T1ce/DWI	Use ROI of B0, FA, MD, and T1ce as input, then predict genotyping of IDH, MGMT, 1p19q, and TERT by CNN network.	ACC: 0.946, 0.790 ACC: 0.881, 0.660
[85]	FLAIR/T1/T1ce/T2	Simultaneous segmentation and IDH genotyping of glioma using SGPNet multi-task network.	AUC: 0.949 ACC: 0.895
[81]	DTI/DKI/NODDI/MAP	Identification of IDH genotyping by using advanced multimodal MRI tumor histogram information.	AUC: 0.820 ACC: 0.810

and genotyping tasks to improve performance and propose a multi-task learning network. For example, Liu et al. [83] proposed a cascade deep neural network, which automatically segmented brain stem gliomas first and then predicted the mutation of the H3 K27M gene. Bangalore et al. [84] trained a multi-class segmentation network to classify and predict pixels according to genotyping tags, then determined the mutation type of the IDH gene by majority voting method, achieving an AUC classification performance of 0.95. Wang et al. [85] proposed a multi-task network SGPNet, which can simultaneously perform glioma segmentation and IDH genotyping. Although some progress has been made in predicting glioma genotyping, it is still necessary to break through with better generalization performance for how to fuse multimodal conventional MRI images and further provide a reliable basis for clinical practice. Table 3.4 summarizes the above research methods of glioma genotyping.

2.3.6 SURVIVAL ANALYSIS OF GLIOMA

Glioblastoma (GBM) is still the most aggressive primary malignant brain tumor in adults. The median survival time after initial diagnosis is only 15 months, and the five-year survival rate is about 5% [87]. Clinically, almost all GBM patients will relapse, although the comprehensive treatment method of maximum safe resection, postoperative radiotherapy combined with temozolomide (TMZ) and adjuvant chemotherapy is provided. At present, the treatment of glioma needs the cooperation of neurosurgery, neuroimaging department, radiotherapy department, neurooncology department, pathology department, and neurorehabilitation department. According to the principle of evidence-based medicine, the treatment decision and plan should be further optimized and standardized with the goal of the individualized comprehensive treatment plan to achieve the maximum treatment benefit for patients, prolong the progression-free survival (PFS) and overall survival (OS) of patients as much as possible, and thus improve their overall health and life. However, spatial and temporal heterogeneity, as well as range and location changes of glioma, are important factors that make it difficult to remove the tumor. In some cases, it is impossible to perform complete tumor resection, even surgery, and deliver bad drugs to the brain, which is the main reason for the lack of effective treatment and poor prognosis [88].

MRI images play an important role in the initial diagnosis of brain tumors and the treatment of response evaluation. They are also used as a non-invasive prediction tool. The latest research shows that MRI can provide valuable information different from pathological and clinical data and can be used to predict survival. By extracting quantitative features such as tumor intensity, volume, shape, and texture changes, a survival prediction algorithm is designed and established to find the characteristics associated with the survival and prognosis of patients. This process is called radiology [89]. At present, much work has been done to study the survival analysis of glioma by using the image group method to extract qualcomm image features from preoperative brain images or to explore the prognosis of patients through the relationship between genes and clinical phenotypes. Many studies have explored the WHO classification, image phenotypic characteristics, and the relationship between clinical features and overall survival of gliomas. Early studies have revealed that the survival of malignant tumors is related to patients' age, quality of life score (KPS), total resection rate, and the size of necrotic and enhanced areas in preoperative MRI images [90]. Bisdas et al. revealed that relative cerebral blood volume (rCBV) can be used as a biomarker for the recurrence and 1-year survival rate of astrocytoma [91]. However, it cannot be applied to the prognosis and survival prediction of other high-grade gliomas.

In order to fully reveal the heterogeneity of tumor survival and prognosis, researchers began to explore the prognosis and survival analysis of glioma patients using multimodal MRI images. For example, Chang et al. combined the preoperative and postoperative image features of T1 and FLAIR mode to establish a survival prediction model to provide clinical decision-making [92]. Sun et al. first segmented the tumor area of multimodal MRI images by using the deep learning segmentation model and divided the patient's survival time into three categories: short, medium, and long [93]. Then, a random forest prediction model was established by using the imaging characteristics of tumor areas, and the classification accuracy was 61% on the BraTS 2018 challenge data set. In addition, some scholars use the Cox proportional hazard (Cox) model to find the relationship between patient survival and predictive variables [94]. For example, Lao et al. developed the least absolute shrinkage and selection operator Cox (LASSO-Cox) regression to select important features from high-dimensional imaging data for predicting the overall survival rate of glioblastoma patients [95]. Hu et al. used the elastic-Cox proportional hazard model to predict the prognosis of glioma patients with polygenic characteristics [96]. These multimodal data provide essential value for the study of preoperative survival and prognosis of glioma.

Most of the above-mentioned research on survival analysis is based on artificial definitions or prior knowledge. This cannot often use the potential value of MRI image data because artificial definition or prior knowledge is often limited by specific domain knowledge. Recent studies have incorporated deep learning algorithms into survival prediction, replacing the traditional Cox model with the fully connected layer for modeling. At present, most studies using this strategy are based on pathological images and gene expression data [97–100]. For example, [97] put forward a survival convolutional neural network, which integrates histological images and genomic biomarkers into a unified framework to predict the survival of glioma patients. Similarly, Chen et al. proposed an interpretable framework that used the fusion of pathological images and genetic features to predict survival [99]. These works are based on the imaging modality of biopsy, and the acquisition cost is expensive. Braman et al. devised a deep orthogonal fusion (DOF) model. It learns to combine embeddings from each modality via attention-gated tensor fusion and introduces a multimodal orthogonalization (MMO) loss term that increases model performance by incentivizing constituent embeddings to be more complementary [100]. Therefore, it is of great clinical significance to predict the survival of glioma by using multimodal MRI images with non-invasive characteristics.

2.3.7 CONCLUSION

With precision medicine becoming an important trend of medical development, the application and research of data fusion based on multimodality or multi-omics is becoming increasingly obvious in the medical field. As an essential means of developing a medical assistant diagnosis, artificial intelligence technology, with its distinct and unique advantages, has achieved some good results in automatic segmentation, grading diagnosis, preoperative genetic and molecular characteristics prediction, and prognosis evaluation of glioma. However, in the face of the complexity and challenges in the actual clinical process, it will take time to apply these research results to clinical auxiliary diagnosis, and it is still necessary to carry out in-depth exploration and research on specific clinical practical problems and challenges.

1. Design and construct a multimodal fusion diagnosis model. In clinical work, different scanning imaging modalities can often reflect different phenotypic signs of lesions. For the differential diagnosis or grading diagnosis of glioma, even experienced imaging doctors must refer to various modality images to draw more accurate diagnosis conclusions. Currently used multimodal MRI data is conventional, and some high-level imaging modalities such as diffusion-weighted imaging (DWI), perfusion imaging (PWI), diffusion tensor imaging (DTI), magnetic resonance spectroscopy imaging (MRS), functional magnetic resonance imaging (fMRI) and positron emission computed tomography (PET) are not included. These high-level imaging modalities are of great significance and value for the differential diagnosis and therapeutic evaluation of glioma. Therefore, the intelligent diagnosis model of glioma can imitate the thinking mode of human experts and make joint diagnosis decisions with heterogeneous multimodal data as input, which is expected to improve the performance of the intelligent diagnosis model of glioma further.
2. Study the intelligent diagnosis model under the condition of missing modes. In clinical practice, due to the differences in medical institutions, scanning equipment, scanning protocols, image collectors, and other factors, it is usually difficult to obtain a relatively complete multimodal MRI image, and then a large number of low-quality and missing modal samples are produced, which can not be directly used or discarded. On the one hand, this is a waste of data resources for deep model research. On the other hand, missing modes have a great impact on the performance of deep learning models. How to make full and effective use of missing modal data to establish a robust deep-learning model has become a hot issue in the field of medical image multimodal research. At present, there are two ways to solve this problem. One is to build a generation model [101] using the full-modal image information to generate the missing modal image. Although this method can get missing images, it is cumbersome and inflexible. Another solution is constructing a deep learning model [102] that can directly adapt to the missing modal

data and realize the missing modal feature compensation by learning the shared feature representation between modes. This solution is flexible, but it has some challenges to the design and training of the algorithm.

3. Design and propose an intelligent diagnosis model of federated learning. The lack of tag data samples makes it difficult for deep learning models to achieve ideal prediction performance. At the same time, due to privacy, ethics, and other factors, the data of independent medical institutions can not be shared, and the data is distributed in an information island state. It has become an inevitable trend to apply federated learning with privacy protection to the intelligent assistant diagnosis of glioma. The intelligent diagnosis model based on federated learning aims at ensuring data security and privacy, sharing model training parameters in different institutions or physical nodes without transmitting data information so as to build a universal medical intelligent diagnosis model. In recent years, NVIDIA and King's College London have proposed a brain tumor segmentation algorithm based on federated learning [103]. At the same time, the School of Artificial Intelligence of Huazhong University of Science and Technology, together with authoritative scientific research institutions at home and abroad, jointly proposed an open-source medical artificial intelligence computing framework based on federated learning, which was applied to the intelligent diagnosis of COVID-19 [104]. These algorithms provide a foundation for the federated learning application of medical images. Therefore, the intelligent diagnosis model based on federated learning can further help to improve the auxiliary diagnosis performance of glioma.

In summary, MRI image segmentation of glioma is important for quantitatively evaluating glioma auxiliary diagnosis. As an essential means of developing a medical assistant diagnosis, AI technology, with its distinct and unique advantages, has achieved considerable progress in automatic segmentation, grading diagnosis, preoperative genetic and molecular characteristics prediction, and prognosis evaluation of glioma. Combining the key technologies in artificial intelligence with MRI images of brain gliomas to solve practical clinical problems scientifically, reasonably, and accurately is significant for developing individualized diagnosis and treatment in China's medical undertakings. However, in the face of the complexity and challenges in the actual clinical scenarios, it will take time to apply these research findings to clinical auxiliary diagnosis, and it is still necessary to carry out in-depth exploration and research on specific clinical practical problems and challenges.

REFERENCES

[1] Md Ishtyaq Mahmud, Muntasir Mamun and Ahmed Abdelgawad. 2023. A deep analysis of brain tumor detection from MR images using deep learning networks. Algorithms. 16(4): 176.

[2] Hyuna Sung, J. Ferlay, R.L. Siegel, M. Laversanne, Isabelle Soerjomataram, Ahmedin Jemal, et al. 2021. Global cancer statistics 2020: GLOBOCAN estimates of incidence and mortality worldwide for 36 cancers in 185 countries. CA: A Cancer Journal for Clinicians. 71(3): 209–249.

[3] David N. Louis, Arie Perry, Guido Reifenberger, Andreas von Deimling, Dominique Figarella-Branger, Webster K. Cavenee, et al. 2016. World Health Organization classification of tumors of the central nervous system: A summary. Acta Neuropathologica. 131(6): 803–820.

[4] David N. Louis, Arie Perry, Pieter Wesseling, Daniel J. Brat, Ian A. Cree, Dominique Figarella-Branger, et al. 2021. The 2021 WHO classification of tumors of the central nervous system: a summary. Neuro-oncology. 23(8): 1231–1251.

[5] Kaustav Bera, N. Braman, Amit Gupta, Vamsidhar Velcheti and Anant Madabhushi. 2022. Predicting Cancer Outcomes with Radiomics and Artificial Intelligence in Radiology. Nature Reviews Clinical Oncology. 19(2): 132–146.

[6] Robert J. Gillies, Paul E. Kinahan and Hedvig Hricak. 2016. Radiomics: images are more than pictures, they are data. Radiology. 278(2): 563–577.

[7] Sérgio Pereira, Pinto Adriano, Victor Alves and Carlos A Silva. 2016. Brain tumor segmentation using convolutional neural networks in MRI images. IEEE Transactions on Medical Imaging. 35(5): 1240–1251.

[8] Qian Sun, Rui Xu, Hongbo Xu, Gengming Wang, Xueming Shen and Hao Jiang. 2017. Extracranial metastases of high-grade glioma: The clinical characteristics and mechanism. World Journal of Surgical Oncology. 15: Article number: 181.

[9] Shigao Huang, Jie Yang, Simon Fong and Qi Zhao. 2019. Mining prognosis index of brain metastases using artificial intelligence. Cancers. 11(8): 1140.

[10] Elizabeth Huynh, Ahmed Hosny, C. Guthier, Danielle S. Bitterman, Steven F. Petit, Daphne A. Haas-Kogan, et al. 2020. Artificial intelligence in radiation oncology. Nature Reviews Clinical Oncology. 17(12): 771–781.

[11] Ahammed Muneer K.V., V.R. Rajendran, and Paul Joseph K. 2019. Glioma tumor grade identification using artificial intelligent techniques. Journal of Medical Systems. 43: 1–12.

[12] Viet Huan Le, Tran Nguyen Tuan Minh, Quang H. Kha and Nguyen Q. Khanh Le. 2023. A transfer learning approach on MRI-based radiomics signature for overall survival prediction of low-grade and high-grade gliomas. Medical and Biological Engineering and Computing. 61(10): 2699–2712.

[13] Sirvan Khalighi, Kartik Reddy, Abhishek Midya, Krunal Balvantbhai Pandav, Anant Madabhushi and Malak Abedalthagafi. 2024. Artificial intelligence in neuro-oncology: Advances and challenges in brain tumor diagnosis, prognosis, and precision treatment. NPJ Precision Oncology. 8(1): 80.

[14] Zhihua Liu, Lei Tong, Long Chen, Zheheng Jiang, Feixiang Zhou, Qianni Zhang, et al. 2023. Deep learning based brain tumor segmentation: a survey. Complex and Intelligent Systems. 9(1): 1001–1026.

[15] Laifa Ma, Zheng Xiao, Kenli Li, Shengli Li, Jianlin Li and Xiaoping Yi. 2020. Game theoretic interpretability for learning based preoperative gliomas grading. Future Generation Computer Systems. 112: 1–10.

[16] Faizan Ullah, Muhammad Nadeem, Muhammad Abrar, Farhan Amin, Abdu Salam and Amerah Alabrah. 2023. Evolutionary model for brain cancer-grading and classification. IEEE Access. 11: 126182–126194.

[17] Satrajit Chakrabarty, Pamela LaMontagne, Joshua Shimony, Daniel S Marcus and Aristeidis Sotiras. 2023. MRI-based classification of IDH mutation and 1p/19q codeletion status of gliomas using a 2.5D hybrid multi-task convolutional neural network. Neuro-Oncology Advances. 5(1): vdad023.

[18] Chandan G. Bangalore Yogananda, Bhavya R. Shah, Frank F. Yu, Marco C. Pinho, Sahil S. Nalawade, Gowtham K. Murugesan, et al. 2020. A novel fully automated MRI-based deep-learning method for classification of 1p/19q co-deletion status in brain gliomas. Neuro-oncology Advances 2. Supplement_4: iv42–iv48.

[19] Shumpei Onishi, Masato Kojima, F. Yamasaki, Vishwa J. Amatya, Ushio Yonezawa, Akira Taguchi, et al. 2024. T2-FLAIR mismatch sign, an imaging biomarker for CDKN2A-intact in non-enhancing astrocytoma, IDH-mutant. Neurosurgical Review. 47(1): 412.

[20] Jacob S. Young, Ramin A. Morshed, Shawn L. Hervey-Jumper and M.S. Berger. 2023. The surgical management of diffuse gliomas: Current state of neurosurgical management and future directions. Neuro-oncology. 25(12): 2117–2133.

[21] Xiangrui Li, Paul S. Morgan, John Ashburner, Jolinda Smith and Christopher Rorden. 2016. The first step for neuroimaging data analysis: DICOM to NIfTI conversion. Journal of Neuroscience Methods. 264: 47–56.

[22] Torsten Rohlfing, Natalie M. Zahr, Edith V. Sullivan and Adolf Pfefferbaum. 2010. The SRI24 multichannel atlas of normal adult human brain structure. Human Brain Mapping. 31(5): 798–819.

[23] Nobuyuki Otsu. 1975. A threshold selection method from gray-level histograms. Automatica. 11(285–296): 23–27.

[24] Hidetomo Suzuki and Jun-ichiro Toriwaki. 1991. Automatic segmentation of head MRI images by knowledge guided thresholding. Computerized Medical Imaging and Graphics. 15(4): 233–240.

[25] Gordon J. Harris, P.E. Barta, L.W. Peng, S. Lee, P.D. Brettschneider, A. Shah, J.D. Henderer, et al. 1994. MR volume segmentation of gray matter and white matter using manual thresholding: dependence on image brightness. American Journal of Neuroradiology. 15(2): 225–230.

[26] Rolf Adams and Leanne Bischof. 1994. Seeded region growing. IEEE Transactions on Pattern Analysis and Machine Intelligence. 16(6): 641–647.

[27] Andrew Mehnert and Paul Jackway. 1997. An improved seeded region growing algorithm. Pattern Recognition Letters. 18(10): 1065–1071

[28] Yang Wang, Kia-Fock Loe, and Jian-Kang Wu. 2007. A dynamic conditional random field model for foreground and shadow segmentation. IEEE Transactions on Pattern Analysis and Machine Intelligence. 28(2): 279–289.

[29] Stan Z. Li. 1994. Markov random field models in computer vision. *In*: Computer Vision—ECCV'94: Third European Conference on Computer Vision Stockholm, Sweden, May 2–6 1994 Proceedings, Volume II 3. Springer. 361–370.

[30] Zhao Yu-qian, Gui Wei-hua, Chen Zhen-cheng, Tang Jing-tian and Li Ling-yun. 2006. Medical images edge detection based on mathematical morphology. *In*: 2005 IEEE Engineering in Medicine and Biology 27th Annual Conference. IEEE. 6492–6495.

[31] Yun-Chang Sung, Ki-Sun Han, Chang-Jun Song, Seung-Moo Noh and Jong-Won Park. 2000. Threshold estimation for region segmentation on MR image of brain having the partial volume artifact. *In*: WCC 2000-ICSP 2000. 2000 5th

International Conference on Signal Processing Proceedings. 16th World Computer Congress 2000. IEEE. 2: 1000–1009.

[32] Andreas Stadlbauer, Ewald Moser, S. Gruber, Rolf Buslei, Christopher Nimsky, Rudolf Fahlbusch, et al. 2004. Improved delineation of brain tumors: An automated method for segmentation based on pathologic changes of 1H-MRSI metabolites in gliomas. Neuroimage. 23(2): 454–461.

[33] Thomas M Hsieh, Yi-Min Liu, Chun-Chih Liao, Furen Xiao, I-Jen Chiang and Jau-Min Wong. 2011. Automatic segmentation of meningioma from non-contrasted brain MRI integrating fuzzy clustering and region growing. BMC Medical Informatics and Decision Making. 11(1): 54.

[34] Dipak Kumar Kole and Amiya Halder. 2012. Automatic brain tumor detection and isolation of tumor cells from MRI images. International Journal of Computer Applications. 39(16): 26–30.

[35] Jingxin Nie, Z. Xue, T. Liu, G.S. Young, K. Setayesh, L. Guo, et al. 2009. Automated brain tumor segmentation using spatial accuracy-weighted hidden Markov Random Field. Computerized Medical Imaging and Graphics. 33(6): 431–441.

[36] Ines Njeh, Lamia Sallemi, Ismail Ben Ayed, Khalil Chtourou , Stephane Lehericy, Damien Galanaud et al. 2015. 3D multimodal MRI brain glioma tumor and edema segmentation: a graph cut distribution matching approach. Computerized Medical Imaging and Graphics. 40: 108–119.

[37] Valentina Pedoia, Sergio Balbi and Elisabetta Binaghi. 2015. Fully automatic brain tumor segmentation by using competitive EM and graph cut. *In*: Image Analysis and Processing—ICIAP 2015: 18th International Conference, Genoa, Italy. Proceedings, Part I 18. Springer. 568–578.

[38] Spyridon Bakas, Hamed Akbari, Aristeidis Sotiras, M. Bilello, Martin Rozycki, Justin S. Kirby, et al. 2017. Advancing the Cancer Genome Atlas glioma MRI collections with expert segmentation labels and radiomic features. Scientific Data. 4(1): 1–13.

[39] Debojyoti Pal, Tanushree Meena, Dwarikanath Mahapatra and Sudipta Roy. 2023. AW-Net: A novel fully connected attention-based medical image segmentation model. *In*: Proceedings of the IEEE/CVF International Conference on Computer Vision. 2532–2541.

[40] Olaf Ronneberger, Philipp Fischer and Thomas Brox. 2015. U-net: Convolutional networks for biomedical image segmentation. *In*: Medical Image Computing and Computer-assisted Intervention–MICCAI 2015: 18th International Conference, Munich, Germany. Proceedings, Part III 18. Springer. 234–241.

[41] Bjoern H. Menze, Andras Jakab, Stefan Bauer, Jayashree Kalpathy-Cramer, Keyvan Farahani and Justin Kirby. 2014. The multimodal brain tumor image segmentation benchmark (BRATS). IEEE Transactions on Medical Imaging. 34(10): 1993–2024.

[42] Konstantinos Kamnitsas, Enzo Ferrante, Sarah Parisot, C. Ledig, Aditya V. Nori, Antonio Criminisi, et al. 2016. DeepMedic for brain tumor segmentation. *In*: Brainlesion: Glioma, Multiple Sclerosis, Stroke and Traumatic Brain Injuries: Second International Workshop, BrainLes 2016, with the Challenges on BRATS, ISLES and mTOP 2016, Held in Conjunction with MICCAI 2016, Athens, Greece, October 17, 2016, Revised Selected Papers 2. Springer. 138–149.

[43] Adrià Casamitjana, Santi Puch, Asier Aduriz, Elisa Sayrol and Veronica Vilaplana. 2016. 3D convolutional networks for brain tumor segmentation. *In*: Proceedings of the MICCAI challenge on Multimodal Brain Tumor Image Segmentation (BRATS). 2016: 65–68.

[44] Lucas Fidon, Wenqi Li, Luis C. Garcia-Peraza-Herrera, Jinendra Ekanayake, Neil Kitchen, Sebastien Ourselin, et al. 2017. Scalable multimodal convolutional networks for brain tumour segmentation. *In*: Medical Image Computing and Computer Assisted Intervention-MICCAI 2017: 20th International Conference, Quebec City, QC, Canada. Proceedings, Part III 20. Springer. 285–293.

[45] Guotai Wang, Wenqi Li, Sébastien Ourselin and Tom Vercauteren. 2017. Automatic brain tumor segmentation using cascaded anisotropic convolutional neural networks. *In*: Brainlesion: Glioma, Multiple Sclerosis, Stroke and Traumatic Brain Injuries: Third International Workshop, BrainLes 2017, Held in Conjunction with MICCAI 2017, Quebec City, QC, Canada. Revised Selected Papers 3. Springer. 178–190.

[46] Fabian Isensee, Philipp Kickingereder, Wolfgang Wick, Martin Bendszus and Klaus H. Maier-Hein. 2017. Brain tumor segmentation and radiomics survival prediction: Contribution to the BRATS 2017 challenge. *In*: Brainlesion: Glioma, Multiple Sclerosis, Stroke and Traumatic Brain Injuries: Third International Workshop, BrainLes 2017, Held in Conjunction with MICCAI 2017, Quebec City, QC, Canada. Revised Selected Papers 3. Springer. 287–297.

[47] Fabian Isensee, Jens Petersen, Andre Klein, David Zimmerer, Paul F. Jaeger, Simon Kohl, et al. 2018. nnu-net: Self-adapting framework for U-Net-based medical image segmentation. arXiv preprint arXiv:1809(10486).

[48] David N. Louis, Hiroko Ohgaki, Otmar D. Wiestler, Webster K. Cavenee, Peter C. Burger, Anne Jouvet, et al. 2007. The 2007 WHO classification of tumours of the central nervous system. Acta Neuropathologica. 114(2): 97–109.

[49] Yang Chen, Zhenyu Yang, Jingtong Zhao, Justus Adamson, Yang Sheng, Fang-Fang Yin, et al. 2023. A radiomics-incorporated deep ensemble learning model for multi-parametric MRI-based glioma segmentation. Physics in Medicine and Biology. 68(18): 185025.

[50] Gagandeep Singh, S. Manjila, Nicole Sakla, Alan True, A.H. Wardeh, Niha Beig, et al. 2021. Radiomics and radiogenomics in gliomas: A contemporary update. British Journal of Cancer. 125(5): 641–657.

[51] Evangelia I. Zacharaki, Sumei Wang, S. Chawla, Dong Soo Yoo, Ronald Wolf and Elias R. Melhem. 2009. MRI-based classification of brain tumor type and grade using SVM-RFE. *In*: 2009 IEEE International Symposium on Biomedical Imaging: From Nano to Macro. IEEE. 1035–1038.

[52] A. Vamvakas, S.C. Williams, K. Theodorou, E. Kapsalaki, K. Fountas, C. Kappas, et al. 2019. Imaging biomarker analysis of advanced multiparametric MRI for glioma grading. Physica Medica. 60: 188–198.

[53] Hwan-ho Cho, Seung-hak Lee, Jonghoon Kim and Hyunjin Park. 2018. Classification of the glioma grading using radiomics analysis. PeerJ. 6: e5982.

[54] Syed M.S. Reza, M.D. Samad, Z.A. Shboul, K.A. Jones and K.M. Iftekharuddin. 2019. Glioma grading using structural magnetic resonance imaging and molecular data. Journal of Medical Imaging. 6(2): 024501–024501.

[55] Guohua Zhao, Panpan Man, Jie Bai, Longfei Li, Peipei Wang and Guan Yang. 2021. AI-powered radiomics algorithm based on slice pooling for the glioma grading. IEEE Transactions on Industrial Informatics. 18(8): 5383–5393.

[56] Tao Chen, Feng Xiao, Zunpeng Yu, Mengxue Yuan, Haibo Xu and Long Lu. 2021. Detection and grading of gliomas using a novel two-phase machine learning method based on MRI images. Frontiers in Neuroscience. 15: 650629.

[57] Ying Zhuge, Holly Ning, P. Mathen, J.Y. Cheng, A.V. Krauze, Kevin Camphausen, et al. 2020. Automated glioma grading on conventional MRI images using deep convolutional neural networks. Medical Physics. 47(7): 3044–3053.

[58] Aikaterini Kotrotsou, Ahmed Elakkad, Jia Sun, Ginu A. Thomas, Dongni Yang, Srishti Abrol, et al. 2019. Multi-center study finds postoperative residual non-enhancing component of glioblastoma as a new determinant of patient outcome. Journal of Neuro-oncology. 139: 125–133.

[59] Ji Eun Park, Ho Sung Kim, Youngheun Jo, Roh-Eul Yoo, Seung Hong Choi, Soo Jung Nam, et al. 2020. Radiomics prognostication model in glioblastoma using diffusion- and perfusion-weighted MRI. Scientific Reports. 10(1): 4250.

[60] A. Lasocki and F. Gaillard. 2019. Non-contrast-enhancing tumor: A new frontier in glioblastoma research. American Journal of Neuroradiology. 40(5): 758–765.

[61] Yang Yang, Lin-Feng Yan, Xin Zhang, Yu Han, Hai-Yan Nan, Yu-Chuan Hu, et al. 2018. Glioma grading on conventional MR images: A deep learning study with transfer learning. Frontiers in Neuroscience. 12: 804.

[62] Taohui Xiao, Wenqing Hua, Cheng Li and Shanshan Wang. 2019. Glioma grading prediction by exploring radiomics and deep learning features. *In*: Proceedings of the Third International Symposium on Image Computing and Digital Medicine. 208–213.

[63] Mohamed A. Naser and M. Jamal Deen. 2020. Brain tumor segmentation and grading of lower-grade glioma using deep learning in MRI images. Computers in Biology and Medicine. 121: 103758.

[64] Milan Decuyper, Stijn Bonte, Karel Deblaere and Roel Van Holen. 2021. Automated MRI based pipeline for segmentation and prediction of grade, IDH mutation and 1p19q co-deletion in glioma. Computerized Medical Imaging and Graphics. 88: 101831.

[65] Fan Zhang, S.C. Karayumak, Nico Hoffmann, Yogesh Rathi, Alexandra J. Golby and Lauren J. O'Donnell. 2020. Deep white matter analysis (DeepWMA): Fast and consistent tractography segmentation. Medical Image Analysis. 65: 101761.

[66] Man He, Kangfu Han, Yu Zhang and Wufan Chen. 2021. Hierarchical-order multimodal interaction fusion network for grading gliomas. Physics in Medicine and Biology. 66(21): 215016.

[67] Prasun Chandra Tripathi and Soumen Bag. 2022. A computer-aided grading of glioma tumor using deep residual networks fusion. Computer Methods and Programs in Biomedicine. 215: 106597.

[68] Jialin Ding, Rubin Zhao, Qingtao Qiu, Jinhu Chen, Jinghao Duan, Xiujuan Cao, et al. 2022. Developing and validating a deep learning and radiomic model for glioma grading using multiplanar reconstructed magnetic resonance contrast-enhanced T1-weighted imaging: A robust, multi-institutional study.Quantitative Imaging in Medicine and Surgery. 12(2): 1517.

[69] Jianhong Cheng, Min Gao, Jin Liu, Hailin Yue, Hulin Kuang and Jun Liu. 2021. Multimodal disentangled variational autoencoder with game theoretic interpretability for glioma grading. IEEE Journal of Biomedical and Health Informatics. 26(2): 673–684.

[70] Ken Chang, Harrison X. Bai, Hao Zhou, Chang Su, Wenya Linda Bi and Ena Agbodza. 2018. Residual convolutional neural network for the determination of IDH status in low-and high-grade gliomas from MR imaging. Clinical Cancer Research. 24(5): 1073–1081.

[71] Lauren R. Schaff and Ingo K. Mellinghoff. 2023. Glioblastoma and other primary brain malignancies in adults: A review. Jama. 329(7): 574–587.

[72] Sohil H. Patel, Laila M. Poisson, Daniel J. Brat, Yueren Zhou, Lee Cooper and Matija Snuderl. 2017. T2–FLAIR mismatch, an imaging biomarker for IDH and 1p/19q status in lower-grade gliomas: A TCGA/TCIA project. Clinical Cancer Research. 23(20): 6078–6085.

[73] Martinus P.G. Broen, Marion Smits, Maarten M.J. Wijnenga, Hendrikus J. Dubbink, Monique H.M.E Anten, Olaf E.M.G. Schijns, et al. 2018. The T2-FLAIR mismatch sign as an imaging marker for non-enhancing IDH-mutant, 1p/19q-intact lower-grade glioma: A validation study. Neuro-oncology. 20(10): 1393–1399.

[74] Eric Aliotta, Sunil W. Dutta, Xue Feng, Nicholas J. Tustison, Prem P. Batchala, David Schiff, et al. 2020. Automated apparent diffusion coefficient analysis for genotype prediction in lower grade glioma: Association with the T2-FLAIR mismatch sign. Journal of Neuro-oncology. 149(2): 325–335.

[75] Derek R. Johnson, T.J. Kaufmann, S.H. Patel, Andrew S. Chi, Matija Snuderl and Rajan Jain. 2019. There is an exception to every rule—T2-FLAIR mismatch sign in gliomas. Neuroradiology. 61(2): 225–227.

[76] Chia-Feng Lu, Fei-Ting Hsu, K. Li-Chun Hsieh, Yu-Chieh J. Kao, Sho-Jen Cheng, Justin Bo-Kai Hsu, et al. 2018. Machine learning–based radiomics for molecular subtyping of gliomas. Clinical Cancer Research. 24(18): 4429–4436.

[77] Sebastian R. van der Voort, F. Incekara, Maarten M.J. Wijnenga, Georgios Kapas, Mayke Gardeniers and Joost W. Schouten. 2019. Predicting the 1p/19q codeletion status of presumed low-grade glioma with an externally validated machine learning algorithm. Clinical Cancer Research. 25(24): 7455–7462.

[78] Martin A. Lewis, B. Ganeshan, Anna Barnes, Sotirios Bisdas, Zane Jaunmuktane, Sebastian Brandner, et al. 2019. Filtration-histogram based magnetic resonance texture analysis (MRTA) for glioma IDH and 1p19q genotyping. European Journal of Radiology. 113: 116–123.

[79] John Maynard, Sachi Okuchi, Stephen Wastling, A. Al Busaidi, Ofran Almossawi, Wonderboy Mbatha, et al. 2020. World Health Organization grade II/III glioma molecular status: prediction by MRI morphologic features and apparent diffusion coefficient. Radiology. 296(1): 111–121.

[80] Zhenyu Tang, Yuyun Xu, Lei Jin, A. Aibaidula, Junfeng Lu and Zhicheng Jiao. 2020. Deep learning of imaging phenotype and genotype for predicting overall survival time of glioblastoma patients. IEEE Transactions on Medical Imaging. 39(6): 2100–2109.

[81] Ankang Gao, Huiting Zhang, Xu Yan, Shaoyu Wang, Q. Chen and Eryuan Gao. 2022. Whole-tumor histogram analysis of multiple diffusion metrics for glioma genotyping. Radiology. 302(3): 652–661.

[82] Jianhong Cheng, Jin Liu, Hulin Kuang and Jianxin Wang. 2022. A fully automated multimodal MRI-based multi-task learning for glioma segmentation and IDH genotyping. IEEE Transactions on Medical Imaging. 41(6): 1520–1532.

[83] Jia Liu, Fang Chen, Changcun Pan, Mingyu Zhu, Xinran Zhang and Liwei Zhang. 2018. A cascaded deep convolutional neural network for joint segmentation and genotype prediction of brainstem gliomas. IEEE Transactions on Biomedical Engineering. 65(9): 1943–1952.

[84] Chandan G.B. Yogananda, B.R. Shah, Frank F. Yu, M.C. Pinho, S.S. Nalawade, Gowtham K. Murugesan, et al. 2020. A novel fully automated MRI-based deep-

learning method for classification of 1p/19q co-deletion status in brain gliomas. Neuro-oncology Advances. 2(Supplement_4): iv42–iv48.

[85] Yao Wang, Yan Wang, Chunjie Guo, Shuangquan Zhang and Lili Yang. 2021. SGPNet: A three-dimensional multitask residual framework for segmentation and IDH genotype prediction of gliomas. Computational Intelligence and Neuroscience. 2021(1): 5520281.

[86] Kyu Sung Choi, Seung Hong Choi and Bumseok Jeong. 2019. Prediction of IDH genotype in gliomas with dynamic susceptibility contrast perfusion MR imaging using an explainable recurrent neural network. Neuro-oncology. 21(9): 1197–1209.

[87] Pawel Jarmuzek, K. Kozlowska, P. Defort, M. Kot and Agnieszka Zembron-Lacny. 2023. Prognostic values of systemic inflammatory immunological markers in glioblastoma: A systematic review and meta-analysis. Cancers. 15(13): 3339.

[88] Bhargav Mallampati, Abid Ishaq, Furqan Rustam, Venu Kuthala, Sultan Alfarhood, and Imran Ashraf. 2023. Brain tumor detection using 3D-UNet segmentation features and hybrid machine learning model. IEEE Access. 11: 135020–135034.

[89] Ahmad Chaddad, M.J. Kucharczyk, Paul Daniel, Siham Sabri, B.J. Jean-Claude, Tamim Niazi, et al. 2019. Radiomics in glioblastoma: Current status and challenges facing clinical implementation. Frontiers in Oncology. 9: 374.

[90] Michel Lacroix, Dima Abi-Said, Daryl R. Fourney, Ziya L. Gokaslan, Weiming Shi, Franco DeMonte, et al. 2001. A multivariate analysis of 416 patients with glioblastoma multiforme: prognosis, extent of resection, and survival. Journal of Neurosurgery. 95(2): 190–198.

[91] S. Bisdas, M. Kirkpatrick, P. Giglio, C. Welsh, M.V. Spampinato and Z. Rumboldt. 2009. Cerebral blood volume measurements by perfusion weighted MR imaging in gliomas: ready for prime time in predicting short-term outcome and recurrent disease? American Journal of Neuroradiology. 30(4): 681–688.

[92] Ken Chang, Biqi Zhang, Xiaotao Guo, Min Zong, R. Rahman, David Sanchez, et al. 2016. Multimodal imaging patterns predict survival in recurrent glioblastoma patients treated with bevacizumab. Neuro-oncology. 18(12): 1680– 1687.

[93] Li Sun, Sontao Zhang, Hang Chen and Liu Luo. 2019. Brain tumor segmentation and survival prediction using multimodal MRI scans with deep learning. Frontiers in Neuroscience. 13: 810.

[94] David R. Cox. 1972. Regression models and life-tables. Journal of the Royal Statistical Society: Series B (Methodological). 34(2): 187–202.

[95] Jiangwei Lao, Yinsheng Chen, Zhi-Cheng Li, Qihua Li, Ji Zhang, Jing Liu, et al. 2017. A deep learning-based radiomics model for prediction of survival in glioblastoma multiforme. Scientific Reports. 7(1): 10353.

[96] Xin Hu, Emmanuel Martinez-Ledesma, Siyuan Zheng, Hoon Kim, Floris Barthel, Tao Jiang, et al. 2017. Multigene signature for predicting prognosis of patients with 1p19q co-deletion diffuse glioma. Neuro-oncology. 19(6): 786–795.

[97] Pooya Mobadersany, Safoora Yousefi, Mohamed Amgad, David A. Gutman, Jill S. Barnholtz-Sloan, José E. Velázquez Vega, et al. 2018. Predicting cancer outcomes from histology and genomics using convolutional networks. Proceedings of the National Academy of Sciences. 115(13): E2970–E2979.

[98] Sören Richard Stahlschmidt, Benjamin Ulfenborg and Jane Synnergren. 2022. Multimodal deep learning for biomedical data fusion: A review. Briefings in Bioinformatics. 23(2): bbab569.

[99] Richard J. Chen, Ming Y. Lu, Jingwen Wang, Drew F.K. Williamson, Scott J. Rodig and Neal I. Lindeman. 2020. Pathomic fusion: an integrated framework for fusing histopathology and genomic features for cancer diagnosis and prognosis. IEEE Transactions on Medical Imaging. 41(4): 757–770.

[100] Nathaniel Braman, Jacob W.H. Gordon, Emery T. Goossens, Caleb Willis, Martin C. Stumpe and Jagadish Venkataraman. 2021. Deep orthogonal fusion: Multimodal prognostic biomarker discovery integrating radiology, pathology, genomic, and clinical data. Medical Image Computing and Computer Assisted Intervention–MICCAI 2021: 24th International Conference, Strasbourg, France. Proceedings, Part V 24. Springer. 667–677.

[101] Dongwook Lee, Won-Jin Moon and Jong Chul Ye. 2020. Assessing the importance of magnetic resonance contrasts using collaborative generative adversarial networks. Nature Machine Intelligence. 2(1): 34–42.

[102] Mengmeng Ma, Jian Ren, Long Zhao, Sergey Tulyakov, Cathy Wu and Xi Peng. 2021. Smil: Multimodal learning with severely missing modality. *In*: Proceedings of the AAAI Conference on Artificial Intelligence. 35(3): 2302–2310.

[103] Wenqi Li, Fausto Milletarì, Daguang Xu, Nicola Rieke, J. Hancox, Wentao Zhu, et al. 2019. Privacy-preserving federated brain tumour segmentation. *In*: Machine Learning in Medical Imaging: 10th International Workshop, MLMI 2019, Held in Conjunction with MICCAI 2019, Shenzhen, China. Proceedings 10. Springer. 133–141.

[104] Xiang Bai, Hanchen Wang, Liya Ma, Yongchao Xu, Jiefeng Gan, Ziwei Fan, et al. 2021. Advancing COVID-19 diagnosis with privacy-preserving collaboration in artificial intelligence. Nature Machine Intelligence. 3(12): 1081– 1089.

Chapter **2.4**

Graph-based Deep Learning for MRI-based Brain Network Analysis

Jiazhou Chen[1], Li Zhang[2], Xiaoqi Sheng[3] and Hongmin Cai[3,4*]

[1]School of Computer Science and Technology, Guangdong University of Technology, Guangzhou, Guangdong, China

[2]School of Biomedical Engineering, Medical School, Shenzhen University, Shenzhen, Guangdong, China

[3]School of Future Technology, South China University of Technology, Guangzhou, Guangdong, China

[4]School of Computer Science and Engineering, South China University of Technology, Guangzhou, Guangdong, China

2.4.1 INTRODUCTION

Magnetic Resonance Imaging (MRI) of the brain stands as a sophisticated imaging technique extensively employed in the medical domain, offering researchers a vital tool for comprehending the intricate structures and functions of the brain. This technology is broadly categorized into two main types: functional MRI (fMRI) and structural MRI (sMRI). Functional MRI delves into the study of brain function by monitoring the blood oxygen level-dependent (BOLD) changes. Through functional MRI images, researchers can investigate cognitive functions, emotional regulation, and motor control, aiding in unraveling the mechanisms and patterns of brain activity [1, 2]. On the other hand, structural MRI focuses on

*For Correspondence: hm-cai@scut.edu.cn

DOI: 10.1201/9781003518754-9

unveiling the anatomical structures and tissue characteristics of the brain. With structural MRI imaging, high-resolution images of brain structures, including the cortex, gray matter, white matter, hippocampus, and other regions, can be obtained, furnishing detailed insights essential for diagnosing brain disorders, evaluating structural changes, and exploring brain development and aging processes [3, 4].

Brain MRI images are pivotal in mapping brain networks, revealing the connections and interactions between different brain regions [5–7]. This process typically involves several key steps: (1) extracting functional or structural features of various brain regions from brain MRI images; (2) establishing a brain network based on these features with nodes representing different brain regions and edges denoting connections between these regions; and (3) employing network analysis techniques such as graph theory and complex network analysis to study the topological structure, functional features, and dynamic changes of brain networks. Brain network research is gaining increasing favor among researchers due to the close association between brain network alterations and the progression of brain diseases like Parkinson's disease [8, 9], Alzheimer's disease [10–13], major depressive disorder [14, 15], and others [16, 17]. By delving into the relationship between brain networks and brain diseases, more precise methods and strategies can be developed for early disease diagnosis, treatment, and prevention.

Recently, graph-based deep learning methods have found widespread application in analyzing brain networks as a prominent network analysis technique. This cutting-edge artificial intelligence technology concentrates on processing and analyzing data with intricate relationships, such as social networks [18], protein interaction networks [19], and brain networks [20]. While traditional deep learning methods typically represent data as vectors or matrices, graph-based deep learning is adept at handling unstructured data, effectively capturing relationships and interactions between entities. A graph comprises nodes representing entities and edges symbolizing the relationships between these entities. Graph-based deep learning methods model and analyze complex data by utilizing the topological structure of graphs and connection information between nodes. Among these methods, Graph Neural Networks (GNNs) [1] serve as a critical branch of graph-based deep learning methods, capable of learning feature representations at both the node and graph levels, facilitating information inference and prediction across the entire graph. Within the realm of brain network analysis, graph-based deep learning methods are extensively utilized to identify hub nodes in brain networks [21, 22], explore connection patterns between different brain regions [23, 24], and discover neuropathological propagation patterns [25, 26]. These techniques not only aid in comprehending brain function complexity but also offer fresh perspectives and tools for diagnosing and researching brain diseases, thereby contributing to the advancement of precision medicine.

In this chapter, we first briefly illustrate the fundamental concepts and methodologies of graph-based deep learning in Section 2.4.2. Furthermore, we explore their applications in brain network analysis in Section 2.4.3. It delves into how graph-based deep learning techniques are leveraged to process extensive brain network data, unveil the structure and function of brain networks, and apply this information to the study and clinical practice of brain diseases, presenting readers with the latest developments in neuroscience. Finally, we conclude this chapter by summarizing the research content and providing potential research directions in network neuroscience in Section 2.4.4.

2.4.2 OVERVIEW OF GRAPH-BASED DEEP LEARNING

In this section, we review graph-based deep learning methods. First, we discuss the fundamental graph neural network models, which profoundly impacted the field of graph-based deep learning. Most studies build upon these basic graph neural network models. Following that, we explore important methods derived from these basic models, focusing on two aspects: graph representation learning and graph structure learning.

2.4.2.1 Graph Basic Models

Fundamental graph neural network models represent a class of widely applied classical frameworks in the domain of graph-based deep learning. These models are commonly utilized as foundational architectures for deriving variants or baselines for evaluating performance. In this section, we focus on discussing four primary models: GCN, GraphSAGE, GAT, and GAE. Certain variants of GAT and GAE are also included in our discussion.

GCN

The Graph Convolutional Network (GCN) [1] is a neural network that, unlike CNNs, is designed to handle graph-structured data. Before the introduction of GCN, graph convolution theories [27] were already based on the definition of convolution operators in the spectral domain. First, the graph signal x is transformed into the spectral domain through the Fourier transform, where convolution is performed, and the result is transformed back using the inverse graph Fourier transform. The graph Fourier transform is expressed as:

$$\mathcal{F}(x) = U^T x, \mathcal{F}^{-1}(x) = Ux, \tag{1}$$

where U is the eigenvector matrix of the normalized graph Laplacian $L = I_N - D^{-\frac{1}{2}} A D^{-\frac{1}{2}}$ with D as the degree matrix and A as the adjacency matrix of the graph. The normalized graph Laplacian is a symmetric positive semi-definite matrix, allowing it to be decomposed as $L = U\Lambda U^T$, where Λ is a diagonal matrix of eigenvalues. The graph convolution operation can thus be defined as:

$$g \star x = \mathcal{F}^{-1}(\mathcal{F}(g) \odot \mathcal{F}(x)) = U(U^T g \odot U^T x), \tag{2}$$

where $U^T g$ represents the filter in the spectral domain and denotes the Hadamard product. If a learnable diagonal matrix g_w is used as the filter, the basic spectral convolution method is expressed as:

$$g \star x = U g_w U^T x. \tag{3}$$

The matrix g_w operates on the eigenvalues of the Laplacian matrix, which is computationally expensive. To reduce this cost, [28] proposed constructing g_w using K-order Chebyshev polynomials:

$$g_w \approx \sum_{k=0}^{K} w_k T_k(\tilde{L}), \tag{4}$$

where $\tilde{L} = \frac{2}{\lambda_{\max}} L - I_N$, and $\lambda_{\max}$ is the largest eigenvalue of L. The coefficients $w_k \in \mathbb{R}^K$ are the Chebyshev coefficients, and the Chebyshev polynomial is defined as $T_k(x) = 2xT_{k-1}(x) - T_{k-2}(x)$, with $T_0(x) = 1$ and $T_1(x) = x$.

To further simplify computation, [1] set K = 1 in Eqn. 4 and approximated $\lambda_{\max} \approx 2$, reducing the equation to:

$$g_w \star x \approx w_0 x + w_1 \left(L - I_N\right) x = w_0 x - w_1 D^{-\frac{1}{2}} A D^{-\frac{1}{2}} x, \tag{5}$$

where, by setting $w = w_0 = -w_1$, the expression simplifies to:

$$g_w \star x \approx w\left(I_N + D^{-\frac{1}{2}} A D^{-\frac{1}{2}}\right) x. \tag{6}$$

Rewriting $I_N + D^{-\frac{1}{2}} A D^{-\frac{1}{2}}$ as $\tilde{D}^{-\frac{1}{2}} \tilde{A} \tilde{D}^{-\frac{1}{2}}$, with $\tilde{A} = A + I_N$ and $\tilde{D}_{ii} = \sum_j \tilde{A}_{ij}$, we arrive at the final form of GCN:

$$H = \tilde{D}^{-\frac{1}{2}} \tilde{A} \tilde{D}^{-\frac{1}{2}} X W, \tag{7}$$

where $X \in \mathbb{R}^{N \times d}$ is the input matrix, $W \in \mathbb{R}^{d \times d'}$ is a learnable parameter matrix, and $H \in \mathbb{R}^{N \times d'}$ is the output matrix after convolution. The dimensions d and d' represent the input and output dimensions, respectively. Eqn. 7 describes a single GCN layer, and stacking multiple layers leads to the expression for the l-th layer:

$$H_l = \tilde{D}^{-\frac{1}{2}} \tilde{A} \tilde{D}^{-\frac{1}{2}} X_{l-1} W. \tag{8}$$

GraphSAGE

GraphSAGE (Sample and AggreGatE) is an algorithm designed to learn node embeddings for inductive unsupervised learning tasks, extending the GCN framework beyond fixed-graph transductive settings [29]. It generalizes the GCN approach by introducing trainable aggregation functions, surpassing simple convolutions. GraphSAGE is a versatile framework capable of inductive node embedding learning, meaning it can learn embeddings for unseen nodes based on known node features. For graphs without node features, it can leverage structural information to infer node features. The following equations summarize the sampling and aggregation process of Graph SAGE:

$$h_{\mathcal{N}_v}^{t+1} = AGG_{t+1}(h_t^u \mid \forall u \in \mathcal{N}_v), h_v^{t+1} = \sigma\left(W^{t+1} \cdot \left[h_v^t \parallel h_{\mathcal{N}_v}^{t+1}\right]\right), \tag{9}$$

where h_t^u is the node feature at layer t, $u \in \mathcal{N}_v$ denotes the sampled neighbors of node v, and W^{t+1} represents the aggregation function's parameters. As shown, GraphSAGE does not aggregate all neighboring nodes but instead samples a fixed number of neighbors for aggregation. The aggregation function AGG_{t+1} can include mean aggregation, LSTM aggregation, and pooling aggregation. GraphSAGE with mean aggregation can be viewed as an inductive version of GCN. Additionally, GraphSAGE is conceptually inspired by the Weisfeiler-Lehman (WL) algorithm for testing graph isomorphism. Under certain conditions, GraphSAGE can be viewed as an instance of the WL test, which can determine whether two input subgraphs are isomorphic. Although the goal of GraphSAGE is to learn node representations rather than test graph isomorphism, the strong representational power of the WL test theoretically supports GraphSAGE's ability to capture node neighborhood topology.

GAT

Graph Attention Network (GAT) is a neural network architecture designed to operate on graph-structured data [30]. Inspired by the attention mechanism, it computes the hidden representations of each node in a graph by focusing on its neighbors and following a self-attention strategy. Like GraphSAGE, GAT directly applies to inductive learning problems, allowing it to generalize to completely unseen graphs.

First, the attention coefficient α_{ij} between two nodes is computed based on their features:

$$\alpha_{ij} = \frac{\exp\left(\text{LeakyReLU}\left(\vec{a}^T\left[W\vec{h}_i \,\|\, W\vec{h}_j\right]\right)\right)}{\sum_{k\in\mathcal{N}_i}\exp\left(\text{LeakyReLU}\left(\vec{a}^T\left[W\vec{h}_i \,\|\, W\vec{h}_k\right]\right)\right)}, \tag{10}$$

where $\vec{h} \in \mathbb{R}^F$ is the input node feature, $W \in \mathbb{R}^{F\times F'}$ is the weight matrix, $\vec{a} \in \mathbb{R}^{2F'}$ is the weight vector, and || represents the concatenation operation. The normalized attention coefficients are then used to compute the new node features:

$$\vec{h}_i' = \sigma\left(\sum_{j\in\mathcal{N}_i} \alpha_{ij} W\vec{h}_j\right), \tag{11}$$

where σ is a non-linear activation function. After adding multi-head attention, Eqn. 11 becomes:

$$\vec{h}_i' = \Big\Vert_{k=1}^{K} \sigma\left(\sum_{j\in\mathcal{N}_i} \alpha_{ij}^k W^k \vec{h}_j\right), \tag{12}$$

where K represents the number of attention heads, and $\vec{h}_i'$ is the updated node feature. One advantage of GAT is that it allows the implicit assignment of different importance to different nodes in the neighborhood while handling neighborhoods of varying sizes without relying on prior knowledge of the entire graph structure. This versatile architecture has also inspired various extensions for other graph learning domains.

HAN

Heterogeneous graph Attention Network (HAN) [31] is a neural network that generates node embeddings for heterogeneous graphs using hierarchical attention. First, it is important to define heterogeneous graphs: these are graphs with different types of nodes and edges. For instance, in a movie dataset, nodes may represent movies, actors, and directors. Based on meta-paths, nodes of the same type can be connected. The relationships between nodes connected through a meta-path are aggregated to learn node embeddings. Different attention is assigned to neighbors based on different meta-paths, which is achieved through node-level attention in HAN, as shown below:

$$z_i^{\Phi} = \sigma\left(\sum_{j \in \mathcal{N}_i^{\Phi}} \alpha_{ij}^{\Phi} \cdot h_j'\right). \tag{13}$$

Here, Φ represents a meta-path, and α_{ij}^{Φ} is the normalized attention coefficient computed using Eqn. 10, while z_i^{Φ} is the node embedding for node i based on meta-path Φ.

The node embeddings generated from different meta-paths are aggregated to form the final node embedding. During this process, different meta-path-based node embeddings have varying importance under different semantics, which is captured by semantic-level attention in HAN:

$$Z = \sum_{p=1}^{P} \beta_{\Phi_p} \cdot Z_{\Phi_p}. \tag{14}$$

Here, $\beta_{\Phi_p} = att_{sem}(Z_{\Phi_p})$ is the weight obtained through the semantic attention network att_{sem} for different meta-paths Φ_p, and Z_{Φ_p} is the aggregation of node embeddings computed from Eqn. 13. This completes the node-level aggregation and semantic-level aggregation in HAN.

GTN

As previously mentioned, HAN relies on meta-paths to convert heterogeneous graphs into meta-path-based homogeneous graphs, but selecting meta-paths requires additional domain knowledge. Graph Transformer Network (GTN) [32], on the other hand, can automatically identify useful meta-paths and multi-hop connections to learn effective node representations on graphs. This is primarily achieved through the following formula:

$$Q = F(\mathbb{A}; W_{\phi}) = \phi(\mathbb{A}; \text{softmax}(W_{\phi})), \tag{15}$$

where ϕ is a convolutional layer, $W_{\phi} \in \mathbb{R}^{1\times1\times K}$ are the parameters of ϕ, and $\mathbb{A}$ is the adjacency matrix of the heterogeneous graph. Given two soft-selected adjacency matrices Q_1 and Q_2, the meta-path adjacency matrix is computed via matrix multiplication Q_1Q_2. This process is referred to as a Graph Transformer (GT) layer. Additionally, GTN can learn meta-paths of arbitrary lengths:

$$A_P = \left(\sum_{t_1 \in \mathcal{T}^e} \alpha_{t_1}^{(1)} A_{t_1} \right) \left(\sum_{t_2 \in \mathcal{T}^e} \alpha_{t_2}^{(2)} A_{t_2} \right) \cdots \left(\sum_{t_l \in \mathcal{T}^e} \alpha_{t_l}^{(l)} A_{t_l} \right), \tag{16}$$

where A_P is the meta-path adjacency matrix, $\mathcal{T}^e$ is a set of edge types, and $\alpha_{t_l}^{(l)}$ is the weight for the edge type t_l in the l-th GT layer. Thus, stacking l GT layers enables GTN to learn meta-paths of different lengths.

After automatically learning meta-paths of varying lengths, GTN converts the heterogeneous graph into a meta-path-based homogeneous graph, enabling GCN to learn the representations of each node.

GAE

Graph AutoEncoder (GAE) is an unsupervised learning framework based on Variational AutoEncoders (VAE) designed for deep learning on graph-structured data. It mainly learns interpretable latent space representations for undirected graphs. First, GAE performs variational inference using a two-layer GCN:

$$q(Z|X, A) = \prod_{i=1}^{N} q(z_i | X, A), \text{ with } q\,(z_i | X, A) = \mathcal{N}(z_i \mid \boldsymbol{\mu}_i, \text{diag}\,(\boldsymbol{\sigma}_i^2)). \tag{17}$$

Here, Z is a matrix of latent variables z_i, $\mu = \text{GCN}_\mu(X, A)$ is the mean matrix, and similarly, $\log \sigma = \text{GCN}_\sigma(X, A)$ is the standard deviation matrix. Both GCN layers are defined as $\text{GCN}(X, A) = \tilde{A}\,\text{ReLU}(\tilde{A}XW_0)W_1$, where $\text{GCN}_\mu(X, A)$ and $\text{GCN}_\sigma(X, A)$ share the parameter W_0.

Through variational inference, the model samples the mean and standard deviation from the original graph data and obtains the approximate distribution $q(Z|X, A)$ and the latent variables Z using the reparameterization trick. Next, it regenerates the adjacency matrix based on Z:

$$p(A|Z) = \prod_{i=1}^{N} \prod_{j=1}^{N} p(A_{ij} | z_i, z_j), \text{ with } p(A_{ij} = 1 \mid z_i, z_j) = \sigma(z_i^T z_j), \tag{18}$$

where σ is the logistic sigmoid function.

The final loss function is:

$$\mathcal{L} = \mathbb{E}_{q(Z|X,A)}[\log p(A \mid Z)] - \text{KL}[q(Z \mid X, A) \,\|\, p(Z)], \tag{19}$$

where $\text{KL}[q(\cdot) \| p(\cdot)]$ is the Kullback-Leibler divergence, measuring the closeness between the distributions $q(\cdot)$ and $p(\cdot)$. The Gaussian prior is defined as

$$p(Z) = \prod_i p(z_i) = \prod_i \mathcal{N}(z_i \mid 0, I).$$

In simple terms, GAE learns an approximate distribution and latent variables from the graph data to reconstruct the adjacency matrix, making it close to the true adjacency matrix while ensuring that the learned distribution approximates the Gaussian prior distribution. This approach enables the model to capture effective features of the graph data. However, the original GAE has certain limitations, such as focusing more on learning structural information and ignoring node content. Additionally, the method for aligning latent variables with the prior distribution in Eqn. 19 can be further improved. Below, we discuss two GAE variants that address these issues.

Marginalized GAE

To address the issue of GAE primarily learning the graph structure, [34] proposed the Marginalized GAE (MAGAE). Unlike the original GAE, MAGAE introduces a reconstruction loss to constrain the reconstructed graph and consider node content rather than merely reconstructing the adjacency matrix. The reconstruction loss is given by:

$$\left\|X - f(\tilde{X}, A)\right\|^2, \tag{20}$$

where $f(\cdot)$ represents the encoder composed of GCNs, and $\tilde{X}$ is the node content with random dropout applied. In addition, to enable the encoder to learn richer node content, multiple different versions of $\tilde{X}$ can be generated through m different random dropouts, and the encoder can process them. Thus, the final loss function is:

$$\frac{1}{m}\sum_{i=1}^{m}\left\|X - f(\tilde{X}, A)\right\|^2 + \lambda\|W\|_F^2, \tag{21}$$

where $\|W\|_F^2$ is the L2 regularization term, and W is the parameter matrix. The reconstructed graph from MAGAE is then learned through multiple layers of GCNs to obtain the final representation.

Adversarially Regularized GAE

In Eqn. 19, the latent variables Z are made to approximate the prior distribution using the Kullback-Leibler divergence $\mathrm{KL}[q(Z|X,A)\|p(Z)]$. However, [35] proposed an approach inspired by GANs [36]. In this approach, the random variable Z', which follows the prior distribution p, is used as a positive example, while the latent variable Z serves as a negative example. A discriminator built from an MLP is trained to distinguish between them, with the encoder acting as a generator. The objective function is optimized to allow the encoder to learn latent variables that approximate the prior distribution:

$$\min_{\mathcal{G}}\max_{\mathcal{D}} \mathbb{E}_{z\sim p_z}\left[\log \mathcal{D}(Z)\right] + \mathbb{E}_{x\sim p(x)}\left[\log\left(1-\mathcal{D}\left(\mathcal{G}(X,A)\right)\right)\right], \tag{22}$$

where $\mathcal{G}(X, A)$ and $\mathcal{D}(Z)$ are the generator and discriminator, respectively.

2.4.2.2 Graph Representation Learning

This section discusses several representative models in the field of graph representation learning. The distinction between graph representation and node representation is not strictly defined because the process of converting effective node representations to graph representations is often simple and not the primary focus of most studies. Most tasks aimed at obtaining graph representations focus on researching more efficient node representations. Therefore, the graph representation learning algorithms discussed in this section include both node representation learning and graph representation learning.

Graph Contrastive Learning

Graph Contrastive Learning (GCL) is an unsupervised method inspired by contrastive learning tailored for graph-structured data. Given a training graph, GCL aims to encode similar graph instances (positive sample pairs) close to each other and distant from dissimilar ones (negative sample pairs). Since this approach does not require labeled data, GCL allows for self-supervised learning of graph representations. The general framework of GCL can be summarized into three parts: view generation, graph encoder, and learning objective [37].

View generation creates positive and negative sample pairs required for contrastive learning. Typically, two views from the same graph instance are considered positive sample pairs, while views from different graph instances are treated as negative pairs. View generation methods can be divided into operations in feature space and structural space. The next major section will discuss structural space operations, while feature space operations are the focus here. Feature space refers to node and graph features, and any view generated without altering the graph structure can be considered a feature space operation, such as masking node features [38], where node feature vectors are replaced with constants or random values. Similarly, the Dropout method [39] randomly masks neurons in the encoder network to generate new views, which, in effect, impacts certain dimensions of the node features. Another technique [40] manipulates encoder neurons by varying neuron count, propagation depth, and arrangement across views. In essence, the goal of view generation is to perturb the graph while making the encoder robust to such perturbations, thus learning robust graph representations. The choice of graph encoder varies with context but primarily focuses on learning node representations. Common encoders include foundational models discussed earlier, with the option to include a readout step to generate graph-level representations as needed for downstream tasks.

The design of the learning objective is the core task in contrastive learning. It determines how positive and negative sample pairs are identified and how their similarity is measured. Typically, as mentioned earlier, views of the same graph instance are considered positive sample pairs, while views of different graph instances are treated as negative pairs. In node classification tasks, the instances being compared are nodes. Positive sample pairs consist of the same node across different views, while negative sample pairs are different nodes across views. However, this method may overlook the similarity between a node and its neighboring nodes, leading to approaches such as in NCLA [41], which treats neighboring nodes in different views as positive sample pairs.

Additionally, the quality of views may vary depending on the perturbation method. In [42], different views are assigned different weights based on their quality, with the goal of amplifying the influence of high-quality views and reducing the impact of low-quality ones. Similarly, soft contrastive learning [43] eliminates the binary distinction between positive and negative sample pairs, instead sampling positive samples based on similarity and pushing them closer to the anchor point to different extents; as for measuring the proximity between sample pairs, the most common method is based on mutual information (MI). MI is an information-theoretic concept that quantifies how much information one variable contains about another and can be interpreted as a measure of similarity between two variables. The formula for mutual information is

$$\mathcal{I}(x,y) = D_{KL}(p(x,y) \,\|\, p(x)p(y)) = \mathbb{E}_{p(x,y)}\left[\log \frac{p(x,y)}{p(x)p(y)}\right], \tag{23}$$

where DKL is the Kullback-Leibler divergence. In contrastive learning, the objects being compared are treated as two random variables, and their mutual information is computed. Standard optimizations for the lower bound of mutual information include Donsker-Varadhan, Jensen-Shannon, and noise-contrastive estimation (InfoNCE) [44], with InfoNCE being the most widely used:

$$\mathcal{L}_i = -\log \frac{\exp\left(\mathrm{sim}(z_i, z_i^+)/\tau\right)}{\sum_{j=1}^{N} \exp\left(\mathrm{sim}(z_i, z_j)/\tau\right)}, \tag{24}$$

where z_i is the embedding of sample i, z_i^+ is the corresponding positive sample, and z_j are negative samples. The term sim (z_i, z_j) represents the similarity between z_i and z_j (e.g., cosine similarity), and τ is a temperature parameter.

GCN-based Methods

Earlier, we introduced the GCN as a powerful graph neural network (GNN), but it has some limitations. For example, it cannot be stacked too deeply, which leads to over-smoothing [45]. Additionally, GCN's ability to distinguish non-isomorphic graphs has been criticized [46]. Therefore, improvements to GCN have been continuously proposed, and we list several representative ones here.

Multi-Hop Methods

A key assumption of GCN is that $K = 1$ in Equation 4, meaning it aggregates only information from 1-hop neighbors. This is known as 1-hop message passing. While it reduces computational costs, it introduces the challenge of distinguishing non-isomorphic graphs. One obvious solution is to extend 1-hop message passing to k-hop, allowing nodes to aggregate information from higher-order neighbors. MixHop [47] is a representative method aggregating information from multi-hop neighbors. It considers information from both 1-hop and 2-hop neighbors, applying different linear transformations to encode information from different hops, which are then concatenated for mixing. In KP-GNN [48], not only are different hops considered, but also peripheral subgraphs within those hops. Multi-hop GCNs can also be integrated with contrastive learning. In [49], a GCN is run with L

different hops on the same input graph, and the L resulting graph representations are treated as L views. Representations of the same node across different views are treated as positive samples, while representations of different nodes across views are treated as negative samples, allowing node representations to capture global structural features.

GIN

The Graph Isomorphism Network (GIN) [50] provides another approach to improving GCN's ability to distinguish non-isomorphic graphs. GIN is a highly expressive GNN that generalizes the Weisfeiler-Lehman (WL) test, achieving maximum discriminative power among GNNs. The update rule for node representation in GIN is:

$$h_v^{(k)} = \mathrm{MLP}^{(k)}\left((1+\varepsilon^{(k)})\cdot h_v^{(k-1)} + \sum_{u\in\mathcal{N}(v)} h_u^{(k-1)}\right). \tag{25}$$

Here, ε is a learnable parameter, which can also be a fixed scalar, and MLP is a multilayer perceptron. To provide a more intuitive comparison, we write out the spatial form of GCN:

$$h_v^{(k)} = \sigma\left(\Theta^{k-1}\cdot \mathrm{Mean}\left(h_v^{(k-1)} + \sum_{u\in\mathcal{N}(v)} h_u^{(k-1)}\right)\right). \tag{26}$$

where σ is the activation function, Φ^{k-1} represents the learnable parameters, and $\mathrm{Mean}(\cdot)$ refers to the mean operation. As seen, GIN removes the $\mathrm{Mean}(\cdot)$ from GCN and replaces it with an MLP. This modification is proven in [50] to be the key for GIN to achieve an expressiveness equivalent to the WL test. Theoretically, $\mathrm{Mean}(\cdot)$ can be considered a special case of MLP, meaning that the spatial form of GCN is a special case of GIN.

Frequency Adaptive Methods

The previous section discussed methods to improve the ability of GCN to distinguish non-isomorphic graphs. Now, we will discuss how to address the over-smoothing issue in GCN. It is important to clarify that, from the spectral perspective, GCN performs low-pass filtering on the graph [51], which explains why deeper GCNs tend to lead to over-smoothing. A natural idea is to enable GCN to aggregate both low-frequency and high-frequency information. In [52], this is achieved by first applying low-pass and high-pass filtering to nodes in the spectral domain and then aggregating the low-frequency and high-frequency information based on coefficients obtained through a self-gating mechanism.

2.4.2.3 Graph Structure Learning

Let us revisit the basic components of a graph: nodes, edges, adjacency matrix, and node/edge attributes (if present). The characteristics of a graph reflected by the adjacency matrix and edges are referred to as the graph structure. In the previous sections, we primarily discussed deep learning methods for nodes, including node-level and graph-level representations, with little exploration of graph structure learning. These methods typically rely on a predefined graph structure, which is suitable in some cases where only node information needs to be considered. However, in other cases, the predefined graph structure may be unreliable [53], potentially containing noisy connections. Graph representations learned from such unreliable structures may be less effective for downstream tasks, affecting model performance. In such situations, graph structure learning becomes particularly important. This can be done by assigning different weights to edges, as in GAT, modifying the adjacency matrix, or even extracting subgraphs (referred to as causal subgraphs, which will be discussed later) from the original graph. We have already discussed GAT in Section 2.4.2.1. Next, we will explore two aspects of graph structure learning: graph augmentation through adjacency matrix modification and causal subgraph discovery. The main content of this section is illustrated in Figure 4.1.

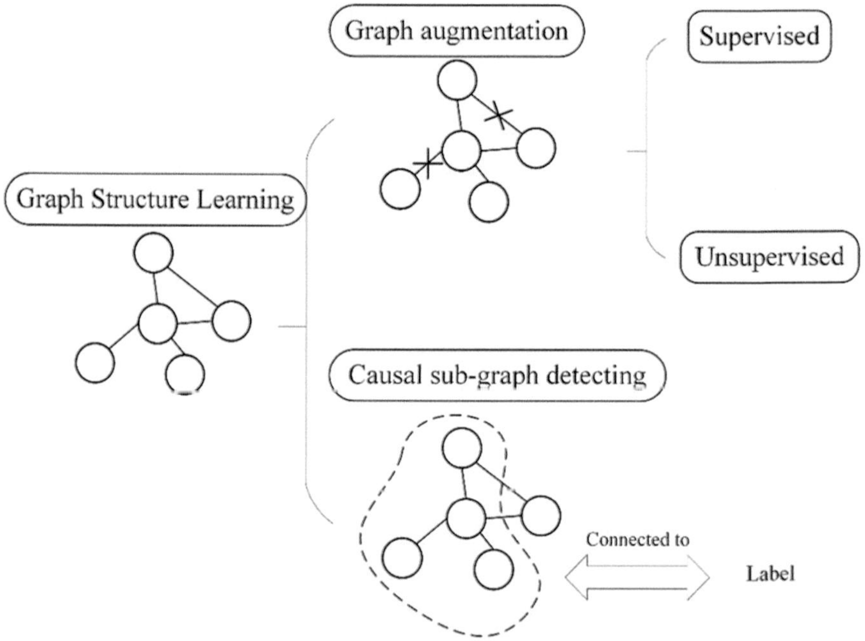

Figure 4.1 Main content of graph structure learning.

Graph Augmentation

Graph augmentation was previously mentioned in Section 2.4.2.2 as a method for generating views. Here, we focus on graph augmentation specifically related to operations on the adjacency matrix, which can also be referred to as edge dropping. It can be divided into supervised and unsupervised categories.

Supervised Methods

Supervised graph augmentation primarily involves adaptive learning of the adjacency matrix based on downstream task labels. For example, in [54], the proposed DGG module adaptively generates the neighborhood size and selects neighboring nodes for each node based on the downstream task. There are also methods based on the information bottleneck principle [55], which maximize the mutual information between the augmented graph and the downstream labels while minimizing the mutual information between the augmented and original graphs. This effectively discards redundant information in the original graph irrelevant to the downstream task, approaching the information bottleneck. The optimization objective is shown in Eqn. 27:

$$\min \mathcal{J}(G_{IB}, G) - \beta \mathcal{I}(G_{IB}, Y),$$

where $\mathcal{J}$ represents mutual information between variables, G_{IB} is the augmented graph, G is the original graph, and Y is the downstream label.

In addition to spatial operations, there are also spectral augmentation methods. For instance, [56] proposed a spectral augmentation method for graph contrastive learning, where for each view, the low-rank approximation of each feature map is estimated and subtracted from the graph to obtain its complement; meanwhile, [35] proposed Spectral Augmentation for Graph Domain Adaptation (SA-GDA), a method for graph node classification with domain adaptation capabilities, enabling knowledge transfer between different graph domains.

Unsupervised Methods

Supervised augmentation methods rely on downstream labels, making it difficult to perform effective graph augmentation in cases of missing or inaccurate labels, potentially even damaging the truly valuable information in the graph. Correspondingly, unsupervised graph augmentation methods are label-independent. The information bottleneck principle mentioned earlier is not limited to maximizing mutual information with downstream labels. For example, DGI [57] maximizes the mutual information between graph-level representations and graphs while treating corrupted graphs as objects for mutual information minimization. A corruption function is used to perform random perturbations, similar to the discriminator principle in GANs [36]. In ADGCL [58], node features are concatenated and fed into an MLP to learn Bernoulli distribution parameters, with each edge being dropped based on its connected nodes. Unlike DGI's discriminator, ADGCL performs mutual information maximization and minimization adversarially.

Causal Sub-Graph Detection

Let us revisit the goal of graph structure learning and discover effective connections within the graph to learn a structure beneficial for downstream tasks. These effective connections refer to the invariant basic information in the graph, which can also be viewed as causal variables [59], as opposed to environmental variables that change depending on the environment (e.g., datasets, application scenarios) or non-causal variables. Therefore, graph structure learning is essentially about exploring these causal variables or causal subgraphs.

Earlier, we discussed graph augmentation methods that focus on the adjacency matrix or spectral domain, but these approaches are believed to be less effective at discovering invariant causal variables [60]. Using causal inference to uncover causal subgraphs is an important approach to graph structure learning. Causal inference typically employs structural causal models (SCM), as seen in [61], which proposes a causal relationship generation model based on SCM to explore causal relationships in dynamic GNNs; at the same time, [62] combines the reasoning capabilities of large language models based on metadata with the data-driven modeling of deep structural causal models (DSCM) to propose a Causal Modeling Agent (CMA) for causal discovery, applying it to gain deeper insights into causal relationships between biomarkers of Alzheimer's disease.

Causal subgraph discovery is sometimes referred to as invariant learning for graphs [60, 63]. Besides removing unreliable connections to learn more effective graph representations, causal subgraph discovery has a specific advantage in dealing with out-of-distribution (OOD) data. Distribution shifts in graph data are common in real-world scenarios, and most existing methods struggle to handle OOD data [63]. According to the theory of invariant learning [59], all graphs contain a certain amount of invariant information, and the graph labels are only related to this invariant information. It is intuitive that if a model is stable across data from multiple environments, it can effectively handle OOD data. Therefore, one can artificially create multiple environments—using causal inference to divide graphs into causal and non-causal subgraphs and then recombine causal and non-causal subgraphs from different graphs. A common method for such recombination is mixup [64].

2.4.3 APPLICATIONS IN BRAIN NETWORK ANALYSIS

The human brain is an exceptionally intricate system comprised of a vast network of interacting neurons, which poses significant challenges for comprehending its structure, function, and dynamics. In this context, network science has emerged as a crucial tool for exploring such interconnected systems, offering a robust framework for integrating data across multiple scales and managing the inherent complexities involved. Recent advancements in brain network analysis techniques have significantly improved the interpretation of functional imaging studies, enabling researchers to visualize and quantify intricate brain connectivity patterns with greater precision [65]. Moreover, the latest developments in contemporary neuroscience not only leverage these advanced network analysis methods but are also deeply connected to the analysis and modeling of complex biological systems, including proteomics and genomics [66, 67]. This interdisciplinary approach enhances our understanding of the brain by integrating diverse biological data. Additionally, the multimodal fusion of various types of neural data presents a unique opportunity to harness complementary information that may be overlooked when examining single modalities. By combining insights from different sources, researchers can gain a more comprehensive understanding of brain function and dysfunction, ultimately paving the way for more effective interventions and therapies.

2.4.3.1 Multi-Modal Brain Network Analysis

Numerous multimodal fusion approaches have emerged in cognitive and clinical studies, reflecting the growing interest in integrating diverse data types. As highlighted by [68], many of these approaches tend to focus on simplistic and linear relationships between modalities. However, research has shown that the interplay between different data types is far more intricate. For instance, while brain structure and function are closely interconnected, neither can fully elucidate the complex organizational principles of the human brain on its own. Previous studies, such as those by Honey [69] and Li [70], indicate that robust structural connectivity is often associated with strong functional connectivity; however, the reverse is not necessarily true. This suggests a nuanced relationship where alterations in brain structure can lead to changes in functional connectivity and vice versa. For example, when a structural connection between two brain regions diminishes, those regions may compensate by increasing neuronal activity, thereby maintaining communication despite the structural deficit. This dynamic interplay underscores the importance of adopting sophisticated multimodal fusion techniques to capture these complex relationships, ultimately enhancing our understanding of brain function and organization. Emerging research on deep neural network-based machine learning methods, as highlighted by Hinton and Salakhutdinov [71], shows promise in capturing the complex, non-linear relationships between brain structure and function through multimodal fusion. The advancements in deep learning have transformed various domains, including artificial intelligence and machine learning, significantly enhancing fields such as computer vision [72, 73] and beyond [74, 75]. Convolutional neural networks (CNNs), one of the most widely used deep learning models [76], have achieved notable success in neuroimaging tasks, including detection [77], reconstruction [78], segmentation [79], and computer-aided diagnosis [80]. However, applying CNNs to brain network analysis presents challenges. CNNs are primarily designed for regular Euclidean data, such as 2D image pixels or 3D voxel grids, whereas the human brain operates as a highly intricate and interconnected network. This network efficiently coordinates regional specialization and segregation [81–83]. Connectivity, which encompasses influences from distant brain areas through structural links or functional interactions, is the physiological basis for information representation and processing within the brain [84–87]. Consequently, traditional CNN approaches often overlook the interrelated and hidden structures, such as modularity [82], that extend beyond regular grid neighbors.

Furthermore, most existing deep neural network methods focus on single-modal data, such as structural, diffusion, or functional MRI. Few studies have explored multimodal data fusion at the network level using deep learning techniques. Although some models have been developed to handle multimodal data, the scope and number of these studies remain limited. Thus, further research is essential to uncover the potential "deep relationships" between brain structure and function and to create disorder-specific deep modeling architectures. For instance, [88] developed a graph-based deep neural network that simultaneously models brain structure and function in individuals with Mild Cognitive Impairment (MCI).

This innovative approach initializes the graph topology using structural networks derived from diffusion MRI and iteratively updates it by integrating functional information from functional MRI. This process enhances the model's ability to distinguish MCI patients from elderly normal controls, resulting in a novel connectome that elucidates the "deep relations" between brain structure and function in MCI patients, a concept referred to as the Deep Brain Connectome.

2.4.3.2 Multi-Modal Imaging Genetic Analysis

Brain imaging genetics presents remarkable opportunities for advancing our understanding of brain function and the underlying mechanisms of brain diseases. A significant breakthrough in this domain is the efficient integration of multimodal data, which provides deeper insights into complex brain functions and pathological processes. Effective multimodal data fusion involves accurately combining information from various sources, including structural and functional brain imaging, genomic data, and environmental factors. This integration relies on advanced multimodal fusion techniques designed to enhance the accuracy and depth of analysis [89]. One of the primary challenges in multimodal data fusion is identifying and integrating features from heterogeneous data modalities, particularly when considering the relationships between edge features and joint representations. Deep learning techniques have emerged as powerful tools in this context due to their exceptional capability for automatic feature extraction and representation learning. These models excel in parsing complex unstructured data and can efficiently handle large datasets through end-to-end training. However, they often require substantial computational resources and time, and their relative lack of interpretability can hinder their practical application in clinical settings.

On the other hand, traditional machine learning methods offer notable advantages regarding computational efficiency and speed of training, especially when working with smaller datasets. These methods typically provide higher levels of model interpretability, making them more accessible for researchers and clinicians. However, they often depend on manual feature engineering, which may limit their efficacy in capturing the complexities inherent in unstructured data and achieving effective multimodal fusion. This limitation can restrict the potential for discovering valuable information and intricate relationships within the data. Therefore, selecting the appropriate fusion method necessitates carefully evaluating the specific objectives of the research, the characteristics of the data involved, and the available computational resources. In studies focused on multimodal data fusion within brain imaging genetics, three key levels of integration are typically employed [90]: data layer fusion, feature layer fusion, and decision layer fusion. Each level plays a crucial role in synthesizing diverse information sources to understand brain function and disease pathology comprehensively.

Data layer fusion is the foundation for multi-modal analysis, aiming to integrate raw data from various imaging modalities and genetic datasets into a cohesive framework. One of the primary advantages of data layer fusion is its straightforwardness; it eliminates the need to make complex design choices regarding extracting marginal representations. Despite this simplicity, data layer fusion strategies can learn cross-modal relationships directly from low-level features. Key efforts in this area focus on data preprocessing, alignment, and standardization, essential for ensuring compatibility and consistency across diverse data sources. For instance, [91] introduced a structured, sparse, low-rank regression model designed to untangle complex relationships between imaging phenotypes and genotypes. This method effectively captures the underlying structural features of the data by employing low-rank decomposition techniques, allowing researchers to discern intricate patterns that might otherwise remain obscured. Additionally, [92] developed a temporal structure learning model to predict disease phenotypes by analyzing longitudinal genotype-phenotype relationships. In part, the success of DL can be attributed to learning well from large data sets even when the number of features is high [72]. However, data sets within the biomedical domain often have small sample sizes, especially compared to their dimensionality.

Nonetheless, one approach to early fusion is to concatenate the input features of different modalities, formally $x_{\text{concat}} = x_1 \parallel x_2 \parallel \cdots \parallel x_m$, where x_i is the input vector of one modality. Another commonly applied approach to learning from x concat is to find a joint latent representation of the lower dimension that contains the necessary information to reconstruct the original input. AEs and variational AEs are architectures that can learn such embeddings z from input x through an encoder function $f(x)$ and a decoder function $g(z)$ in an unsupervised manner. This approach reveals the dynamic interplay between genetic and imaging data over time but also enhances our understanding of how these relationships evolve. While these methodologies provide a robust groundwork for data layer fusion, they have limitations. Specifically, they may struggle to fully capture higher-level abstract patterns and deeper relational insights that are not immediately apparent in the raw data.

Although data layer fusion is ignorant of the modality from which a feature originates, intermediate fusion strategies take advantage of this prior knowledge. Marginal representations of each modality are learned to discover within-modality correlations before using these to either learn joint representations or make predictions directly. Feature layer fusion is mainly concerned with extracting representative features from the fused data and performing feature selection and dimensionality reduction. The key to this layer is how to extract the most valuable information from complex multi-modal data to reveal potential associations between different data modalities. Deep learning techniques perform particularly well in feature layer fusion because they can automatically learn and integrate data features from different modalities by constructing deep network structures. [93] proposed a three-stage deep feature learning framework, which significantly improves the joint representation of multimodal data by learning the potential features of each modality layer by layer and performing inter-modal feature fusion in the middle layer. Meanwhile, [94] designed a feed-forward neural network additive model based on stochastic weights, effectively capturing the nonlinear relationship between neuroimaging data and genetic data, thus providing more accurate phenotype prediction results. These innovative approaches in feature layer fusion fully demonstrate the advantages of deep learning techniques to extract more precise and comprehensive features from complex data.

Decision-level fusion synthesizes the independent analysis results of each modality to achieve more accurate and comprehensive decision-making. This stage integrates the results of each modality's analysis by weighting them to produce a comprehensive output that reflects the unique characteristics of each modality while integrating all of their information. This approach allows the model to extract edge features from each modality as each submodel focuses on modality-specific feature learning. Since the errors of the sub-models are usually independent, this approach effectively exploits the complementary effects of the errors, thus improving the robustness and accuracy of the overall model [95]. Also, [96] proposed a decision layer fusion method based on deep learning, which can dynamically adjust the weight ratio of image and gene features. The method performs brain disease analysis and recognition from multiple perspectives through an adaptive learning mechanism, significantly improving the classification performance and biomarker recognition accuracy in multimodal brain image genetics. In addition, [97] proposed a hybrid machine learning strategy that fuses fMRI and SNP data for classifying schizophrenia patients. They constructed multiple models, including the SNPs-SVME model, Voxel-SVME model, and ICA-SVMC model, and applied the majority voting integrated learning method for final classification. Although the method improved the classification results to a certain extent, the final models still have deficiencies in learning the multimodal effects of data and feature levels and have failed to exploit the complex interactions between modalities fully.

2.4.4 CONCLUSION

This chapter briefly introduces the fundamental concepts of the most popular graph-based deep learning models and discusses their applications in brain networks, including functional and structural brain network analysis and multi-modal brain network integration analysis. It is worth noting that incorporating prior or domain knowledge can effectively enhance the model's performance, such as considering the unique topological characteristics of brain networks. Generally, graph-based deep learning techniques outperform traditional deep learning methods, like brain networks, in handling irregular data. With the advancement of artificial intelligence technology, we can explore adopting next-generation graph-based deep learning methods (such as graph foundation models) for analyzing multi-modal brain networks.

REFERENCES

[1] Kipf, T.N. and Welling, M. 2017. Semi-supervised classification with graph convolutional networks. arXiv preprint arXiv: 1609.02907.

[2] Glover, G.H. 2011. Overview of functional magnetic resonance imaging. Neurosurgery Clinics. 22(2): 133–139.

[3] Erhart, S.M., A.S. Young, S.R. Marder J. and Mintz. 2005. Clinical utility of magnetic resonance imaging radiographs for suspected organic syndromes in adult psychiatry. Journal of Clinical Psychiatry. 66(8): 968–973.

[4] Helms, G. 2016. Segmentation of human brain using structural MRI. Magnetic Resonance Materials in Physics, Biology and Medicine. 29(2): 111–124.

[5] Buckner, R.L., F.M. Krienen and B.T.T. Yeo. 2013. Opportunities and limitations of intrinsic functional connectivity MRI. Nature Neuroscience. 16(7): 832–837.

[6] Wang, H., X. Jin, Y. Zhang and J. Wang. 2016. Single-subject morphological brain networks: connectivity mapping, topological characterization and test–retest reliability. Brain and Behavior. 6(4): e00448.

[7] Sebenius, I., J. Seidlitz, V. Warrier, R.A. Bethlehem, A. Alexander-Bloch, T.T. Mallard, et al. 2023. Robust estimation of cortical similarity networks from brain MRI. Nature Neuroscience. 26(8): 1461–1471.

[8] Olde Dubbelink, K.T., A. Hillebrand, D. Stoffers, J.B. Deijen, J.W. Twisk, C.J. Stam, et al. 2014. Disrupted brain network topology in Parkinson's disease: a longitudinal magnetoencephalography study. Brain. 137(1): 197– 207.

[9] Filippi, M., S. Basaia, E. Sarasso, T. Stojkovic, I. Stankovic, A. Fontana, et al. 2021. Longitudinal brain connectivity changes and clinical evolution in Parkinson's disease. Molecular Psychiatry. 26(9): 5429–5440.

[10] Greicius, M.D., G. Srivastava, A.L. Reiss and V. Menon. 2004. Default-mode network activity distinguishes Alzheimer's disease from healthy aging: Evidence from functional MRI. Proceedings of the National Academy of Sciences. 101(13): 4637–4642.

[11] Pievani, M., N. Filippini, M.P. Van Den Heuvel, S.F. Cappa and G.B. Frisoni. 2014. Brain connectivity in neurodegenerative diseases—from phenotype to proteinopathy. Nature Reviews Neurology. 10(11): 620–633.

[12] Wu, J.W., S.A. Hussaini, I.M. Bastille, G.A. Rodriguez, A. Mrejeru, K. Rilett, et al. 2016. Neuronal activity enhances tau propagation and tau pathology in vivo. Nature Neuroscience. 19(8): 1085–1092.

[13] Sepulcre, J., M.J. Grothe, F. d'Oleire Uquillas, L. Ortiz-Terán, I. Diez, H.S. Yang, et al. 2018. Neurogenetic contributions to amyloid beta and tau spreading in the human cortex. Nature Medicine. 24(12): 1910–1918.

[14] Otte, C., S.M. Gold, B.W. Penninx, C.M. Pariante, A. Etkin, M. Fava, et al. 2016. Major depressive disorder. Nature Reviews Disease Primers. 2(1): 1–20.

[15] Yan, C.G., X. Chen, L. Li, F.X. Castellanos, T.J. Bai, Q.J. Bo, et al. 2019. Reduced default mode network functional connectivity in patients with recurrent major depressive disorder. Proceedings of the National Academy of Sciences. 116(18): 9078–9083.

[16] Rubinov, M. and E. Bullmore. 2013. Schizophrenia and abnormal brain network hubs. Dialogues in Clinical Neuroscience. 15(3): 339–349.

[17] Van Den Heuvel, M.P. and A. Fornito. 2014. Brain networks in schizophrenia. Neuropsychology Review. 24: 32–48.

[18] Li, X., L. Sun, M. Ling and Y. Peng. 2023. A survey of graph neural network based recommendation in social networks. Neurocomputing. 549: 126441.

[19] Gao, Z., C. Jiang, J. Zhang, X. Jiang, L. Li, P. Zhao, et al. 2023. Hierarchical graph learning for protein–protein interaction. Nature Communications. 14(1): 1093.

[20] Bessadok, A., M.A. Mahjoub and I. Rekik, I.. 2022. Graph neural networks in network neuroscience. *In*: IEEE Transactions on Pattern Analysis and Machine Intelligence. 45(5): 5833–5848.

[21] Yang, D., J. Chen, C. Yan, M. Kim, P.J. Laurienti, M. Styner, et al. 2021. Group-wise hub identification by learning common graph embeddings on Grassmannian manifold. *In*: IEEE Transactions on Pattern Analysis and Machine Intelligence. 44(11): 8249–8260.

[22] Yang, D., X. Zhu, C. Yan, Z. Peng, M. Bagonis, P.J. Laurienti, et al. 2021. Joint hub identification for brain networks by multivariate graph inference. Medical Image Analysis. 73: 102162.

[23] Gu, Y., S. Peng, Y. Li, L. Gao and Y. Dong. 2025. FC-HGNN: A heterogeneous graph neural network based on brain functional connectivity for mental disorder identification. Information Fusion. 113: 102619.

[24] Li, Y., X. Zhang, J. Nie, G. Zhang, R. Fang, X. Xu, et al. 2022. Brain connectivity based graph convolutional networks and its application to infant age prediction. *In*: IEEE Transactions on Medical Imaging. 41(10): 2764–2776.

[25] Chen, J., G. Han, H. Cai, D. Yang, P.J. Laurienti, M. Styner, et al. 2020. Learning common harmonic waves on Stiefel manifold–A new mathematical approach for brain network analyses. *In*: IEEE Transactions on Medical Imaging. 40(1): 419–430.

[26] Cai, H., R. Deng, D. Yang, F. Zhang, G. Wu and J. Chen. 2024. Harmonic Wavelet Neural Network for Discovering Neuropathological Propagation Patterns in Alzheimer's Disease. IEEE Journal of Biomedical and Health Informatics. 29(1): 608–619.

[27] Shuman, D.I., S.K. Narang, P. Frossard, A. Ortega and P. Vandergheynst. 2013. The emerging field of signal processing on graphs: Extending high-dimensional data analysis to networks and other irregular domains. *In*: IEEE Signal Processing Magazine. 30(3). Cited by: 3094; All Open Access, Green Open Access. 83–98. doi: 10.1109/MSP.2012.2235192. url: https://www.scopus.com/inward/record.uri?eid=2-s2.0-85032751310&doi=10.1109%2fMSP.2012. 2235192&partnerID=40&md5=b16 4ded04be86734baf9b60035e842b6.

[28] Hammond, D.K., P. Vandergheynst and R. Gribonval. 2011. Wavelets on graphs via spectral graph theory. *In*: Applied and Computational Harmonic Analysis 30(2). Cited by: 1583; All Open Access, Green Open Access, pp. 129–150. doi: 10.1016/j.acha.2010.04.005. url: https://www.scopus.com/inward/record.uri?eid=2-s2.0-78751582295&doi=10.1016%2fj.acha.2010.04.005&partnerID=40&md5=23ab 681c616a91db3f1dae27d66605b2.

[29] Hamilton, W.L., R. Ying and J. Leskovec. 2018. Inductive Representation Learning on Large Graphs. arXiv:1706.02216 [cs, stat]. Sept. 2018. url: http://arxiv.org/abs/1706.02216 (visited on 06/17/2024).

[30] Veličković, P., G. Cucurull, A. Casanova, A. Romero, P. Lio and Y. Bengio. 2018. Graph Attention Networks. arXiv:1710.10903 [cs, stat]. Feb. 2018. url: http://arxiv.org/abs/1710.10903 (visited on 06/17/2024).

[31] Wang, X., H. Ji, C. Shi, B. Wang, Y. Ye, P. Cui, et al. 2021. Heterogeneous Graph Attention Network. arXiv:1903.07293 [cs]. url: http://arxiv.org/abs/1903.07293 (visited on 06/18/2024).

[32] Yun, S., M. Jeong, R. Kim, J. Kang and H.J. Kim. 2019. Graph Transformer Networks [J]. Advances in neural information processing systems. 32.

[33] Jeong, C., S. Jang, E. Park and S. Choi. 2019. A context-aware citation recommendation model with BERT and graph convolutional networks. Scientometrics. 124: 1907–1922. url: https://api.semanticscholar.org/CorpusID:80628443.

[34] Wang, C., S. Pan, G. Long, X. Zhu and J. Jiang. 2017. MGAE: Marginalized graph autoencoder for graph clustering. *In*: Proceedings of the 2017 ACM on Conference on Information and Knowledge Management. CIKM'17. Singapore, Singapore: Association for Computing Machinery. 889–898. isbn: 9781450349185. doi: 10.1145/3132847 .3132967. url: https://doi.org/10.1145/3132847.3132967.

[35] Pang, J., Z. Wang, J. Tang, M. Xiao and N. Yin. 2023. SA-GDA: Spectral augmentation for graph domain adaptation. *In*: Proceedings of the 31st ACM International Conference on Multimedia. MM'23. Ottawa ON, Canada: Association for Computing Machinery. 309–318. isbn: 9798400701085. doi: 10.1145/3581783.3612264. url: https://doi.org/10.1145/3581783.3612264.

[36] Goodfellow, I.J., J. Pouget-Abadie, M. Mirza, B. Xu, D. Warde-Farley, S. Ozair, et al. 2014. Generative Adversarial Nets. Neural Information Processing Systems. url: https://api.semanticscholar.org/CorpusID:261560300.

[37] Xie, Y., Z. Xu, J. Zhang, Z. Wang and S. Ji. 2023. Self-supervised learning of graph neural networks: A unified review. *In*: IEEE Transactions on Pattern Analysis and Machine Intelligence. 45(2): 2412–2429. doi: 10.1109/TPAMI.2022. 3170559.

[38] You, Y., T. Chen, Y. Sui, T. Chen, Z. Wang and Y. Shen 2020. Graph Contrastive Learning with Augmentations. ArXiv abs/2010.13902. url: https://api.semanticscho lar.org/CorpusID: 225076220.

[39] Hinton, G.E., N. Srivastava, A. Krizhevsky, I. Sutskever and R.R. Salakhutdinov. 2012. Improving neural networks by preventing co-adaptation of feature detectors. ArXiv abs/1207.0580. url: https://api.semanticscholar.org/CorpusID:14832074.

[40] Gong, X., C. Yang and C. Shi. 2023. MA-GCL: Model Augmentation Tricks for Graph Contrastive Learning. en. *In*: Proceedings of the AAAI Conference on Artificial Intelligenc.e 37(4): 4284–4292. issn: 2374-3468, 2159-5399. doi: 10.1609/aaai. v37i4.25547. url: https://ojs.aaai.org/index.php/AAAI/article/view/25547 (visited on 02/20/2024).

[41] Shen, X., D. Sun, S. Pan, X. Zhou and L.T. Yang. 2023. Neighbor Contrastive learning on learnable graph augmentation. *In*: Proceedings of the AAAI Conference on Artificial Intelligence. 37(8): 9782–9791. ISSN: 2374-3468, 2159-5399. doi: 10.1609/aaai.v37i8.26168. url: https://ojs.aaai.org/index.php/AAAI/article/ view/26168 (visited on 02/20/2024).

[42] Xu, J., S. Chen, Y. Ren, X. Shi, H. Shen, G. Niu, et al. 2023. Self-weighted contrastive learning among multiple views for mitigating representation degeneration. *In*: Thirty-seventh Conference on Neural Information Processing Systems. url: https:// openreview.net/forum?id=X8dbFcAox2.

[43] Qian, S., D. Xue, Q. Fang and C. Xu. 2022. Integrating multi-label contrastive learning with dual adversarial graph neural networks for cross-modal retrieval. *In*: IEEE Transactions on Pattern Analysis and Machine Intelligence. 1–18. ISSN: 0162- 8828, 2160-9292, 1939-3539. doi: 10.1109/TPAMI.2022.3188547. url: https:// ieeexplore.ieee.org/document/9815553/ (visited on 03/01/2024).

[44] Oord, A., Y. Li and O. Vinyals. 2018. Representation Learning with Contrastive Predictive Coding. ArXiv abs/1807.03748. url: https://api.semanticscholar.org/ CorpusID:49670925.

[45] Rusch, T.K., M.M. Bronstein and S. Mishra. 2023. A Survey on Oversmoothing in Graph Neural Networks. ArXiv abs/2303.10993. url: https://api.semanticscholar.org/CorpusID:257632346.

[46] Maron, H., H. Ben-Hamu, H. Serviansky and Y. Lipman. 2019. Provably Powerful Graph Networks. ArXiv abs/1905. 11136. url: https://api.semanticscholar.org/CorpusID:166228757.

[47] Abu-El-Haija, S., B. Perozzi, A. Kapoor, N. Alipourfard, K. Lerman, H. Harutyunyan, et al. 2019. MixHop: Higher-order graph convolutional architectures via sparsified neighborhood mixing. International Conference on Machine Learning. url: https://api.semanticscholar.org/CorpusID:141460877.

[48] Feng, J., Y. Chen, F. Li, A. Sarkar and M. Zhang. 2022. How powerful are K-hop message passing graph neural networks. ArXiv abs/2205.13328. url: https://api.semanticscholar.org/CorpusID: 249097935.

[49] Ding, K., Y. Wang, Y. Yang and H. Liu. 2023. Eliciting structural and semantic global knowledge in unsuper vised graph contrastive learning. *In*: Proceedings of the AAAI Conference on Artificial Intelligence. 37(6): 7378–7386. ISSN: 2374-3468, 2159-5399. doi: 10.1609/aaai.v37i6.25898. url: https://ojs.aaai.org/index.php/AAAI/article/view/25898 (visited on 02/20/2024).

[50] Xu, K., W. Hu, J. Leskovec and S. Jegelka. 2018. How powerful are graph neural networks? ArXiv abs/1810.00826. url: https://api.semanticscholar.org/CorpusID:52895589.

[51] Wu, F., A. Souza, T. Zhang, C. Fifty, T. Yu and K. Weinberger. 2019. Simplifying graph convolutional networks. International Conference on Machine Learning. url: https://api.semanticscholar.org/Corpus ID:67752026.

[52] Bo, D., X. Wang, C. Shi and H. Shen. 2021. Beyond low-frequency information in graph convolutional networks. *In*: Proceedings of the AAAI Conference on Artificial Intelligence. 35(5): 3950–3957. issn: 2374-3468, 2159-5399. doi: 10.1609/aaai.v35i5.16514. url: https://ojs.aaai.org/index.php/AAAI/article/view/16514 (visited on 02/20/2024).

[53] Drton, M. and M.H. Maathuis. 2019. Structure learning in graphical modeling. arXiv: Methodology. url: https://api.semanticscholar.org/CorpusID:6395 6329.

[54] Saha, A., O. Mendez, C. Russell and R. Bowden. 2023. Learning adaptive neighborhoods for graph neural networks. *In*: 2023 IEEE/CVF International Conference on Computer Vision (ICCV). Paris, France: IEEE. 22484–22493. isbn: 9798350307184. doi: 10.1109ICCV51070.2023. 02060. url: https://ieeexplore.ieee.org/document/10376873/(visited on 03/01/2024).

[55] Sun, Q., J. Li, H. Peng, J. Wu, X. Fu, C. Ji, et al. 2022. Graph structure learning with variational information bottleneck. *In*: Proceedings of the AAAI Conference on Artificial Intelligence. 36(4): 4165–4174. ISSN: 2374-3468, 2159-5399. doi: 10.1609/aaai.v36i4.20335. url: https://ojs.aaai.org/index.php/AAAI/article/view/20335 (visited on 02/20/2024).

[56] Zhang, Y., H. Zhu, Z. Song, P. Koniusz and I. King. 2023. Spectral feature augmentation for graph contrastive learning and beyond. *In*: Proceedings of the AAAI Conference on Artificial Intelligence. 37(9): 11289–11297. doi: 10.1609/aaai.v37i9.26336. url: https://ojs.aaai.org/index.php/AAAI/article/view/26336.

[57] Veličković, P., W. Fedus, W.L. Hamilton, P. Liò, Y. Bengio and R.D. Hjelm. 2018. Deep graph infomax. ArXiv abs/1809.10341. url: https://api.semanticscholar.org/CorpusID:52877454.

[58] Suresh, S., P. Li, C. Hao and J. Neville. 2021. Adversarial graph augmentation to improve graph contrastive learning. Advances in Neural Information Processing Systems. 34: 15920–15933.

[59] Arjovsky, M., L. Bottou, I. Gulrajani and D. Lopez-Paz. 2019. Invariant risk minimization. ArXiv abs/1907.02893. url: https://api.semanticscholar.org/CorpusID:195820364.

[60] Mo, Y., X. Wang, S. Fan and C. Shi. 2024. Graph contrastive invariant learning from the causal perspective. arXiv:2401.12564 [cs]. url: http://arxiv.org/abs/2401.12564 (visited on 03/06/2024).

[61] Zhao, K. and L. Zhang. 2024. Causality-inspired spatial-temporal explanations for dynamic graph neural networks. *In*: The Twelfth International Conference on Learning Representations. url: https://openreview.net/forum?id=AJBkfwXh3u.

[62] Abdulaal, A., A. Hadjivasiliou, N. Montana-Brown, T. He, A. Ijishakin, I. Drobnjak, et al. 2024. Causal modelling agents: Causal graph discovery through synergising metadata- and data-driven reasoning. *In*: The Twelfth International Conference on Learning Representations. url: https://openreview.net/ forum?id=pAoqRlTBtY.

[63] Chen, Y., Y. Zhang, Y. Bian, H. Yang, M.A. Kaili, B. Xie, et al. 2022. Learning causally invariant representations for out-of-distribution generalization on graphs. *In*: Neural Information Processing Systems. url: https://api.semanticscholar.org/CorpusID:252815553.

[64] Zhang, H., M. Cisse, Y.N. Dauphin and D. Lopez-Paz. 2018. Mixup: Beyond empirical risk minimization.arXiv:1710.09412 [cs, stat]. url: http://arxiv.org/abs/1710.09412 (visited on 04/13/ 2024).

[65] Barabási, D.L., G. Bianconi, E. Bullmore, M. Burgess, S. Chung, T. Eliassi-Rad, et al. 2023. Neuroscience needs network science. Journal of Neuroscience. 43(34): 5989–5995.

[66] Watson, J.D. 1990. The human genome project: past, present, and future. Science. 248(4951): 44–49.

[67] Collins, F.S., M. Morgan and A. Patrinos. 2003. The human genome project: Lessons from large-scale biology. Science. 300(5617): 286–290.

[68] Plis, S.M., M.F. Amin, A. Chekroud, D. Hjelm, E. Damaraju, H.J. Lee, et al. 2018. Reading the (functional) writing on the (structural) wall: Multi-modal fusion of brain structure and function via a deep neural network based translation approach reveals novel impairments in schizophrenia. NeuroImage. 181: 734–747.

[69] Honey, C.J., O. Sporns, L. Cammoun, X. Gigandet, J.P. Thiran, R. Meuli, et al. 2009. Predicting human resting-state functional connectivity from structural connectivity. Proceedings of the National Academy of Sciences. 106(6): 2035–2040.

[70] Li, K., L. Guo, C. Faraco, D. Zhu, F. Deng, T. Zhang, et al. 2012. Individual functional ROI optimization via maximization of group-wise consistency of structural and functional profiles. Neuroinformatics. 10: 225–242.

[71] Hinton, G.E. and R.R. Salakhutdinov. 2006. Reducing the dimensionality of data with neural networks. Science. 313(5786): 504–507.

[72] LeCun, Y., Y. Bengio and G. Hinton. 2015. Deep learning. Nature. 521(7553): 436–444.

[73] He, K., X. Zhang, S. Ren and J. Sun. 2016. Deep residual learning for image recognition. *In*: Proceedings of the IEEE Conference on Computer Vision and Pattern Recognition. 770–778.

[74] Monti, F., M. Bronstein and X. Bresson. 2017. Geometric matrix completion with recurrent multi-graph neural networks. Advances in Neural Information Processing Systems. 30.

[75] Ying, R., R. He, K. Chen, P. Eksombatchai, W.L. Hamilton and J. Leskovec. 2018. Graph convolutional neural networks for web-scale recommender systems. *In*: Proceedings of the 24th ACM SIGKDD International Conference on Knowledge Discovery and Data Mining. 974–983.

[76] LeCun, Y., B. Boser, J. Denker, D. Henderson, R. Howard, W. Hubbard, et al. 1989. Handwritten digit recognition with a back-propagation network. Advances in Neural Information Processing Systems. 2.

[77] Sirinukunwattana, K., S.E.A. Raza, Y.W. Tsang, D.R. Snead, I.A. Cree and N.M. Rajpoot. 2016. Locality sensitive deep learning for detection and classification of nuclei in routine colon cancer histology images. IEEE Transactions on Medical Imaging. 35(5): 1196–1206.

[78] Sun, L., Z. Fan, X. Ding, Y. Huang and J. Paisley. 2019. Region-of-interest undersampled MRI reconstruction: A deep convolutional neural network approach. Magnetic Resonance Imaging. 63: 185– 192.

[79] Wang, L., Y. Gao, F. Shi, G. Li, J.H. Gilmore, W. Lin, et al. 2015. LINKS: Learning-based multi-source Integration framework for segmentation of infant brain images. NeuroImage. 108: 160–172.

[80] Roth, H.R., L. Lu, J. Liu, J. Yao, A. Seff, K. Cherry, et al. 2015. Improving computer -aided detection using convolutional neural networks and random view aggregation. IEEE Transactions on Medical Imaging. 35(5): 1170–1181.

[81] Tononi, G., O. Sporns and G.M. Edelman. 1994. A measure for brain complexity: Relating functional segregation and integration in the nervous system. Proceedings of the National Academy of Sciences. 91(11): 5033–5037.

[82] Bullmore, E. and O. Sporns. 2009. Complex brain networks: Graph theoretical analysis of structural and functional systems. Nature Reviews Neuroscience. 10(3): 186–198.

[83] Fornito, A., A. Zalesky and M. Breakspear. 2015. The connectomics of brain disorders. Nature Reviews Neuroscience. 16(3): 159–172.

[84] Sporns, O., D.R. Chialvo, M. Kaiser and C.C. Hilgetag. 2004. Organization, development and function of complex brain networks. Trends in Cognitive Sciences. 8(9): 418–425.

[85] Fries, P. 2005. A mechanism for cognitive dynamics: neuronal communication through neuronal coherence. Trends in Cognitive Sciences. 9(10): 474–480.

[86] Petersen, S.E. and O. Sporns. 2015. Brain networks and cognitive architectures. Neuron. 88(1): 207–219.

[87] Lynn, C.W. and D.S. Bassett. 2019. The physics of brain network structure, function and control. Nature Reviews Physics. 1(5): 318–332.

[88] Zhang, L., L. Wang, J. Gao, S.L. Risacher, J. Yan, G. Li, et al. 2021. Deep fusion of brain structure-function in mild cognitive impairment. Medical Image Analysis. 72: 102082.

[89] Sui, J., S. Qi, T.G. van Erp, J. Bustillo, R. Jiang, D. Lin, et al. 2018. Multimodal neuromarkers in schizophrenia via cognition-guided MRI fusion. Nature Communications. 9(1): 3028.

[90] Venugopalan, J., L. Tong, H.R. Hassanzadeh and M.D. Wang. 2021. Multimodal deep learning models for early detection of Alzheimer's disease stage. Scientific Reports. 11(1): 3254.

[91] Zhu, X., H.I. Suk, H. Huang and D. Shen. 2016. Structured sparse low-rank regression model for brain-wide and genome-wide associations. *In*: Medical Image Computing and Computer-Assisted Intervention–MICCAI 2016: 19th International Conference, Athens, Greece. Proceedings, Part I 19. Springer. 344–352.

[92] Wang, X., J. Yan, X. Yao, S. Kim, K. Nho, S.L. Risacher, et al. 2017. Longitudinal genotype-phenotype association study via temporal structure auto-learning predictive model. *In*: Research in Computational Molecular Biology: 21st Annual International Conference, RECOMB 2017, Hong Kong, China. Proceedings 21. Springer. 287–302.

[93] Zhou, T., K.H. Thung, X. Zhu and D. Shen. 2019. Effective feature learning and fusion of multimodality data using stage-wise deep neural network for dementia diagnosis. Human brain mapping 40(3): 1001–1016.

[94] Wang, X., H. Chen, J. Yan, K. Nho, S.L. Risacher, A.J. Saykin, et al. 2018. Quantitative trait loci identification for brain endophenotypes via new additive model with random networks. Bioinformatics. 34(17): i866–i874.

[95] Ramachandram, D. and G.W. Taylor. 2017. Deep multimodal learning: A survey on recent advances and trends. IEEE Signal Processing Magazine. 34(6): 96–108.

[96] Lyu, Y., X. Yu, L. Zhang and D. Zhu. 2021. Classification of mild cognitive impairment by fusing neuroimaging and gene expression data: Classification of mild cognitive impairment by fusing neuroimaging and gene expression data. *In*: Proceedings of the 14th Pervasive Technologies Related to Assistive Environments Conference. 26–32.

[97] Yang, H., J. Liu, J. Sui, G. Pearlson and V.D. Calhoun. 2010. A hybrid machine learning method for fusing fMRI and genetic data: Combining both improves classification of schizophrenia. Frontiers in Human Neuroscience. 4: 192.

Chapter 2.5

AI in Stroke Segmentation Study

Liangliang Liu*
College of Information and Management Science,
Henan Agricultural University, Zhengzhou, Henan 450046, China

2.5.1 INTRODUCTIONS

Stroke is a medical condition characterized by the sudden loss of blood circulation to an area of the brain, resulting in a corresponding loss of neurologic function. Stroke is currently the second leading cause of death and the third leading cause of disability worldwide [1]. As per the World Stroke Organization, around 15 million people suffer from stroke annually; out of these 15 million, about 43% lose their lives, and of the survivors, roughly two-thirds have some disability [2]. Stroke is mainly caused by two types: ischemic and hemorrhagic. Ischemic stroke is the most common type of stroke, accounting for approximately 87% of all stroke cases. Stroke patients typically undergo neuroimaging techniques to distinguish between ischemic and hemorrhagic strokes. This differentiation can be achieved through magnetic resonance imaging (MRI) and computed tomography (CT), each offering distinctive insight into the condition of the brain [3]. MRI offers excellent soft tissue contrast for the brain, and when diagnosis is uncertain, it can be more informative than CT [4–6], providing information on stroke location [7], timing [8], and mechanism [9]. Diffusion-weighted imaging (DWI) and perfusion-weighted imaging (PWI) within the MRI protocol offer valuable information on the extent and impact of stroke on brain tissue [10].

*For Correspondence: liangliu@henau.edu.cn

DOI: 10.1201/9781003518754-10

Stroke segmentation holds significant importance in the diagnosis and management of stroke disease by enabling precise delineation of ischemic or hemorrhagic lesions in the brain, which is crucial for accurate diagnosis and clinical decision-making. By providing exact boundaries of stroke lesions, stroke segmentation allows for the precise localization and quantification of these lesions, leading to better-informed treatment plans tailored to the individual needs of patients. This precision is essential for planning interventions such as thrombolysis, thrombectomy, or surgical procedures, thereby improving outcomes and reducing risks associated with these treatments.

In summary, stroke segmentation is vital in diagnosing and managing stroke disease by providing accurate and reproducible delineation of lesions, enhancing treatment planning, monitoring disease progression, and supporting research and clinical trials. Its significance extends to improving patient outcomes, reducing diagnosis variability, and facilitating advancements in stroke care through better data integration and analysis. As AI and imaging technologies continue to evolve, the precision and utility of stroke segmentation are expected to enhance the effectiveness of stroke diagnosis and treatment further, ultimately leading to more effective and reliable diagnostic tools that can significantly improve patient care.

2.5.2 RESULTS

The study utilized the Google Scholar search engine; 253 articles in the field of stroke seg- mentation were retrieved with the search string ("stroke" and "Segmentation") as of July 30, 2024. These articles covered core topics such as stroke segmentation and the application of segmentation in diagnosing stroke diseases. Through quantitative analysis, the research revealed patterns of interrelations among authors, journals, institutions, and countries. By mining the core ideas of clustered authors, the study explored the current status, perspectives, and future directions of this interdisciplinary field. This study analyzed the development trend, method types, relevant data sets, and existing challenges of stroke segmentation research, aiming to explore the topic's evolution and future research direction.

2.5.2.1 Research Development Trends

In the last decade, machine and deep learning development has grown exponentially. The field of artificial intelligence in ischemic stroke segmentation research is rapidly evolving, with significant advancements in both traditional and AI-based techniques. The integration of AI in medical imaging offers the potential to enhance diagnostic accuracy, streamline workflows, and ultimately improve patient outcomes. Despite challenges in data quality, model interpretability, and clinical integration, the future of AI in stroke care looks promising, driven by continuous technological innovations and collaborative efforts. Deep learning methods are used for automated stroke classification and rehabilitation prediction [11]. However, at the heart of these processes is lesion segmentation, a term used to define the process of tracing lesion outlines by categorizing each voxel as a lesion or non-lesion in a medical image [12]. Segmented lesions can allow the model to learn the anatomical features and their impact on the prediction. The gold standard for lesion segmentation is manual segmentation [13]. Computer-aided diagnostics tools and techniques, such as 3D Slicer [14], ITK-SNAP [15], Amira [16], and MIPAV [17], are some of the open-source and commercially available tools that are helpful for lesion segmentation, analysis, and visualization. However, some human intervention and verification are still required. It is also time-consuming and laborious to segment the lesions layer by layer [18], and the chances of error and bias are also high as lesions could be of irregular size and shape in each layer [19], which necessitates the development of automated techniques.

Traditional stroke segmentation methods—including thresholding, region growing, and atlas-based approaches—have been fundamental in medical image analysis for stroke diagnosis. Thresholding classifies pixels based on intensity values, but its manual threshold setting leads to inconsistencies and inaccuracies. Region growing expands from an initial seed point based on intensity similarity, but the manual seed placement and sensitivity to image noise limit its effectiveness. Atlas-based methods utilize anatomical templates to guide segmentation but struggle with inter-patient variability and computational intensity. Despite their foundational role, these methods often require manual intervention and are sensitive to image quality, limiting their generalizability. Deep learning has significantly advanced stroke segmentation by leveraging convolutional neural networks (CNNs) and their variants, such as U-Net and its derivatives, to achieve high accuracy and robustness in delineating stroke lesions from imaging data. Techniques like Generative Adversarial Networks (GANs) have been used to generate realistic segmentations, while Recurrent Neural Networks (RNNs) and Long Short-Term Memory (LSTM) networks model the temporal evolution of lesions. Hybrid models combining CNNs with traditional methods and transfer learning approaches have enhanced performance by utilizing pre-trained networks and anatomical knowledge. Despite these advancements, challenges remain, including the need for large annotated datasets, high computational demands, and model interpretability issues.

2.5.2.2 Summary of Supervised Learning-based Stroke Segmentation Methods

Supervised learning-based stroke segmentation methods leverage neural networks to accurately identify stroke lesions from medical images. Convolutional Neural Networks (CNNs), such as U-Net and its variants (3D U-Net, Attention U-Net, and Residual U-Net), are widely used due to their encoder-decoder structures that enable precise localization and feature extraction. Specialized networks like DeepMedic and V-Net process multi-scale inputs and volumetric data, respectively, to capture local and global contexts. Hybrid models like SegNet improve spatial localization using max-pooling indices, while attention mechanisms enhance focus on relevant regions. Multi-modal networks process different imaging modalities through separate pathways, combining their features to improve segmentation accuracy. The training process for these models involves data augmentation, using various loss functions to handle class imbalance, and optimization algorithms like Adam or SGD. Evaluation metrics such as the Dice Similarity Coefficient (DSC), Hausdorff Distance (HD), sensitivity, and specificity assess model performance. These methods are crucial for early diagnosis, treatment planning, and monitoring of disease progression. CNNs are central to supervised learning approaches for stroke segmentation. They consist of multiple layers that extract features from the input images, enabling precise segmentation. The most prominent CNN architecture used is the U-Net, which features an encoder-decoder structure with skip connections to combine high-level and low-level features for accurate segmentation. The typical architectures of the stroke segmentation method are as follows.

U-Net and Its Variants

U-Net: Originally designed for biomedical image segmentation, U-Net consists of a contracting path to capture context and a symmetric expanding path that enables precise localization. This model has been widely used for stroke lesion segmentation due to its robustness and accuracy.

3D U-Net: This variant extends the U-Net architecture to three dimensions, making it suitable for volumetric data such as MRI scans. Processing 3D data captures spatial context more effectively, improving segmentation performance on stroke lesions.

Attention U-Net: Incorporates attention mechanisms to focus on relevant regions in the image. This helps the model ignore irrelevant background noise and enhance the accuracy of lesion segmentation.

Residual Networks (ResNets)

ResNet: Uses residual blocks with shortcut connections to train deep networks efficiently. These connections help mitigate the vanishing gradient problem, enabling the model to learn more complex features and improve segmentation accuracy.

ResUNet: Combines the U-Net architecture with residual blocks to leverage the strengths of both models, resulting in improved segmentation performance for stroke lesions.

Hybrid Models

CNN+ Conditional Random Fields (CRFs): Integrates CNNs with CRFs to refine segmentation boundaries by modeling spatial dependencies. This combination enhances the accuracy of delineating stroke lesions, particularly at the edges.

Atlas-based CNNs: Utilizes anatomical templates (atlases) alongside CNNs to guide the segmentation process. This approach leverages prior anatomical knowledge to improve segmentation accuracy and robustness.

Transfer Learning

Pre-Trained CNNs: Models pre-trained on large, publicly available datasets (such as ImageNet) are fine-tuned on stroke-specific datasets. Transfer learning leverages pre-learned features, significantly improving performance even with limited labeled data.

Challenges and Future Directions

Despite their success, supervised learning-based methods face several challenges, including the need for large annotated datasets, high computational costs, and the potential for overfitting. Variability in imaging protocols and patient populations can also affect model generalizability. Future research aims to develop more efficient architectures, enhance data augmentation techniques, and explore semi-supervised and unsupervised learning methods to leverage unlabeled data. Additionally, improving the interpretability of deep learning models is crucial for gaining clinical trust and integrating these technologies into routine clinical practice.

2.5.2.3 Unsupervised Learning-based Methods

Unsupervised learning-based stroke segmentation methods utilize algorithms that do not require labeled training data, relying instead on inherent data structures and characteristics. Key methods include clustering techniques like K-Means and Mean Shift, which group pixels based on intensity values; Gaussian Mixture Models (GMM) using Expectation-Maximization (EM) to model image data with multiple Gaussian distributions; and graph-based methods such as Normalized Cuts and Graph Cuts that partition images based on similarity and dissimilarity. Statistical approaches, including Histogram-Based Thresholding and texture analysis using Gabor Filters and Local Binary Patterns (LBP), are employed to segment regions based on intensity and texture differences. Dimensionality reduction methods like Principal Component Analysis (PCA) and region-growing techniques expand regions from seed points based on pixel similarity. Self-organizing maps (SOM) also cluster pixels into distinct regions using unsupervised learning, providing a diverse set of tools for effective stroke segmentation when labeled data is unavailable. The typical architectures are as follows.

Clustering-based Methods

K-Means Clustering: This method partitions the imaging data into K clusters based on the similarity of pixel intensities. The cluster centers can be identified by analyzing regions corresponding to stroke lesions. Although simple, K-Means can effectively segment stroke lesions when the lesion intensity differs significantly from surrounding tissues.

Gaussian Mixture Models (GMM): GMM assumes that the data is generated from a mixture of several Gaussian distributions. By fitting a GMM to the pixel intensity distribution, the method can probabilistically assign each pixel to a cluster, aiding in the segmentation of stroke lesions.

Autoencoders

Variational Autoencoders (VAEs): VAEs are a type of autoencoder that learns a probabilistic latent space representation of the input data. By reconstructing the input images, VAEs can highlight regions with anomalies, such as stroke lesions. This method is particularly useful for identifying subtle differences between normal and abnormal tissue.
Sparse Autoencoders: These models enforce sparsity in the hidden layers, encouraging the network to learn a compressed representation of the input data. Sparse autoencoders can effectively capture the underlying structure of brain images, aiding in identifying stroke lesions without the need for labeled data.

Generative Models

Generative Adversarial Networks (GANs): GANs consist of a generator and a discriminator that are trained adversarially. The generator creates synthetic images that resemble the input data, while the discriminator distinguishes between real and generated images. By analyzing the discrepancies, GANs can identify and segment stroke lesions. CycleGANs, a variant of GANs, can transform images from one domain (e.g., healthy brain) to another (e.g., stroke-affected brain), facilitating unsupervised lesion segmentation.

Deep Convolutional GANs (DCGANs): These models use deep convolutional layers to improve the quality and realism of generated images. DCGANs can be trained to generate healthy brain images from stroke-affected images, with the difference highlighting the lesions.

Self-Supervised Learning

Contrastive Learning: This approach trains the model to distinguish between similar and dissimilar image patches. By maximizing the similarity of patches from the same region and minimizing the similarity of patches from different regions, the model learns to identify and segment stroke lesions. Methods like SimCLR and MoCo have been adapted for medical image segmentation tasks, showing promising results in stroke lesion detection.

Challenges and Future Directions

Unsupervised learning-based methods face several challenges, including the difficulty of evaluating segmentation accuracy without labeled data and the potential for poor performance in the presence of noise and artifacts. Additionally, these methods may struggle to capture the complex variability in lesion appearance across different patients and imaging modalities. Unsupervised learning-based stroke segmentation methods offer a promising avenue for identifying stroke lesions without requiring extensive labeled datasets. By leveraging clustering, autoencoders, generative models, and self-supervised learning, these approaches can uncover hidden patterns in imaging data, contributing to more accurate and efficient stroke diagnosis and treatment.

2.5.2.4 Semi-Supervised Learning-based Methods for Stroke Segmentation

Semi-supervised learning-based stroke segmentation methods integrate labeled and unlabeled data to improve model performance. Key approaches include self-training, where a model initially trained on labeled data iteratively refines its predictions by adding confident pseudo-labels from unlabeled data. Consistency regularization enforces prediction stability under perturbations, enhancing robustness. Generative models like VAEs and GANs generate additional samples to augment training data, while pseudo-labeling involves adding model-generated labels to the training set. Multi-view learning leverages multiple data representations or modalities, and graph-based methods use graph structures to propagate labels from labeled to unlabeled data. Semi-supervised variants of CNNs adapt network architectures to handle both types of data, and contrastive learning focuses on learning robust feature representations by contrasting positive and negative data pairs. These methods collectively enhance segmentation accuracy by effectively utilizing labeled and unlabeled data. The typical architectures are as follows.

Consistency-based Methods

Mean Teacher Model: This model involves two networks: a student network and a teacher network. The teacher network is an exponential moving average of the student network's weights. During training, the student network learns from labeled and unlabeled data, while the teacher network provides stable targets for the student by enforcing consistency between the predictions on augmented versions of the same image. This approach helps the model generalize better by utilizing the unlabeled data effectively.

Temporal Ensembling: Like the mean teacher model, temporal ensembling maintains a running average of the network's predictions over multiple training epochs. The model can generate more stable and reliable targets for the unlabeled data by averaging these predictions, improving segmentation performance.

Adversarial Learning

Semi-Supervised GANs (SS-GANs): These models extend generative adversarial networks (GANs) to the semi-supervised setting. The generator creates synthetic brain images, while the discriminator classifies images as real or fake and predicts the segmentation labels for real images. SS-GANs can utilize unlabeled data to improve segmentation accuracy by training the discriminator to perform both tasks. The adversarial training helps the model learn robust features that generalize well to new data.

Auxiliary Classifier GANs (AC-GANs): AC-GANs add an auxiliary classifier to the discriminator, which predicts the segmentation labels. This approach allows the model to leverage labeled and unlabeled data, with the generator and discriminator working together to improve the segmentation performance.

Graph-based Methods

Graph Convolutional Networks (GCNs): GCNs can incorporate relational information from labeled and unlabeled data. By constructing a graph where nodes represent image patches and edges represent similarities between them, GCNs can propagate label information from labeled nodes to unlabeled ones. This method enhances the model's ability to segment stroke lesions by leveraging the structural relationships in the data.

Laplacian Regularization: This technique involves adding a Laplacian regularization term to the loss function, encouraging the model to produce similar predictions for similar data points. This regularization helps the model learn smoother and more consistent segmentations, improving the utilization of unlabeled data.

Self-Training

Pseudo-Labeling: This method generates pseudo-labels for the unlabeled data using the model's current predictions. These pseudo-labels are then treated as true labels and used to retrain the model. By iteratively refining the pseudo-labels and retraining the model, pseudo-labeling can effectively leverage unlabeled data to improve segmentation performance.

Entropy Minimization: This approach minimizes the entropy of the model's predictions on the unlabeled data, encouraging the network to make confident predictions. By reducing the uncertainty in the model's predictions, entropy minimization helps the model learn better representations and improve segmentation accuracy.

Challenges and Future Directions

Semi-supervised learning-based methods face several challenges, including a careful balance between the supervised and unsupervised components, the potential for propagating errors from incorrect pseudo-labels, and the difficulty of ensuring that the model learns meaningful features from the unlabeled data. Additionally, these methods may require sophisticated training procedures and hyperparameter tuning to achieve optimal performance. Semi-supervised learning-based stroke segmentation methods offer a promising avenue for improving the accuracy and robustness of stroke lesion segmentation by utilizing both labeled and unlabeled data. By employing consistency-based methods, adversarial learning, graph-based techniques, and self-training approaches, these methods can overcome the limitations of purely supervised or unsupervised approaches, paving the way for more effective stroke diagnosis and treatment.

2.5.3 DATASETS

In this section, we introduced available datasets for stroke infarct segmentation, encompassing both ischemic and hemorrhagic strokes across CT and MRI modalities. Each dataset comprises various modalities with a different number of cases. Table 5.1 provides a summary of these datasets.

Table 5.1 Summary of stroke datasets

Dataset Name	Modality	Sample Number	Disease
ISLES 2015-SISS	MRI	64	Subacute ischemic stroke
ISLES 2015-SPES	MRI	50	Acute ischemic stroke
ISLES 2017	MRI	75	Acute ischemic stroke
ISLES 2018	CT	103	Acute ischemic stroke
ISLES 2022	MRI	400	Acute and subacute ischemic stroke
ATLAS v2.0	MRI	1,271	Acute, subacute, and chronic ischemic stroke
MNI	MRI	267	Acute, subacute, and chronic ischemic stroke
LONI	MRI	30,000	Acute, subacute, and chronic ischemic stroke
AISD	CT	397	Acute ischemic stroke
APIS	CT	96	Ischemic stroke
IHS	CT	36	Hemorrhagic stroke
INSTANCE	CT	200	Hemorrhagic stroke

2.5.3.1 Summary of ISLES (Ischemic Stroke Lesion Segmentation) Challenge Datasets

The ISLES (Ischemic Stroke Lesion Segmentation) Challenge Datasets are a collection of benchmark datasets designed to facilitate and advance research in the automatic segmentation of ischemic stroke lesions from medical imaging data. These datasets are used in annual challenges that combine the research community to compare and improve various segmentation methods. The ISLES datasets provide standardized data and evaluation metrics, promoting the development of robust and accurate segmentation algorithms. Below are the key datasets from the ISLES challenges and their research contents and contributions.

ISLES 2015 Dataset

The ISLES 2015 dataset consists of multimodal MRI scans, including Diffusion-Weighted Imaging (DWI), Fluid-Attenuated Inversion Recovery (FLAIR), and Time-of-Flight (TOF) angiography images from acute ischemic stroke patients. It includes 28 training and 36 testing cases. This dataset enabled researchers to develop and benchmark new methods for acute stroke lesion segmentation. It emphasized the importance of multimodal data integration for accurate lesion identification and segmentation. The challenge results highlighted the potential of machine learning methods to improve segmentation accuracy compared to traditional techniques.

ISLES 2016 Dataset

The ISLES 2016 dataset expanded to include two sub-challenges: the SISS (Sub-acute Ischemic Stroke Lesion Segmentation) and SPES (Stroke Perfusion Estimation). The SISS dataset contains MRI scans with follow-up FLAIR images, while the SPES dataset includes perfusion maps from CT and MRI. The 2016 challenge encouraged the development of methods that can handle different stages of stroke, from acute to sub-acute phases. It highlighted the importance of temporal information and follow-up imaging in improving segmentation accuracy. Including perfusion data in the SPES sub-challenge promoted research into perfusion-based assessment of stroke severity and outcomes.

ISLES 2017 Dataset

The ISLES 2017 dataset focused on chronic stroke lesions, providing multimodal MRI scans, including DWI, FLAIR, and T1-weighted images. It includes 43 training and 32 testing cases with chronic stroke lesions annotated. This dataset addressed the challenges of chronic stroke lesion segmentation, which often involves characteristics different from acute and sub-acute lesions. It facilitated the development of algorithms capable of identifying long-term brain tissue damage. The results underscored the importance of combining structural and diffusion imaging for effective chronic lesion segmentation.

ISLES 2018 Dataset

The ISLES 2018 challenge introduced the combination of acute stroke lesions with tissue outcome prediction. The dataset includes multimodal MRI scans from acute stroke patients, with follow-up FLAIR images to assess tissue outcome. This challenge bridged the gap between acute lesion segmentation and outcome prediction, encouraging methods that not only segment lesions but also predict long-term tissue viability. The dataset promoted the integration of segmentation and prediction tasks, leading to more comprehensive stroke assessment tools.

ISLES 2022 Dataset

The ISLES 2022 challenge featured high-resolution MRI scans from acute stroke patients, including DWI, ADC (Apparent Diffusion Coefficient), and perfusion-weighted imaging (PWI). It provided a larger number of cases for training and testing, aiming to improve generalizability. The 2022 challenge emphasized the need for high-resolution imaging data to capture finer details of stroke lesions. It highlighted advancements in deep learning techniques, particularly convolutional neural networks (CNNs) and attention mechanisms, which significantly improved segmentation accuracy. The results demonstrated the potential of advanced neural network architectures to handle complex medical imaging tasks.

2.5.3.2 Summary of ATLAS v2.0 (Anatomical Tracings of Lesions After Stroke) Dataset

The ATLAS v2.0 dataset, an extension of the Anatomical Tracings of Lesions After Stroke project, is a comprehensive resource designed to facilitate research in stroke imaging and recovery. The dataset is meticulously curated to provide high-quality, manually segmented brain lesion data, which are critical for developing and validating automated methods for lesion detection and segmentation. ATLAS v2.0 includes a variety of neuroimaging modalities, with a primary focus on T1-weighted MRI scans. These scans provide detailed anatomical information necessary for accurate lesion delineation. ATLAS v2.0 has significantly contributed to developing advanced lesion segmentation techniques, particularly those employing machine learning and deep learning. The manual segmentations provide a reliable benchmark for evaluating the accuracy of these automated methods.

2.5.3.3 Summary of MNI (Montreal Neurological Institute) Dataset

The Montreal Neurological Institute (MNI) Stroke Dataset is a valuable resource for researchers and clinicians focused on understanding and improving the diagnosis and treatment of stroke. The MNI Stroke Dataset comprises a wide range of neuroimaging modalities, including high-resolution structural MRI, diffusion-weighted imaging (DWI), and perfusion-weighted imaging (PWI). The dataset includes scans from patients with different types of stroke, including ischemic and hemorrhagic strokes, covering various stages from acute to chronic phases. The MNI Stroke Dataset has been instrumental in developing and benchmarking various segmentation algorithms, particularly those leveraging machine learning and deep learning techniques. It provides a robust foundation for training and validating models that accurately delineate stroke lesions from MRI scans.

2.5.3.4 Summary of LONI (Laboratory of Neuro Imaging) Stroke Dataset

The Laboratory of Neuro Imaging (LONI) Stroke Dataset is an essential resource for the neuroimaging community, aimed at advancing research on stroke diagnosis, treatment, and recovery. The LONI Stroke Dataset includes a variety of neuroimaging modalities, such as T1-weighted MRI, T2-weighted MRI, diffusion-weighted imaging (DWI), and perfusion-weighted imaging (PWI). The dataset encompasses scans from patients with different types and stages of stroke, including acute ischemic stroke, hemorrhagic stroke, and chronic stroke conditions. The LONI Stroke Dataset has been pivotal in developing and benchmarking segmentation algorithms, particularly those using machine learning and deep learning techniques. Researchers have used this dataset to train and validate models that accurately delineate stroke lesions in various imaging modalities.

2.5.3.5 Summary of AISD (Acute Ischemic Stroke Dataset)

The Acute Ischemic Stroke Dataset (AISD) is a valuable resource for researchers and clinicians focused on studying and managing acute ischemic stroke (AIS). This dataset is designed to support developing and validating algorithms for stroke detection, segmentation, and outcome prediction, leveraging various imaging modalities and comprehensive clinical data. The AISD includes multiple neuroimaging modalities critical for stroke research, such as non-contrast computed tomography (NCCT), magnetic resonance imaging (MRI), including T1-weighted, T2-weighted, diffusion-weighted imaging (DWI), and perfusion-weighted imaging (PWI). The AISD has been instrumental in developing and benchmarking lesion segmentation algorithms, particularly those utilizing machine learning and deep learning techniques. Researchers use this dataset to improve the accuracy and reliability of automated stroke detection and segmentation methods.

2.5.3.6 Summary of APIS (Automated Processing of Ischemic Stroke)

The Automated Processing of Ischemic Stroke (APIS) dataset is a significant resource in stroke research and medical imaging. It is designed to support the development and evaluation of automated methods for ischemic stroke detection, segmentation, and analysis using advanced imaging techniques and comprehensive clinical data. The APIS dataset includes a variety of neuroimaging modalities crucial for the study of ischemic stroke. These typically encompass non-contrast CT (NCCT), MRI sequences such as T1-weighted, T2-weighted, FLAIR, diffusion-weighted imaging (DWI), and perfusion imaging (PWI). The APIS dataset has been pivotal in developing robust lesion segmentation algorithms, particularly those leveraging machine learning and deep learning techniques. Researchers utilize this dataset to enhance the precision and reliability of automated stroke detection and segmentation tools.

2.5.3.7 Summary of IHS (International Stroke Study)

The International Stroke Study (IHS) is a prominent and comprehensive dataset dedicated to stroke research. It plays a crucial role in advancing the understanding, diagnosis, and treatment of stroke by providing a rich collection of imaging and clinical data from a diverse population of stroke patients. The IHS dataset encompasses a variety of neuroimaging modalities essential for stroke research, including non-contrast computed tomography (NCCT), magnetic resonance imaging (MRI) sequences such as T1-weighted, T2-weighted, FLAIR, diffusion-weighted imaging (DWI), and perfusion-weighted imaging (PWI). The IHS dataset has been instrumental in developing accurate and robust lesion segmentation algorithms, particularly those based on machine learning and deep learning techniques. Researchers leverage this dataset to enhance the precision and reliability of automated tools for detecting and delineating ischemic lesions.

2.5.3.8 Summary of INSTANCE (Ischemic Stroke Lesion Segmentation Challenge)

The INSTANCE (Ischemic Stroke Lesion Segmentation Challenge) dataset is a valuable resource in the realm of ischemic stroke research, designed to facilitate the development and evaluation of automated methods for segmenting ischemic stroke lesions from medical imaging data. This dataset is crucial for researchers aiming to improve the accuracy and reliability of stroke lesion segmentation algorithms. The INSTANCE dataset includes a range of imaging modalities typically used in stroke diagnosis and treatment. These modalities include non-contrast computed tomography (NCCT) and magnetic resonance imaging (MRI) sequences such as T1-weighted, T2-weighted, FLAIR, and diffusion-weighted imaging (DWI). The INSTANCE dataset includes a range of imaging modalities typically used in stroke diagnosis and treatment. These modalities include non-contrast computed tomography (NCCT) and magnetic resonance imaging (MRI) sequences such as T1-weighted, T2-weighted, FLAIR, and diffusion-weighted imaging (DWI). The variety of modalities provides comprehensive data to capture different aspects of ischemic stroke lesions.

2.5.4 LIMITATIONS

Artificial intelligence (AI) in stroke segmentation research has achieved notable advancements, but several limitations remain that impact its effectiveness and applicability. The quality and quantity of data pose significant challenges; many datasets suffer from limited annotations and imbalances in stroke types or lesion sizes, which can affect the performance of AI models. Additionally, generalizing AI models across different populations and imaging modalities is problematic, as models trained on specific datasets may not perform well on diverse or global populations or different imaging protocols. The complexity of stroke lesions—varying in size, shape, and intensity—further complicates accurate segmentation, especially when lesions overlap with other brain abnormalities.

Interpretability remains a critical issue, as many AI models, particularly deep learning networks, operate as "black boxes," making it difficult for clinicians to understand their decision-making processes and trust their outputs. Integration into clinical workflows presents logistical challenges, including compatibility with existing systems and addressing regulatory and ethical concerns related to data privacy, consent, and liability. Model robustness is also a concern. AI systems are sensitive to image noise, artifacts, and adversarial attacks, which can impact their reliability. Furthermore, a lack of standardization in imaging protocols and segmentation practices makes it challenging to compare and evaluate different AI models consistently. Lastly, the high computational demands of advanced AI models can limit their accessibility in various clinical settings. Addressing these limitations involves improving dataset quality, enhancing model robustness and interpretability, ensuring effective clinical integration, and resolving ethical and regulatory issues to realize the potential of AI in stroke segmentation.

2.5.5 RESULTS AND FUTURE DIRECTIONS

Artificial intelligence (AI) has made significant strides in stroke segmentation research, leading to notable advancements in accuracy, efficiency, and automation.

AI algorithms, especially those based on deep learning techniques like U-Net and convolutional neural networks (CNNs), have demonstrated improved performance in identifying and segmenting stroke lesions compared to traditional methods. These models have enhanced diagnostic capabilities by integrating multi-modal imaging data, such as MRI and CT scans, which allows for more comprehensive stroke assessment and faster analysis. Developing benchmark datasets and challenges, such as the ISLES challenges, has provided standardized resources for evaluating and comparing AI models, advancing the field.

However, despite these achievements, several limitations remain. Current AI models often struggle with generalization across different populations and imaging modalities due to limited and sometimes imbalanced datasets. The variability in stroke lesions and their appearance can affect model performance, and many AI systems still lack interpretability, making it challenging to understand and trust their decision-making processes. Furthermore, integrating AI into clinical workflows presents logistical challenges, including ensuring compatibility with existing systems and addressing regulatory and ethical concerns related to data privacy and model validation.

Looking ahead, researchers expect AI-based stroke segmentation to evolve in several key areas. Efforts will focus on improving model robustness and generalization by creating more diverse and representative datasets. Enhancing interpretability through explainable AI and integrating clinical knowledge will be crucial for aligning AI outputs with medical expertise. Advanced learning techniques, such as semi-supervised and unsupervised learning, are being explored to use limited annotated data better. Additionally, seamless integration into clinical workflows and real-time analysis capabilities will be prioritized to support immediate diagnostic and decision-making processes. Addressing regulatory and ethical considerations will be essential to ensure responsible AI deployment. Overall, the future of AI in stroke segmentation promises further advancements in diagnostic precision and clinical utility, with ongoing research and development aimed at overcoming current limitations and enhancing the impact of AI technologies in stroke care.

2.5.6 CONCLUSIONS

Artificial intelligence (AI) in stroke segmentation has led to significant advancements, offering improved accuracy and efficiency in detecting and analyzing stroke lesions. AI techniques, particularly deep learning models such as convolutional neural networks (CNNs) and U-Net architectures, have demonstrated enhanced performance in automated segmentation tasks compared to traditional methods. These AI systems have facilitated faster and more consistent stroke lesion detection, contributing to better diagnostic capabilities and quicker analysis.

However, challenges persist. AI models often face limitations related to data quality and quantity, including issues with limited annotations, data imbalances, and variability across imaging modalities and patient populations. The complexity and variability of stroke lesions, combined with the "black box" nature of many

AI models, can hinder interpretability and clinical trust. Integration into clinical workflows is also challenging, requiring compatibility with existing systems and addressing regulatory and ethical considerations.

Future directions for AI in stroke segmentation involve improving model robustness and generalization through diverse and well-annotated datasets, enhancing interpretability and alignment with clinical insights, and addressing integration and ethical concerns. Advances in semi-supervised and unsupervised learning, real-time analysis capabilities, and personalized medicine approaches are expected further to enhance the role of AI in stroke care, ultimately leading to more effective and reliable diagnostic tools.

REFERENCES

[1] Valery L. Feigin, Mayowa O. Owolabi, Foad Abd-Allah, Rufus O. Akinyemi, Natalia V. Bhattacharjee, Michael Brainin, et al. 2023. Pragmatic solutions to reduce the global burden of stroke: A World Stroke Organization–Lancet Neurology Commission. The Lancet Neurology. 22(12): 1160–1206.

[2] Valery L. Feigin, Michael Brainin, Bo Norrving, Sheila Martins, Ralph L. Sacco, Werner Hacke, et al. 2022. World Stroke Organization (WSO): Global stroke fact sheet 2022. International Journal of Stroke. 17(1): 18–29.

[3] Larry B. Goldstein and David L. Simel. 2005. Is this patient having a stroke? JAMA. 293(19): 2391–2402.

[4] David Y. Hwang, Gisele S. Silva, Karen L. Furie and David M. Greer. 2012. Comparative sensitivity of computed tomography vs. magnetic resonance imaging for detecting acute posterior fossa infarct. The Journal of Emergency Medicine. 42(5): 559–565.

[5] Julio A. Chalela, Chelsea S. Kidwell, Lauren M. Nentwich, Marie Luby, John A. Butman, Andrew M Demchuk, et al. 2007. Magnetic resonance imaging and computed tomography in emergency assessment of patients with suspected acute stroke: A prospective comparison. The Lancet. 369(9558):293–298.

[6] J.B. Fiebach, P.D. Schellinger, O. Jansen, M. Meyer, P. Wilde, J. Bender, et al. 2002. CT and diffusion-weighted MR imaging in randomized order: diffusion-weighted imaging results in higher accuracy and lower interrater variability in the diagnosis of hyperacute ischemic stroke. Stroke. 33(9): 2206– 2210.

[7] Enrico Flossmann, Jessica N. Redgrave, Dennis Briley and Peter M. Rothwell. 2008. Reliability of clinical diagnosis of the symptomatic vascular territory in patients with recent transient ischemic attack or minor stroke. Stroke. 39(9): 2457–2460.

[8] Junya Aoki, Kazumi Kimura, Yasuyuki Iguchi, Kensaku Shibazaki, Kenichiro Sakai and Takeshi Iwanaga. 2010. FLAIR can estimate the onset time in acute ischemic stroke patients. Journal of the Neurological Sciences 293(1–2): 39–44.

[9] T. Wessels, C. Wessels, A. Ellsiepen, I. Reuter, S. Trittmacher, E. Stolz, et al. 2006. Contribution of diffusion-weighted imaging in determination of stroke etiology. American Journal of Neuroradiology. 27(1): 35–39.

[10] Claus Z. Simonsen, Mette H. Madsen, M.L. Schmitz, I.K. Mikkelsen, Marc Fisher and Grethe Andersen 2015. Sensitivity of diffusion-and perfusion-weighted imaging for diagnosing acute ischemic stroke is 97.5%. Stroke. 46(1): 98–101.

[11] Jian Wang, Hengde Zhu, Shui-Hua Wang and Yu-Dong Zhang. 2021. A review of deep learning on medical image analysis. Mobile Networks and Applications. 26(1): 351–380.

[12] Yue Zhang, Shijie Liu, Chunlai Li and Jianyu Wang. 2022. Application of dee.p learning method on ischemic stroke lesion segmentation. Journal of Shanghai Jiaotong University (Science). 1–13.

[13] Cheng Chen, Kai Yuan, Yuqi Fang, Shichun Bao and Raymond Kai-yu Tong. 2021. Hierarchically spatial encoding module for chronic stroke lesion segmentation. *In*: 2021 10th International IEEE/EMBS Conference on Neural Engineering (NER). IEEE. 1000–1003.

[14] Steve Pieper, Michael Halle and Ron Kikinis. 2004. 3D Slicer. *In*: 2004 2nd IEEE international symposium on biomedical imaging: Nano to macro (IEEE Cat No. 04EX821). IEEE. 632–635.

[15] Paul A. Yushkevich, Yang Gao and Guido Gerig. 2016. ITK-SNAP: An interactive tool for semi-automatic segmentation of multi-modality biomedical images. *In*: 2016 38th Annual International Conference of the IEEE Engineering in Medicine and Biology Society (EMBC). IEEE. 3342–3345.

[16] Detlev Stalling, Malte Westerhoff and Hans-Christian Hege. 2005. Amira: A highly interactive system for visual data analysis. The Visualization Handbook. 38: 749–767.

[17] Matthew J. McAuliffe, Francois M. Lalonde, Delia McGarry, William Gandler, Karl Csaky and Benes L. Trus. 2001. Medical image processing, analysis and visualization in clinical research. *In*: Proceedings 14th IEEE Symposium on Computer-based Medical Systems. CBMS 2001. IEEE. 381–386.

[18] Xiangchen Zhang, Huan Xu, Yujun Liu, Jiajia Liao, Guorong Cai, Jinhe Su, et al. 2021. A multiple encoders network for stroke lesion segmentation. *In*: Chinese Conference on Pattern Recognition and Computer Vision (PRCV). Springer. 524–535.

[19] Chuanlong Li. 2021. Stroke lesion segmentation with visual cortex anatomy alike neural nets. arXiv preprint arXiv:2105.06544.

Chapter **2.6**

Multi-Scale Feature Fusion-based Sweet Spots Localization from Microelectrode Recordings in STN-DBS Surgery

Linxia Xiao[1]*, Qingqing Zheng[1], Xiangyun Liao[1], Doudou Zhang[2], Weixin Si[1], Yanjie Wei[1,4] and Yi Pan[3,4]

[1]Shenzhen Institute of Advanced Technology, Chinese Academy of Sciences

[2]Department of Neurosurgery, Shenzhen Second People's Hospital

[3]Faculty of Computer Science and Control Engineering, Shenzhen University of Advanced Technology

[4]Shenzhen Key Laboratory of Intelligent Bioinformatics, Shenzhen Institute of Advanced Technology

2.6.1 INTRODUCTIONS

Parkinson's disease (PD) is a common progressive neurodegenerative disorder characterized by motor symptoms such as tremors, muscle rigidity, difficulties in walking, and impaired coordination. These symptoms not only severely affect patients' quality of life but also place a heavy burden on their families and society [1]. Deep brain stimulation of the subthalamic nucleus (STN-DBS) has emerged as a widely used and effective therapeutic approach to alleviate these motor symptoms associated with PD [2]. By delivering accurate electrical

*For Correspondence: lx.xiao@siat.ac.cn

DOI: 10.1201/9781003518754-11

stimulation to the subthalamic nucleus (STN), STN-DBS modulates relevant neural circuits involved in motor control, thereby improving motor function and overall treatment efficacy [3]. The success of STN-DBS surgery hinges critically on accurate sweet spot localization for optimal electrode placement [4]. However, in clinical practice, precisely identifying sweet spots poses significant challenges [5]. Currently, it often relies on a trial-and-error process where multiple attempts are made to assess motor function improvement after electrical stimulation. This method is not only time-consuming but also labor-intensive, increasing the complexity and costs of the surgical procedure. Therefore, developing an efficient sweet spot localization method is crucial for STN-DBS surgery to assist surgeons in making beneficial decisions for patients.

The subthalamic nucleus (STN) is functionally subdivided into the sensorimotor, associative, and limbic zones [6]. For STN-DBS surgery, the closer the electrode is placed to the sensorimotor region, the greater the improvement in motor symptoms for PD patients [7, 8]. However, the sensorimotor zone occupies only a small portion of the STN. Though traditional magnetic resonance imaging (MRI) techniques can provide basic anatomical information about the STN, they are insufficient for precisely identifying the sweet spots for stimulation. Microelectrode recordings (MERs), which monitor real-time electrophysiological activity in specific brain regions during surgery [9], offer a solution. By analyzing MERs, surgeons can detect the unique electrophysiological features of different functional zones, particularly those of the sensorimotor region. Therefore, identifying MER features can assist in accurately localizing sweet spots for effective stimulation.

In recent years, several MER classification methods based on time-series features have been proposed [10]. For example, Karthick et al. [11] used wavelet features combined with a random forest (RF) classifier to recognize MERs. Khosravi et al. [12] employed a convolutional neural network (CNN) for the automatic recognition of MERs to determine the STN and its boundaries. However, these methods primarily focus on STN localization. Ciecierski et al. [13] developed a computer-assisted decision support system for DBS procedures, utilizing attention-based artificial neural networks to classify MERs and determine the optimal stimulation position of electrodes within the STN.

Maged et al. [14] proposed a lightweight deep-learning model to detect MERs for automatically localizing STN. In order to determine the optimal positions for DBS electrode stimulation, some studies have explored MERs-based sweet spot localization [15]. Xiao et al. [16] proposed the use of Gramian Angular Summation Field (GASF) features with CNNs (GASF-CNN) to identify MERs, aiding in sweet spot localization. However, the GASF feature extraction method is less advantageous for atypical high-frequency and high-amplitude MERs [17]. To overcome this challenge, Xiao et al. [18] introduced an amplitude-frequency aware deep fusion network (AFA-DFN), which improved MERs recognition and optimal contact selection. Nevertheless, these MERs feature fusion methods involve simple feature concatenation, which may result in redundant features and fail to capture discriminate features. Therefore, developing a specialized network can simultaneously handle time-frequency and amplitude-sequence feature fusion from MERs and learn the importance of different features. This would enable a more effective extraction of both global and local complementary information between MER features.

We propose a multi-scale feature fusion method for sweet spot localization from MERs in STN-DBS surgery to address these challenges. We first preprocess the MERs to obtain the time-frequency and amplitude-sequence images. Secondly, we propose a dual-branch feature fusion network to extract the multi-scale temporal and spatial features, which are then fused within a Transformer encoder module for accurate sweet spot localization. Experimental results demonstrate that our method outperforms the state-of-the-art methods in achieving accurate sweet spot localization.

2.6.2 METHOD

This chapter proposes a multi-scale feature fusion method for sweet spot localization using MERs in STN-DBS. Our approach consists of three parts, including data preprocessing, dual-branch feature fusion module, and MER classification. The overall architecture of the model is depicted in Figure 6.1.

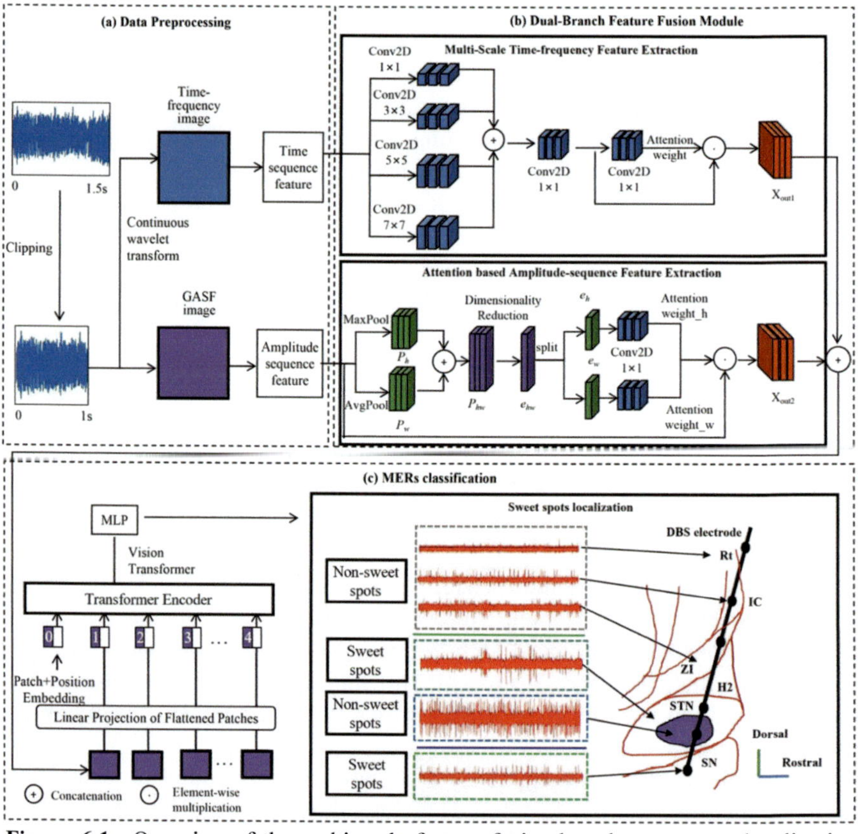

Figure 6.1 Overview of the multi-scale feature fusion-based sweet spots localization method.

2.6.2.1 Materials

The research collected 7,420 segments of MERs from 100 Parkinson's disease patients who underwent successful STN-DBS surgeries in January 2018. These surgeries were conducted using a bipolar electrode setup and assisted by the NeuroNav 223/12 electrophysiological navigation system (Alpha Omega Engineering, Israel) at the local medical center. In order to ensure the stability of the collected MERs, approximately 1 to 5 seconds of raw data were acquired at each electrode position. Considering that longer signal durations might introduce algorithm biases, professional neurosurgeons recommended trimming initial noisy segments and selecting a one-second segment with minimal noise for analysis [19, 20]. All MERs, with a sample rate of 24 kHz and amplified 1,000 times, were followed by digital bandpass filtering using a sixth-order Butterworth filter with a frequency range of 0.5 to 5 kHz, along with a 60 Hz notch filter in Matlab software [21]. Subsequently, the MERs were downsampled to 12 kHz to improve computational efficiency [11].

The microelectrode trajectory in STN-DBS surgery starts from the premotor cortex and extends to the STN [22]. As shown in Figure 1, since the characteristics of MERs vary across different brain structures, experienced clinicians typically classify MERs based on peak, frequency, and amplitude characteristics for precise sweet spot localization. Preoperative T1-weighted images were collected using a 3-T MRI system (Prisma, Siemens, Germany) with a 64-channel head coil, offering a resolution of 1 mm^3 and a repetition time/echo time of 1780 ms/2.32 ms. Postoperative CT scans were collected with a spiral CT system (SO- MATOM Emotion 16/Definition AS/Definition Flash, Siemens, Germany) with a slice thickness of 1 mm. By integrating the MER classification results with anatomical data from preoperative MRI and postoperative CT scans, the sweet spots for DBS electrode placement were identified.

2.6.2.2 Data Preprocessing

Due to the stochastic, multicomponent, and non-stationary nature of MERs, converting MERs into two-dimensional images for visualization better aligns with surgeons' observational habits, making the analysis more intuitive. Therefore, we transform MERs into time-frequency and amplitude-sequence feature images to facilitate more effective analysis.

Continuous Wavelet Transform (CWT) is an effective tool for time-frequency domain analysis, capable of accurately capturing the time-series characteristics of MERs data and visualizing them as time-frequency images [23]. Due to the excellent ability to handle both time and frequency information simultaneously, we choose the complex Morlet wavelet (specifically cmor3-3) [24, 25] as the basis for analyzing MERs data. In order to achieve the optimal trade-off between frequency and time resolution, the length of the amplitude sequence is set to 256. While increasing the sequence length can enhance frequency resolution, excessive length would compromise time resolution. Therefore, the sampling frequency is set to 12 kHz, with each signal lasting one second. By shifting the sampling points along the time axis, time-shift coefficients are obtained, from which wavelet coefficients are calculated, leading to the constructing of a complete time-frequency distribution map. Finally, the time-frequency images are generated using CWT, with a resolution of $100 \times 100 \times 3$.

To obtain the amplitude-sequence features, we utilized GASF to generate the visual images [16]. Given a MERs data $Y = \{y_1, y_2, \ldots, y_n\}$, Y was normalized to the interval [–1, 1]:

$$\tilde{y}_i = \left(\frac{\left(y_i - \max(Y) + (y_i - \min(Y))\right)}{\max(Y) - \min(Y)} \right) \tag{1}$$

where $\max(Y)$ and $\min(Y)$ represents the maximum and minimum values of Y, respectively, the preprocessed MERs were transformed into polar coordinates to facilitate the analysis of temporal correlations across different time intervals through trigonometric summation. The GASF matrix is calculated as:

$$\text{GASF} = [\cos(\phi_i + \phi_j)] \tag{2}$$

where ϕ_i and ϕ_j are the angles in polar coordinates, and cos is the cosine operation. Finally, the GASF images with dimensions $100 \times 100 \times 3$ can be obtained based on the GASF matrix.

2.6.2.3 Dual-Branch Feature Fusion Module

We designed a dual-branch feature fusion module, which can concurrently process and integrate time-frequency and amplitude-sequence feature information, thereby providing a more comprehensive global and local representation. Specifically, one branch of the architecture focuses on capturing temporal features, while the other processes amplitude-sequence features. By fusing information from both branches, this design captures the temporal dynamics and spectral characteristics of MERs, thus improving the accuracy of sweet spot localization.

2.6.2.4 Multi-Scale Time-Frequency Feature Extraction

We develop a multi-scale time-frequency feature extraction framework to extract temporal information effectively. This framework consists of 4 convolutional modules, and each convolutional module contains four convolutional layers with kernel sizes of 1×1, 3×3, 5×5, and 1×7. By utilizing different receptive fields to capture multi-scale time-frequency features, this approach combines low-level and high-level features, resulting in a comprehensive feature representation.

Let the input feature map be X, and the convolution kernel be K_i, and the feature map F_i extracted by the convolution layer can be represented as:

$$F_i = \text{Re}\,LU(Conv(X, K_i)) \tag{3}$$

where Re LU means the Rectified Linear Unit, and $Conv$ means convolution operation.

The extracted multi-scale features F_1, F_2, F_3, F_4 are concatenated along the channel dimension to form F_c, and then a 1×1 convolution layer is used to compress the channels back to the original size, resulting in the fused feature F_c. To further enhance the feature representation, we apply a channel attention mechanism to weight the compressed features, ultimately outputting the refined feature representation X_{out1}:

$$X_{out1} = F_c \odot \sigma(Conv(F_c)), \tag{4}$$

where $\odot$ denotes element-wise multiplication, and σ is the sigmoid activation function. This design enables the input data to be interpreted from multiple perspectives, enhancing the expressiveness and robustness of the model.

2.6.2.5 Attention-based Amplitude-Sequence Feature Extraction

To extract important global and local information from GASF images for classification, we propose an attention-based amplitude-sequence feature extraction method by utilizing the coordinate attention mechanism. As shown in Figure 6.1 (b), for the input feature $X_2 \in \mathbb{R}^{B \times C \times W \times H}$, we first perform global maxpooling and average pooling to generate feature vectors P_h and P_w along the height and width directions, respectively. These two feature vectors are concatenated to obtain the combined feature P_{hw}. Then, a 1×1 convolution module followed by a nonlinear activation function, is applied to the combined feature to generate the combination feature representation e_{hw}, which can generate the feature vectors e_h and e_w along the height and width directions based on the same principles as above. Finally, two three-layer convolution modules with a kernel of 1×1 are used to generate attention weights a_h and a_w for rows and columns, respectively. These attention weights are applied to the input feature X_2 to obtain the enhanced feature representation X_{out2}:

$$a_h = \sigma(Conv(e_h)),\ a_w = \sigma(Conv(e_w)) \tag{5}$$

$$X_{out2} = X_2 \odot a_h \odot a_w \tag{6}$$

Finally, the fusion features X_{out} can be obtained by a combination of the multi-scale time-frequency features X_{out1} and attention-based amplitude-sequence features X_{out2}.

2.6.2.6 MERs Classification

To accurately classify the MERs for sweet spot determination, we integrate a transformer module into our model. The core of the transformer lies in its ability to capture complex dependencies within the input data using multi-head self-attention, allowing it to process information in parallel and improve feature representation, thereby increasing the accuracy of MERs classification.

To input the previously obtained feature representation X_{out} into the Transformer module, we first map it to a fixed-length embedding space via a linear layer. Positional encoding is then added to form the input sequence X. The Transformer encoder is composed of multiple layers, each containing a multi-head self-attention mechanism and a feedforward neural network. The self-attention mechanism computes the attention between the input features as follows:

$$Attention(Q, K, V) = softmax\left(\frac{QK^T}{\sqrt{d_k}}\right) \cdot V \tag{6.7}$$

where Q, K, V are the query, key, and value matrices derived from the input sequence X through linear projections. The values are weighted by the attention weights to produce the output features, which are subsequently processed through the feedforward neural network. The final output is fed into a multilayer perceptron (MLP) to obtain the classification results. Based on the identified MERs results, the sweet spot localization can be determined in conjunction with MRI and postoperative CT to guide the placement of the therapeutic electrodes in STN-DBS.

2.6.3 EXPERIMENTS

To evaluate the performance of our method, we conducted the experiment on the dataset of the MERs from 100 PD patients to identify sweet spots. The raw MERs data was initially preprocessed using MATLAB 2017a on a Windows 10 operating system. For multi-scale feature fusion and MERs classification, the experiments were implemented using PyTorch 2.1.2 on a GeForce RTX 3060 NVIDIA GPU.

2.6.3.1 Model Performance

In this experiment, we employed the ten-fold cross-validation approach to evaluate our method. For each fold, 10% of the training samples were randomly selected for validation, while the remaining samples were used for training. As shown in Table 6.1, the results from the ten-fold cross-validation demonstrate that the proposed method achieved an average accuracy of 99.00%, precision of 98.75%, sensitivity of 98.99%, specificity of 99.08%, and F1-score of 98.78%, underscoring the model's high effectiveness in identifying sweet spots.

Table 6.1 Results (%) of our method using ten-fold cross-validation for sweet spot identification

Method	1	2	3	4	5	6	7	8	9	10	Results
Accuracy	99.08	99.27	98.59	98.91	99.02	99.00	97.53	99.55	99.49	99.53	**99.00±0.39**
Precision	98.47	99.45	98.13	98.62	99.03	99.05	96.74	99.18	99.15	99.64	**98.75±0.60**
Sensitivity	98.93	99.38	99.01	98.86	98.95	99.01	97.34	99.41	99.40	99.58	**98.99±0.37**
Specificity	99.31	99.09	98.02	99.31	99.31	98.98	97.89	99.82	99.80	99.28	**99.08±0.47**
F1-score	98.68	99.23	98.40	98.70	98.98	98.77	97.02	99.27	99.25	99.51	**98.78±0.47**

Table 6.2 Comparison results (%) of different methods for sweet spot identification

Method	Accuracy	Precision	Sensitivity	Specificity	F1-score
KNN	87.65±2.02	87.56±2.87	84.03±2.63	90.54±2.13	85.76±2.75
RF	91.77±2.14	92.35±3.33	88.88±2.52	94.15±2.46	90.56±2.52
SVM	90.76±1.41	91.03±2.23	87.89±2.22	93.10±1.62	89.41±1.67
DT	89.37±1.25	88.57±2.14	86.65±0.90	91.45±1.67	87.60±1.27
CNN	93.99±2.80	95.88±3.51	90.78±2.56	96.94±2.35	93.26±4.21
GASF-CNN [16]	97.68±1.65	95.33±5.22	98.34±1.99	97.57±2.68	96.63±2.63
AFA-DFN [18]	96.78±1.47	97.44±1.10	95.26±3.40	98.07±0.81	96.34±1.66
ResATNet [13]	97.37±0.97	95.18±2.66	97.31±1.82	97.32±1.47	96.21±1.55
Ours	99.00±0.39	98.75±0.60	98.99±0.37	99.08±0.47	98.78±0.47

To further assess the performance of our method, we compared our method with several classic MER classification methods, including machine learning such as k-Nearest Neighbors (KNN, K = 5), Support Vector Machine (SVM), Decision Tree (DT), RF [11], as well as deep learning methods like CNN [12], GASF-CNN [16], AFA-DFN [18] and ResATNet [13]. The results showed that the proposed method outperforms other methods for sweet spot identification, which are depicted in Table 6.2.

2.6.3.2 Ablation Study

To assess the contribution of each component in our proposed model, we conducted ablation experiments and compared the performance across various model configurations. As shown in Table 6.3, experiment results illustrated that the performance of our method outperformed alternative configurations for sweet spot identification. Our method incorporating the multi-scale feature extraction, coordinate attention mechanism, and transformer module achieved the highest performance, with an average accuracy of 99.00%, precision of 98.75%, sensitivity of 98.99%, specificity of 99.08%, and an F1-score of 98.78%.

Table 6.3 Ablation study results from different methods for identifying the sweet spots (%)

Multi-Scale Feature Extraction	Coordinate Attention	Trans-former	Accuracy	Precision	Sensiti-vity	Speci-ficity	F1-score
✓			98.20	97.52	98.63	97.25	98.03
✓	✓		91.73	90.34	93.68	87.36	91.28
✓		✓	96.76	95.71	97.53	95.05	96.49
✓	✓	✓	**99.00**	**98.75**	**98.99**	**99.08**	**98.78**

2.6.4 DISCUSSION

Accurate localization of sweet spots is essential for neurosurgeons performing STN-DBS surgery. Currently, clinicians typically first determine the nucleus position through MRI imaging and then guide the implantation of DBS electrodes based on the characteristics of MERs. However, due to the small size of the sensorimotor area within the STN and the limited precision of MRI for localizing it, this study localizes sweet spots by identifying MERs. Our method leverages powerful pattern recognition capabilities by combining data pre-processing, dual-branch feature fusion modules, and MER classification. Moreover, MERs can be affected by various interferences, such as noise or non-specific discharges, which may compromise the accuracy of sweet spot identification. Our method can effectively remove noise and automatically identify MERs, reducing reliance on expert experience and enhancing the efficiency and consistency of STN-DBS surgery.

Although the proposed method has shown promising results in sweet spot localization, it still has certain limitations. Firstly, the localization of sweet spots depends not only on the clinical electrophysiological information and MRI information but also on the exercise recovery status of the patients, and postoperative adverse reactions can also affect the final outcome of sweet spot localization. Secondly, the current study is based on data from a single center. In order to validate the generalization capability of the proposed method, it is essential to collect and analyze data from multiple centers. Therefore, future work will involve gathering multi-center data from various types of equipment to confirm the effectiveness of our approach.

2.6.5 CONCLUSION

In this study, we propose a multi-scale feature fusion method for sweet spot localization from MERs in STN-DBS surgery. First, we extract time-frequency and amplitude-sequence features. Second, we introduce a dual-branch feature fusion network to integrate multi-scale temporal and spatial information from these features, respectively. Finally, we utilize a Transformer encoder to identify the sweet spots. The experimental results demonstrate that our model surpasses the state-of-the-art methods in sweet spot identification. Our method achieves an average accuracy of 99.00%, precision of 98.75%, sensitivity of 98.99%, specificity of 99.08%, and an F1-score of 98.78%. These results indicate that our approach has great potential to improve the efficiency of DBS surgery and reduce the reliance on the clinician's subjective experience, making it a valuable tool in neuromodulation.

REFERENCES

[1] E. Ray Dorsey, lexis Elbaz, mma Nichols, ooshin Abbasi, Foad Abd-Allah, Ahmed Abdelalim, et al. 2018. Global, regional, and national burden of Parkinson's disease, 1990–2016: A systematic analysis for the Global Burden of Disease Study 2016. The Lancet Neurology. 17(11): 939–953.

[2] W.M.M. Schuepbach, J. Rau, K. Knudsen, J. Volkmann, P. Krack, L. Timmermann, T.D. Hälbig, et al. 2013. Neurostimulation for Parkinson's disease with early motor complications. New England Journal of Medicine. 368(7): 610–622.

[3] J.M. Mann, K.D. Foote, C.W. Garvan, H.H. Fernandez, C.E. Jacobson IV, R.L. Rodriguez, et al. 2009. Brain penetration effects of microelectrodes and DBS leads in STN or GPi. Journal of Neurology, Neurosurgery and Psychiatry. 80(7): 794–798.

[4] Alexandre Boutet, Radhika Madhavan, Gavin J.B. Elias, S.E. Joel, Robert Gramer, Manish Ranjan, et al. 2021. Predicting optimal deep brain stimulation parameters for Parkinson's disease using functional MRI and machine learning. Nature Communications. 12(1): 3043.

[5] Mallory L. Hacker, Nanditha Rajamani, Clemens Neudorfer, Barbara Hollunder, Simon Oxenford, Ningfei Li, et al. 2023. Connectivity profile for subthalamic nucleus deep brain stimulation in early stage Parkinson disease. Annals of Neurology. 94(2): 271–284.

[6] Birgit R. Plantinga, Yasin Temel, Yuval Duchin, Kâmil Uludağ, Rémi Patriat, Alard Roebroeck, et al. 2018. Individualized parcellation of the subthalamic nucleus in patients with Parkinson's disease with 7T MRI. Neuroimage. 168: 403–411.

[7] Peter Novak, Andrzej W. Przybyszewski, Andrei Barborica, Paula Ravin, Lee Margolin and Julie G. Pilitsis. 2011. Localization of the subthalamic nucleus in Parkinson disease using multiunit activity. Journal of the Neurological Sciences. 310(1–2): 44–49.

[8] Jana Peeters, Tine Van Bogaert, Alexandra Boogers, Robin Gransier, Jan Wouters, Philippe De Vloo, et al. 2024. Electrophysiological sweet spot mapping in deep brain stimulation for Parkinson's disease patients. Brain Stimulation. 17(4): 794–801.

[9] Qianli Jia, Luyi Jing, Yuxin Zhu, Meiqi Han, Peiyao Jiao, Yu Wang, et al. 2024. Real-time precise targeting of the subthalamic nucleus via transfer learning in a rat model of Parkinson's disease based on microelectrode arrays. *In*: IEEE Transactions on Neural Systems and Rehabilitation Engineering, vol. 32, pp. 1787–1795.

[10] Kai Rui Wan, Tomasz Maszczyk, Angela An Qi See, Justin Dauwels and Nicolas Kon Kam King. 2019. A review on microelectrode recording selection of features for machine learning in deep brain stimulation surgery for Parkinson's disease. Clinical Neurophysiology. 130(1): 145–154.

[11] P.A. Karthick, Kai Rui Wan, Angela See An Qi, Justin Dauwels and Nicolas Kon Kam King. 2020. Automated detection of subthalamic nucleus in deep brain stimulation surgery for Parkinson's disease using microelectrode recordings and wavelet packet features. Journal of Neuroscience Methods. 343: 108826.

[12] Mahsa Khosravi, S.F. Atashzar, G. Gilmore, M.S. Jog, R.V. Patel Ahmed Maged, Minwei Zhu, et al. 2020. Intraoperative localization of STN during DBS surgery using a data-driven model. IEEE Journal of Translational Engineering in Health and Medicine. 8: 1–9.

[13] Konrad A. Ciecierski and Tomasz Mandat. 2024. Classification of DBS microelectrode recordings using a residual neural network with attention in the temporal domain. Neural Networks. 170: 18–31.

[14] Ahmed Maged, Minwei Zhu, Wenpeng Gao and Mohamed Hosny. 2024. Lightweight deep learning model for automated STN localization using MER in Parkinson's disease. Biomedical Signal Processing and Control. 96: 106640.

[15] John A. Thompson, Salam Oukal, Hagai Bergman, Steven Ojemann, Adam O. Hebb, Sara Hanrahan, et al. 2018. Semi-automated application for estimating subthalamic nucleus boundaries and optimal target selection for deep brain stimulation implantation surgery. Journal of Neurosurgery 130(4): 1224–1233.

[16] Linxia Xiao, Caizi Li, Yanjiang Wang, Weixin Si, Doudou Zhang, Hai Lin, et al. 2021. Automatic identification of sweet spots from MERs for electrodes implantation in STN-DBS. International Journal of Computer Assisted Radiology and Surgery 16(5): 809–818.

[17] Zhiguang Wang and Tim Oates. 2015. Encoding time series as images for visual inspection and classification using tiled convolutional neural networks. *In*: Workshops at the twenty-ninth AAAI conference on artificial intelligence. 1: 000091–000096.

[18] Linxia Xiao, Caizi Li, Yanjiang Wang, Weixin Si, Hai Lin, Doudou Zhang, et al. 2022. Amplitude-frequency-aware deep fusion network for optimal contact selection on STN-DBS electrodes. Science China Information Sciences 65(4): 140404.

[19] Hernán Darío Vargas Cardona, Mauricio A. Álvarez and Álvaro A. Orozco. 2018. Multi-task learning for subthalamic nucleus identification in deep brain stimulation. International Journal of Machine Learning and Cybernetics. 9: 1181–1192.

[20] Thibault Martin, Maxime Peralta, Greydon Gilmore, Paul Sauleau, Claire Haegelen, Pierre Jannin, et al. 2021. Extending convolutional neural networks for localizing the sub-thalamic nucleus from micro-electrode recordings in Parkinson's disease. Biomedical Signal Processing and Control. 67: 102529.

[21] Vikram Rajpurohit, Shabbar F. Danish, Eric L. Hargreaves and Stephen Wong. 2015. Optimizing computational feature sets for subthalamic nucleus localization in DBS surgery with feature selection. Clinical Neurophysiology. 126(5): 975–982.

[22] Akshay T. Rao, Kelvin L. Chou and Parag G. Patil. 2023. Localization of deep brain stimulation trajectories via automatic mapping of microelectrode recordings to MRI. Journal of Neural Engineering. 20(1): 016056.

[23] Lori Mann Bruce, Cliff H. Koger and Jiang Li. 2002. Dimensionality reduction of hyperspectral data using discrete wavelet transform feature extraction. *In*: IEEE Transactions on Geoscience and Remote Sensing. 40(10): 2331–2338.

[24] Yiwei Cheng, Manxi Lin, Jun Wu, Haiping Zhu and Xinyu Shao. 2021. Intelligent fault diagnosis of rotating machinery based on continuous wavelet transform-local binary convolutional neural network. Knowledge-Based Systems. 216: 106796.

[25] Jacob B. Salyers, Yue Dong and Yan Gai. 2018. Continuous wavelet transform for decoding finger movements from single-channel EEG. IEEE Transactions on Biomedical Engineering. 66(6): 1588–1597.

Chapter **2.7**

Intelligent Diagnosis and Classification of Intracerebral Hemorrhage

Ruiquan Ge[1]* and Changmiao Wang[2]
[1]Hangzhou Dianzi University, Hangzhou, China
[2]Shenzhen Research Institute of Big Data, Shenzhen, China

2.7.1 INTRODUCTION

ICH is caused by bleeding within the brain due to the rupture of cerebral blood vessels. It ranks as the second most prevalent type of stroke and is characterized by a significantly high mortality rate [1, 2]. Given its prevalence and the serious health impacts, precise diagnosis and prompt intervention are essential for enhancing patient outcomes. Clinicians typically assess ICH prognosis based on the initial volume of the hemorrhage and the location of the hematoma, which guide treatment strategies. Important prognostic factors encompass hemorrhage volume, Glasgow Coma Scale (GCS) score, and other relevant clinical indicators [3–6]. The Glasgow Outcome Scale (GOS) further assesses functional recovery after brain injury.

Computed tomography (CT) is commonly used to diagnose ICH due to its ability to provide rapid and high-resolution images [7, 8]. In clinical settings, it is essential to promptly and accurately assess the severity of acute cerebral hemorrhage. Traditionally, clinicians use CT images to assess the GCS score, which serves as a basis for predicting the GOS score. However, interpreting CT scans

*For Correspondence: gespring@hdu.edu.cn

DOI: 10.1201/9781003518754-12

requires specialized expertise and is often influenced by the clinician's experience and subjective judgment. Integrating artificial intelligence (AI) into this diagnostic process holds significant promise for improving accuracy and consistency.

2.7.1.1 Experiment Dataset

This study analyzed a dataset of 286 patients diagnosed with spontaneous ICH admitted between August 2013 and May 2021. CT scans were performed utilizing the Philips Brilliance 16-slice and Toshiba Aquilion ONE 320-slice CT imaging systems. To be included in the study, patients had to meet specific criteria: a CT scan within 24 hours of hemorrhage, complete GCS scores at admission, GOS scores at discharge, and clinical details such as age, gender, and location of the bleeding. Clinicians meticulously screened the images to emphasize the bleeding areas and reduce irrelevant data, ensuring that each image accurately represented the affected region, which was crucial given the variability in size and shape among patients.

Following image selection, standardization was done by computing the mean and standard deviation while the dataset underwent validation by expert clinicians. To avoid bias from unrelated structures in the CT images, regions of hyperdense intracranial hemorrhage, threshold segmentation, and connected component screening were applied. These techniques, implemented using the OpenCV library, isolated the bleeding areas and removed non-brain tissues. The final processed images included only relevant brain regions, such as the hemorrhagic region, gray matter, and unaffected brain tissue, ensuring data accuracy for subsequent analysis.

2.7.1.2 Functional Metrics

For the classification task, we employed various metrics to assess model effectiveness, including Accuracy, Recall, Precision, and the Area Under the Curve (AUC). Accuracy determines the fraction of correctly classified instances relative to the total number of instances. Recall, or sensitivity, measures the model's capability to accurately identify positive cases, while precision indicates the fraction of true positives among all predicted positives. AUC offers a comprehensive evaluation by considering the balance between true positive and false positive rates.

For segmentation tasks, we used additional metrics like the Dice Similarity Coefficient (DSC), Jaccard Index, 95% Hausdorff Distance (95HD), and Per-Region-Overlap (PRO). The DSC evaluates the overlap between predicted and actual regions, whereas the Jaccard Index measures the intersection over the union of these regions. The 95HD assesses the largest spatial discrepancy between predicted and actual boundaries, excluding the worst 5% of outliers, thus providing a robust measure of segmentation accuracy. Lastly, PRO examines the overlap of predicted regions with ground truth on a per-region basis, offering detailed insights into the model's spatial accuracy.

2.7.2 GCS-ICHNET: ASSESSMENT OF INTRACEREBRAL HEMORRHAGE PROGNOSIS USING SELF-ATTENTION WITH DOMAIN KNOWLEDGE INTEGRATION

2.7.2.1 Introduction

ICH, resulting from the rupture of weakened cerebral vessels, is the second most prevalent cause of stroke, whereas ischemic stroke is the most prevalent cause, and both are associated with high morbidity and mortality. Accurate and timely prognosis and prompt therapeutic intervention are vital for improving patient outcomes. Traditional prognostic methods, however, often rely on the subjective judgment of clinicians, which can lead to diagnostic inaccuracies and less effective treatments.

Table 7.1 The classification comparisons between GCS-ICHNet and other methods. "Acc" indicates the precision of predicting patient prognosis results, and "AUC" denotes the area under the Receiver Operating Characteristic (ROC) curve. Additionally, "TPR" refers to sensitivity, while "TNR" refers to specificity

Methods	Acc (%)	AUC (10^{-2})	TPR (%)	TNR (%)
ICH score metrics	74	0.80	74	76
Imaging-based classifier	72	0.80	73	71
ML-based classifier	77	0.84	77	76
GCS-ICHNet	**85**	**0.86**	**80**	**83**

To overcome these limitations, we developed GCS-ICHNet, which integrates multimodal data by combining brain CT images with GCS scores as domain-specific knowledge. The baseline prognostic evaluation is based on analyzing brain CT images. We further examined the role of GCS and designed a multilayer perceptron-based GCS module to enhance prognostic predictions. GCS-ICHNet also uses an attention-based gradient-domain multi-modal feature fusion technique to integrate features across different data types effectively.

Experimental results demonstrate that our model, utilizing GCS domain knowledge, outperforms several traditional machine learning-based prognostic methods and achieves greater sensitivity than clinicians with varying levels of expertise [9–11].

2.7.2.2 Method Details

GCS-ICHNet comprises three key components, including the feature extraction module, the feature fusion module, and the final classification. In the feature extraction module, we use a ResNet-50 backbone to derive features from CT slices, which also helps mitigate overfitting due to limited data. Following this, several linear and dropout layers capture the final features extracted from CT slices, resulting in a 128-dimensional vector. We connect GCS scores to the feature extraction module via a multilayer perceptron (MLP) to incorporate domain knowledge. This MLP comprises three hidden layers featuring 32, 128, and 256 neurons, which ultimately output a 64-dimensional vector. The GCS scores and CT slice features are aligned to the same dimensionality to enable seamless fusion.

The initial stepof feture fusion module involves integrating the image features obtained from CT scans with the GCS score features. The merging process is defined by the equation:

$$f_{\text{global}} = unsqueeze(Concat(Conv(x_i), wg_i + b)) \tag{1}$$

where f_{global} represents the combined CT and GCS features, while wg denotes the weights and b denotes biases, separately, with i indicating the dataset index. A decompression function increases the feature dimensionality to be processed by the subsequent encoder.

Table 7.2 Comparison between GCS-ICHNet and assessments by neurosurgeons on CT slices. The "Neurosurgeon1," "Neurosurgeon2," and "Neurosurgeon3," have 2.5, 3.5, and 14 years of relevant work experience, respectively. In this study, "CT" and "CT+GCS" denote the baseline dataset and the GCS-ICHNet dataset, respectively. TPR and TNR mean sensitivity and specificity

Test	**CT (%)**	**TPR (%)**	**TNR (%)**	**CT + GCS (%)**	**TPR (%)**	**TNR (%)**
Neurosurgeon1	57.75	27.40	94.48	54.75	22.79	91.89
Neurosurgeon2	58.00	25.11	97.79	67.25	41.86	96.76
Neurosurgeon3	73.25	**69.14**	77.90	–	–	–
Neurosurgeon Avg.	63.00	40.64	90.05	66.50	45.89	90.45
Baseline	77.75	78.54	76.80	–	–	–
GCS-ICHNet	–	–	–	**88.00**	**85.12**	**91.35**

The combined feature vector is subsequently processed through a transformer encoder, which utilizes a self-attention module with 16 attention heads to integrate features from CT and GCS. The self-attention mechanism captures the relationships between GCS scores and CT images, mathematically expressed as:

$$f_{mix} = concat(head_1, \ldots, head_j)W^O, \tag{2}$$

Meanwhile,

$$head_j = softmax\left(\frac{Q_j K_j^T}{\sqrt{d_k}}\right)V_j, \; j \in (1, 16), \tag{3}$$

where f_{mix} denotes the mixed features, W^O is the output weight matrix, and Q_j, K_j, and V are the results from multiplying the weight matrices corresponding to the various attention heads within f_{global}. Here, d_k is the dimensionality of the key vectors, and j indexes the various attention heads.

Finally, the integrated features are forwarded to a 1D DenseNet-121 classification head, designed to mitigate overfitting and guarantee robust generalization. During training, the Adam optimizer is used, and cross-entropy loss is utilized to compute the error of the predictions.

2.7.2.3 Performance of GCS-ICHNet

We evaluated the performance of GCS-ICHNet against several traditional prognostic classification methods, with the results detailed in Table 7.1. Traditional metrics like the ICH score assess the severity and prognosis of strokes by utilizing clinical features and neuroimaging data collected at the time of admission to predict patient outcomes. The classifier based on imaging predicts prognosis by relying on image texture features, whereas the classifier utilizing ML integrates these features with the ICH score metrics. Our findings show that GCS-ICHNet significantly outperformed these methods, achieving 8% to 13% improvement in accuracy. This enhancement highlights the ability of deep neural networks to effectively harness domain knowledge and CT images to derive valuable, actionable insights.

To further evaluate the clinical utility of our approach, we conducted a study involving two groups: one comprising 400 randomly selected CT slices from 223 unique patients with only the original CT images, and the other including both the CT images and their corresponding GCS scores for the same patients. In order to maintain anonymity, all patient-related information was removed. We engaged neurosurgeons with varying levels of expertise to predict patient outcomes based on these datasets and compared their predictions to those generated by our method. The results of this comparison are summarized in Table 7.2.

Our findings indicate that using GCS scores improved the prognostic accuracy of neurosurgeons by 3.5% compared to the baseline, while GCS-ICHNet increased accuracy by 10.25%. However, for patients with stricter diagnostic criteria, the GCS scores had a limited impact on enhancing prediction accuracy. While GCS scores can be valuable indicators, neurosurgeons may subjectively minimize their importance. Notably, neurosurgeons typically showed high specificity but low sensitivity, and less experienced surgeons often classified all cases as negative, reflecting a significant degree of subjectivity. In contrast, GCS-ICHNet consistently provided more reliable and superior performance.

2.7.3 ICHPRO: INTRACEREBRAL HEMORRHAGE PROGNOSIS CLASSIFICATION VIA JOINT-ATTENTION MECHANISM

2.7.3.1 Introduction

ICH has a mortality rate exceeding 40%, with only about 20% of survivors achieving functional independence. Accurate prognosis prediction is essential for creating effective treatment plans for patients after ICH. Experienced neurosurgeons rely primarily on CT scans, focusing on the hemorrhage's location, volume, and specific clinical details as key evaluation criteria. Other factors include the patient's age, sex, and GCS score. However, this evaluation process relies heavily on the manual assessments of neurosurgeons, making it labor-intensive and susceptible to variability and inaccuracies due to individual experience and subjective biases.

In order to overcome the challenges, pioneering research has explored machine learning algorithms, which have achieved some success but still leave much room for improvement. While cross-modal methods provide richer and more comprehensive information, the application of the method in predicting the prognosis of ICH has encountered significant limitations, including fusion-based and deep learning approaches, have made progress by combining extracted images with clinical features. GCS-ICHNet, in particular, stands out by leveraging a self-attention mechanism to integrate images with specialized domain knowledge seamlessly, thereby boosting its performance. Unfortunately, these methodologies are often deficient in effective fusion mechanisms, which can hinder the establishment of meaningful relationships and inter-modal correlations between CT and clinical modalities.

Our method demonstrates clear superiority over existing approaches, such as the DL-Based Method [12], Multi-Task Method [13], and UniMiSS [14]. ICHPro offers a more comprehensive integration of data, improving the accuracy and reliability of ICH prognosis.

2.7.3.2 Method Details

ICHPro is comprised of three core components that sequentially drive the process: the feature extraction module, the joint-attention fusion module, and the classification module. At the forefront, the feature extraction module leverages the powerful BioClinicalBERT model, which has been pre-trained, to produce comprehensive text representations, denoted as f^t, and the pre-trained 3D ResNet-50 to produce visual representations, f^v. Within the classification module, the pre-trained 1D DenseNet-121 architecture serves as the classification component, tasked with determining the final categories.

Joint-Attention Fusion Module

This module initially processes the text feature f^t through the text representation transformation (TRT) block. Simultaneously, the vision feature f^v is processed through the vision representation transformation (VRT) block. This process produces an integrated, reconstructed text representation f^t and a reconstructed vision representation f^v. These representations are fed into a cross-modal attention fusion (CMAF) block, followed by a multi-head self-attention fusion (MHSAF) block. Ultimately, this sequence of operations results in a text-based vision representation f^{tbv}.

In these processing blocks, we transform f^t and f^v into compatible formats to enhance the semantic connection across both modalities. Within the TRT block, f^t is first multiplied by its transpose, f^{tT}, and processed through a fully connected (FC) layer. This is followed by a reshaping layer, yielding the transformed f^t. Conversely, in the VRT block, f^v transforms an FC layer, which is then followed by four up-sampling layers, resulting in the final form of f^v.

CMAF Block

Drawing partial inspiration from the cross-modal fusion component of the CMAFGAN [15] framework, originally developed for word-to-face generation tasks, we have adapted this approach for fusing modal and tailored it to fit our specific application. To further optimize efficiency, we incorporated a SoftPool layer, which helps decrease computational demands while maintaining essential information. The block's overall framework has undergone reorganization.

We start by reducing the dimensions of the inputs f^v and f^t using an FC layer, labeling the results as x and y. These are then independently mapped into three separate feature domains using 1×1 convolution layers, identified as (V_1, K_1, Q_1) and (V_2, K_2, Q_2), with the weights denoted by ω and corresponding superscripts. Following these transformations, the matching degree can be calculated as follows:

$$\beta_{j,i} = \frac{\exp(S_{ij})}{\sum_{i=1}^{S} \exp(S_{ij})} \quad \text{where } S_{ij} = \omega Q_1 x_i^T \times \omega^{K_2} y_j, \tag{4}$$

$$\rho_{i,j} = \frac{\exp(t_{ij})}{\sum_{i=1}^{S} \exp(t_{ij})} \quad \text{where } t_{ij} = \omega Q_2 y_i^T \times \omega^{K_1} x_j \tag{5}$$

2.7.3.3 Performance of ICHPro

We evaluated ICHPro against a range of sophisticated techniques using our dataset, and the outcomes are concisely presented in Table 7.3. The first four methods listed in the table are tailored for predicting ICH prognosis. In contrast, UniMiSS is a flexible medical image classification network that seamlessly integrates 2D and 3D convolutional approaches. Notably, the 2D GCS-ICHNet, enriched with domain-specific knowledge, attains accuracy levels that rival the 3D multi-task method, which solely relies on imaging data. Intriguingly, it even outperforms the general-purpose 2D + 3D UniMiSS method. Both ICHPro and the deep learning (DL) approach leverage extensive demographic and clinical data, leading to superior AUC scores compared to other methodologies. This highlights the superior robustness of networks.

When compared to the DL method, ICHPro exhibits superior performance across all evaluated metrics, highlighting the efficacy of our joint-attention fusion mechanism. Our approach achieves a notable increase in accuracy by 3.69% and an AUC improvement of 0.0288 over the top-performing metrics of other methods. In summary, our method significantly surpasses the comparison methods, and to our knowledge, it surpasses the performance of existing advanced techniques in classifying ICH prognosis on our dataset.

Table 7.3 Comparisons of ICHPro and other methods

Method	Acc (%)	Recall (%)	Prec (%)	F1 Score	AUC (10^{-2})
Image-Based Method (2D)	74.23	67.11	75.98	0.7127	0.6933
GCS-ICHNet (2D)	85.08	81.88	87.25	0.8448	0.8590
DL-based Method (3D)	81.02	78.52	83.31	0.8084	0.9141
Multi-Task Method (3D)	85.42	79.86	89.80	0.8454	0.8998
UniMiSS (2D+3D)	82.03	78.52	87.59	0.8281	0.8275
ICHPro	**89.11**	**84.56**	**91.02**	**0.8767**	**0.9429**

2.7.4 ICH-SCNET: SEGMENTATION AND PROGNOSIS CLASSIFICATION NETWORK USING CLIP-GUIDED SAM MECHANISM

2.7.4.1 Introduction

ICH is a pressing public health issue, affecting more than 2 million individuals each year and accounting for 10–15% of all stroke incidents. Despite notable advancements in medical imaging technologies, especially with CT scans and continuous research endeavors, a comprehensive treatment option that addresses all stages of ICH remains elusive. As a result, mortality rates and the incidence of long-term disabilities among ICH survivors have not experienced a significant decline.

Effective treatment strategies for ICH critically depend on precise segmentation of ICH lesions and accurate prognosis predictions [16]. Currently, these tasks primarily rely on manual annotations and evaluations conducted by neurosurgeons, which are not only time-consuming but also susceptible to individual biases and variations in expertise. Many existing ICH-related models have limited scope, lack multifunctionality, and fail to leverage non-image data modalities fully. This oversight forgoes the potential benefits of information sharing across different modalities and tasks, which could significantly enhance the overall performance of the models.

In the realm of medical imaging, segmentation tasks demand meticulous pixel-level precision, whereas classification tasks involve assigning categorical labels to entire images. There exists a profound interplay between these two tasks: classification furnishes semantic context that enhances segmentation, while segmentation provides granular details that bolster the accuracy of classification. Acknowledging this mutual dependency can substantially elevate the fidelity of segmentation and bolster the reliability of prognostic predictions, ultimately translating to superior patient outcomes. Despite the adoption of multi-task approaches by some medical imaging networks, those tailored to ICH remain comparatively scant. Consequently, there is a pressing need for a multi-task network capable of concurrently executing ICH segmentation and prognosis classification, effectively harnessing the intrinsic correlations between these tasks.

Another significant challenge is the seamless integration of multifaceted medical information into predictive models. Relying solely on imaging data is frequently insufficient due to the complex nature of medical tasks, necessitating a holistic assortment of data. In biomedical contexts, particularly those pertaining to the brain, it is customary to incorporate non-imaging data, such as domain expertise, diagnostic reports, and patient demographics. Recent methodologies have endeavored to amalgamate image features with auxiliary medical data through rudimentary concatenation techniques, but this approach offers only cursory cross-modal interaction. Efforts to integrate tabular data, domain-specific insights, and textual medical reports are indeed progressing, yet these methodologies still require substantial refinement. In particular, there is a need to establish robust internal dependencies among cross-modal features to enhance the coherence and efficacy of the integrated information.

Our method, ICH-SCNet, leverages the Segment Anything Model (SAM) for segmenting information and Contrastive Language-Image Pre-training (CLIP) for fusing text and images. We argue that combining these two models can effectively address the challenge of merging distinct modalities. Our approach demonstrates comprehensive superiority over existing methods, including image-based approaches [10], DL-PP [12], TOP-GPM [17], AMCons [18], IHA-Net [19], nnU-Net [20], SAM [21], MedSAM [22], ResGANet [23], and SelfMedMAE [24]. Our model consistently outperforms these methods in classification and segmentation tasks, achieving significant improvements across all key performance metrics.

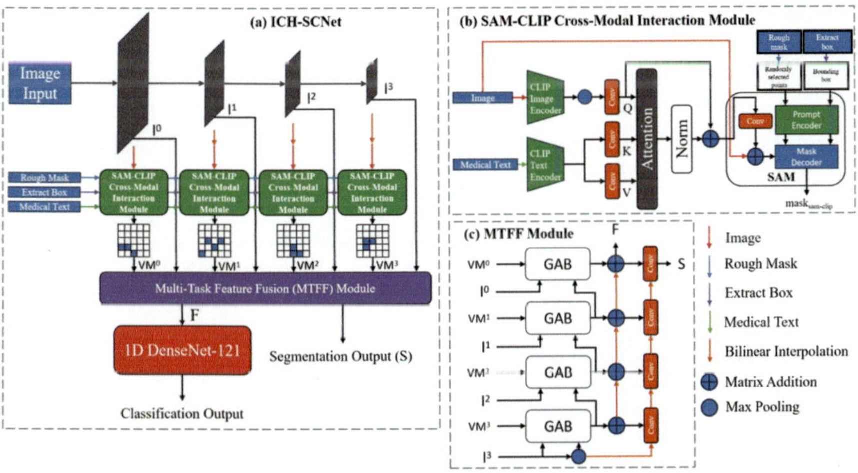

Figure 7.1 (a) Overview of the framework of ICH-SCNet, including depictions of (b) the SAM-CLIP Cross-Modal Interaction module and (c) the MTFF module.

2.7.4.2 Method Details

Our approach starts by employing three down-sampling layers to generate image features at four scales: $\{I_0, I_1, I_2, I_3\}$. In order to accommodate the use of the standard Vision Transformer (ViT) in the SAM image encoder, bilinear interpolation is applied to the features $\{I_1, I_2, I_3\}$, ensuring they are properly resized. These interpolated features are combined with clinical text information, and extracted boxes and rough masks are used as segmentation prompts. Together, these features are then fed into four separate SAM-CLIP cross-modal interaction modules. Each module processes these inputs to produce valid masks at the corresponding scales: $\{VM_0, VM_1, VM_2, VM_3\}$.

After obtaining the multi-scale image features that valid masks have refined, our model incorporates a Multi-Task Feature Fusion (MTFF) module, leveraging group bridge structures to integrate these features effectively. The integrated feature output (**F**) from the previous step is input into a DenseNet-121 classifier. Simultaneously, a segmentation output (S) is produced, representing the definitive segmentation result.

Moreover, a pivotal aspect of our approach is incorporating a multi-task loss function. This function is meticulously crafted to maximize the performance of each individual task while simultaneously acknowledging and exploiting the intrinsic interconnections and correlations between classification and segmentation. It holds a fundamental role in adeptly capturing and harnessing these interdependencies during the model's training phase, thereby enhancing the overall effectiveness of the dual-task network.

SAM-CLIP Cross-Modal Interaction Module

As noted, SAM and CLIP are two foundational models with distinct strengths. SAM-based models are tailored for segmentation tasks, utilizing masks and bounding box prompts, while CLIP-based models excel in interpreting the semantics of text and image data. We propose a SAM-CLIP cross-modal interaction module to harness both advantages. The primary concept is to leverage CLIP's semantic capabilities to produce an initial rough mask, denoted as M_{clip}. This initial mask serves as a guiding constraint for SAM, enabling it to refine and enhance the segmentation outcomes, thus achieving more accurate and reliable results.

At the outset, the CLIP image encoder symbolized as En_{clip}^{img}, processes the incoming image data, whereas the CLIP text encoder, symbolized as En_{clip}^{text}, manages the text input t. Our approach innovatively incorporates a customized attention function, where the text embeddings generated for the query Q^t apply a sequence of operations to the image data. Firstly, a max-pooling layer extracts essential spatial features, followed by a convolutional layer that further refines the representation. Next, distinct convolutional layers are utilized to transform the text features, resulting in the generation of the Key, denoted as K^t, and the Value, denoted as V^t.

An attention mechanism facilitates the interplay between these modalities, further enhanced by residual connections that seamlessly integrate the Q^t with the output from a normalization layer. The rough mask M_{clip} is calculated through this process, providing a foundational guide for refining segmentation results.

$$M_{clip} = Norm(Att(Q^t, K^t, V^t)) + En_{clip}^{img}(v). \tag{6}$$

We refined the rough mask Mclip from the previous step using SAM. This refinement process leverages bounding box and mask prompts to produce a valid mask. Initially, the bounding box prompt is merged with the rough mask to form a bounding box b along with a set of randomly selected points p. These inputs are then processed by the SAM prompt encoder En_{sam}^{pmt}.

The final SAM-CLIP valid mask, referred to as $mask_{sam-clip}$, is generated by the SAM mask encoder En_{sam}^{mk}, which refines the rough segmentation using the original image, adhering to the constraints established by the prompts. Consequently, the valid mask VM is thus represented as follows:

$$VM = En_{sam}^{mk}\left((Conv(M_{clip}) + I), En_{sam}^{pmt}(\beta, \eta)\right). \quad (7)$$

MTFF Module

The variability in size and appearance of medical lesions in CT scans presents a formidable challenge for algorithms, which must be efficient and adaptable for clinical use. To overcome this, we have devised a sophisticated MTFF module capable of managing multiple tasks concurrently. As depicted in Figure 7.1, our MTFF module is structured into four hierarchical levels, ascending from lower to higher resolutions. Taking inspiration from the group bridge structures found in EGE-UNet [25], we have integrated a Group Aggregation Bridge (GAB) to seamlessly blend image feature I at each stage with their respective valid mask VM and the outputs from the preceding stage. These combined features then serve as the input for the subsequent stage.

To generate a predicted mask at each stage, we employ pixel-wise summation of the integrated features and apply a convolutional layer. These predictions are then compared to their corresponding segmentation labels to compute a loss function. Upon completing the process, we obtain two outputs: the segmentation prediction, known as the segmentation output S, and the multi-scale fused features, referred to as the feature output F.

Our GAB is designed with three primary inputs: the image feature, the valid mask, and the lower-level feature. These inputs are first concatenated sequentially within four distinct groups. We then apply dilated convolution to each group, utilizing dilation rates of {1, 3, 5, 7} and a kernel size 3. The outputs from these four groups are then concatenated and passed through an additional convolutional layer to achieve fusion. This innovative approach allows our MTFF module to handle the variability of medical lesions in CT scans with remarkable efficiency and accuracy.

2.7.4.3 Performance of ICH-SCNet

We conducted an exhaustive evaluation of our proposed ICH-SCNet by benchmarking it against a diverse range of state-of-the-art (SOTA) methodologies in the intricate fields of ICH segmentation and prognosis classification. Our initial comparison involved scrutinizing ICH-SCNet against five classification models, encompassing two that rely solely on single-modality data and three cross-modal methods that integrate supplementary medical information. For segmentation tasks, we gauged its performance against two ICH-specific networks and three broad medical segmentation frameworks. Given the rarity of multi-task approaches

Table 7.4 Comparisons with state-of-art (SOTA) methods

No.	Method	Classification				Segmentation			
		Acc (%) (10^{-2})	**Recall (%)**	**Prec (%)**	**AUC**	**DSC (%)**	**Jaccard (%)**	**95HD**	**PRO (%)**
1	Image-based	81.51	76.20	82.85	80.79	–	–	–	–
2	DL-PP	83.32	79.68	83.95	80.74	–	–	–	–
3	GCS-ICHNet	85.08	81.88	85.90	85.90	–	–	–	–
4	TOP-GPM	89.34	84.62	84.61	84.61	–	–	–	–
5	ICHPro	90.71	84.56	91.02	94.29	–	–	–	–
6	AMCCons	–	–		– –	85.18	72.27	4.71	81.88
7	IHA-Net	–	–		– –	84.63	71.70	4.23	80.79
8	nnU-Net	–	–		– –	83.32	71.63	4.68	78.43
9	SAM	–	–		– –	84.99	71.68	5.42	78.55
10	MedSAM	–	–		– –	85.14	72.89	4.89	82.17
11	ResGANet	82.61	75.13	83.06	83.94	81.94	67.54	12.42	82.17
12	SelfMedMAE	84.84	79.99	85.76	85.76	82.36	67.60	10.68	82.06
*	ICH-SCNet	**90.71**	**84.99**	**91.91**	**95.11**	**88.32**	**76.70**	**2.77**	**86.43**

that simultaneously tackle both ICH segmentation and prognosis classification, we incorporated two generic medical multi-task networks into our comparative analysis. The detailed outcomes of these comparisons are presented in Table 7.4.

ICH-SCNet emerged as a standout performer, demonstrating substantial improvements in segmentation and classification capabilities, as evidenced by four segmentation metrics and four classification metrics. In the realm of classification, our method shone brightly in three metrics, trailing only slightly behind the TOP-GPM model. When compared to networks focused exclusively on classification using imaging data, ICH-SCNet offered a decisive edge. Furthermore, the benefits of multi-task information sharing became evident when pitted against other cross-modal methodologies.

In segmentation tasks, ICH-SCNet consistently surpassed rival methods across all four metrics, including those leveraging the SAM approach. The general multi-task methods fell short in competitiveness, potentially due to inadequate mechanisms for task coordination. Overall, ICH-SCNet bolstered classification accuracy by 1.27%, recall by 0.43%, and AUC by 0.82%. For segmentation, it exhibited notable enhancements with a 3.14% increase in the DSC, a 3.81% surge in the Jaccard index, a reduction of 1.43 units in the 95HD, and a 3.75% improvement in PRO.

2.7.5 CONCLUSION

ICH poses a significant threat to human life, making timely detection and treatment essential. Delays and errors in diagnosis can critically impact patient outcomes. This chapter explores three innovative approaches for diagnosing and classifying ICH: GCS-ICHNet, ICH-Pro, and ICH-SCNet. The GCS-ICHNet method combines brain CT images with the GCS scores, integrating them into a multimodal fusion network to enhance diagnostic accuracy. Meanwhile, ICHPro utilizes pre-trained models alongside a joint-attention fusion module, effectively merging image and text features. This approach aims to improve the precision of ICH detection. Moving forward, ICH-SCNet employs SAM-CLIP technology to integrate text and image data, facilitating a multi-task approach to ICH diagnosis. Compared to traditional methods, these three advanced techniques significantly enhance segmentation and classification performance, thereby offering potential improvements in managing ICH cases.

REFERENCES

[1] Emblem, K.E., M.C. Pinho, F.G. Zöllner, P. Due-Tonnessen, J.K. Hald, L.R. Schad, et al. 2015. A generic support vector machine model for preoperative glioma survival associations. Radiology. 275(1): 228–234.

[2] Poon, M.T., S.M. Bell and R. Al-Shahi Salman. 2015. Epidemiology of intracerebral haemorrhage. New Insights in Intracerebral Hemorrhage. 37: 1–12.

[3] Gurevitz, C., E. Auriel, A. Elis and R. Kornowski. 2022. The association between low levels of low density lipoprotein cholesterol and intracerebral hemorrhage: cause for concern? Journal of Clinical Medicine. 11(3): 536.

[4] Shan, X., X. Li, R. Ge, S. Wu, A. Elazab, J. Zhu, et al. 2023. GCS-ICHNet: assessment of intracerebral hemorrhage prognosis using self-attention with domain knowledge integration. International Conference on Bioinformatics and Biomedicine. 2217–2222.

[5] Yu, X., X. Li, R. Ge, S. Wu, A. Elazab, J. Zhu, et al. 2024. ICHPro: Intracerebral hemorrhage prognosis classification via joint-attention fusion-based 3D cross-modal network. International Symposium on Biomedical Imaging. 1–5.

[6] Yu, X., A. Elazab, R. Ge, J. Zhu, L. Zhang, G. Jia, et al. 2025. ICH-PRNet: A cross-modal intracerebral haemorrhage prognostic prediction method using joint-attention interaction mechanism. Neural Networks. 184: 107096.

[7] Lim, M.J.R., A.Y.Y. Neo, G.D. Singh, Y.S.T. Liew, M.F. Rajendram, M.W.X. Tan, et al. 2020. The evaluation of prognostic scores in spontaneous intracerebral hemorrhage in an Asian population: A retrospective study. Journal of Stroke and Cerebrovascular Diseases. 29(12): 105360.

[8] Thierry AGM Huisman. 2005. Intracranial hemorrhage: ultrasound, CT and MRI findings. European Radiology. 15(3): 434–440.

[9] Gregório, T., S. Pipa, P. Cavaleiro, G. Atanásio, I. Albuquerque, P.C. Chaves, et al. 2018. Prognostic models for intracerebral hemorrhage: Systematic review and meta-analysis. BMC Medical Research Methodology. 18: 145.

[10] Wang, H.L., W.Y. Hsu, M.H. Lee, H.H. Weng, S.W. Chang, J.T. Yang, et al. 2019. Automatic machine-learning-based outcome prediction in patients with primary intracerebral hemorrhage. Frontiers in Neurology. 10: 910.

[11] Nawabi, J., H. Kniep, S. Elsayed, C. Friedrich, P. Sporns, T. Rusche, et al. 2021. Imaging-based outcome prediction of acute intracerebral hemorrhage. Translational Stroke Research. 12: 958–967.

[12] Pérez del Barrio, A., A.S. Esteve Domínguez, P. Menéndez Fernández-Miranda, P. Sanz Bellón, D. Rodríguez González, L. Lloret Iglesias, et al. 2023. A deep learning model for prognosis prediction after intracranial hemorrhage. Journal of Neuroimaging. 33(2): 218–226.

[13] Gong, K., Q. Dai, J. Wang, Y. Zheng, T. Shi, J. Yu, et al. 2023. Unified ICH quantification and prognosis prediction in NCCT images using a multi-task interpretable network. Frontiers in Neuroscience. 17: 1118340.

[14] Xie, Y., J. Zhang, Y. Xia and Q. Wu. 2022. Unimiss: Universal medical self-supervised learning via breaking dimensionality barrier. European Conference on Computer Vision. Springer. 558–575.

[15] Luo, X., X. Chen, X. He, L. Qing and X. Tan. 2022. CMAFGAN: A cross-modal attention fusion based generative adversarial network for attribute word-to-face synthesis. Knowledge-Based Systems. 255: 109750.

[16] Yu, X., A. Elazab, R. Ge, H. Jin, X. Jiang, G. Jia, et al. 2024. ICH-SCNet: intracerebral hemorrhage segmentation and prognosis classification network using CLIP-guided SAM mechanism. International Conference on Bioinformatics and Biomedicine. 2795–2800.

[17] Ma, W., C. Chen, J. Abrigo, C.H.K. Mak, Y. Gong, N.Y. Chan, et al. 2023. Treatment Outcome Prediction for Intracerebral Hemorrhage via Generative Prognostic Model

with Imaging and Tabular Data. International Conference on Medical Image Computing and Computer-Assisted Intervention. Springer. 715–725.

[18] Silva-Rodríguez, J., V. Naranjo and J. Dolz. 2022. Constrained unsupervised anomaly segmentation. Medical Image Analysis. 80: 102526.

[19] Ma, Y., F. Ren, W. Li, N. Yu, D. Zhang, Y. Li, et al. 2023. IHA-Net: An automatic segmentation framework for computer-tomography of tiny intracerebral hemorrhage based on improved attention U-net. Biomedical Signal Processing and Control. 80: 104320.

[20] Isensee, F., P.F. Jaeger, S.A. Kohl, J. Petersen and K.H. Maier-Hein. 2021. nnU-Net: A self-configuring method for deep learning-based biomedical image segmentation. Nature Methods. 18(2): 203–211.

[21] Kirillov, A., E. Mintun, N. Ravi, H. Mao, C. Rolland, L. Gustafson, et al. 2023. Segment anything. *In*: Proceedings of the IEEE/CVF International Conference on Computer Vision. 4015–4026.

[22] Ma, J., Y. He, F. Li, L. Han, C. You and B. Wang. 2024. Segment anything in medical images. Nature Communications. 15(1): 654.

[23] Cheng, J., S. Tian, L. Yu, C. Gao, X. Kang, X. Ma, et al. 2022. ResGANet: Residual group attention network for medical image classification and segmentation. Medical Image Analysis. 76: 102313.

[24] Zhou, L., H. Liu, J. Bae, J. He, D. Samaras and P. Prasanna. 2023. Self pre-training with masked autoencoders for medical image classification and segmentation. *In*: 2023 IEEE 20th International Symposium on Biomedical Imaging (ISBI). IEEE. 1–6.

[25] Ruan, J., M. Xie, J. Gao, T. Liu and Y. Fu. 2023. Ege unet: an efficient group enhanced Unet for skin lesion segmentation. *In*: International Conference on Medical Image Computing and Computer-Assisted Intervention. Springer. 481–490.

Chapter 2.8

Prediction and Diagnosis for Autism Spectrum Disorder

Weihao Zheng*, Ying Wang, Mingwen Zhang, Jialong Li and Bin Hu*
School of Information Science and Engineering, Lanzhou University, Lanzhou 730000, China

2.8.1 INTRODUCTION

Autism spectrum disorder (ASD) is a lifelong neurodevelopmental disorder that typically emerges in the first years of life. Individuals with ASD commonly exhibit impaired social abilities, repetitive and stereotyped behaviors, and interests [1]. The clinical diagnosis of ASD can typically be made as early as 18–24 months of age [2]. Rapid developmental changes during infancy and early childhood contribute to the dynamic presentation of ASD symptoms, highlighting the need for reliable tools for early identification and timely intervention. Existing magnetic resonance imaging (MRI) studies have revealed abnormal developmental patterns in brain structure, function, and connectivity in individuals with ASD. However, the clinical phenotypes of ASD remain highly heterogeneous, and the underlying neurobiological mechanisms are not fully characterized. In order to address this, several studies have focused on identifying subtypes through unsupervised clustering algorithms based on morphological measurements and functional connectivity to facilitate ASD diagnosis. In addition, recent advances in machine learning and deep learning methods utilizing multimodal MRI data have shown promise in predicting autistic symptoms.

* For Correspondence: zhengweihao@lzu.edu.cn; bh@lzu.edu.cn

DOI: 10.1201/9781003518754-13

This article integrates multiple modalities, including structural, functional, and diffusion MRI biomarkers, to comprehensively understand autism conditions. We also present a detailed description of subtype classification and prediction models based on multi-modal MRI data, highlighting how these approaches can enhance the diagnostic accuracy of ASD and deepen our understanding of this brain disorder. Finally, we discuss the future directions for improving predictive modeling in ASD.

2.8.2 MRI-DRIVEN BIOMARKERS FOR EARLY DIAGNOSIS OF ASD

The first years of life are crucial for the establishment of subsequent higher-order social, emotional, and communication functions, as well as for early intervention of psychiatric disorders. Existing studies have identified specific neurodevelopmental differences in brain anatomy, functional activity, and connectivity underlying specific autistic symptoms. These differences often manifest before and coincide with the onset of behavioral symptoms in infants later diagnosed with autism.

2.8.2.1 Structural MRI-based Biomarkers

Several prospective studies using structural MRI have suggested that early abnormal variations in brain morphology, microstructure, and connectivity could be important factors in the etiology and prognosis of ASD. In terms of macro-structural development, brain overgrowth has been consistently identified as a risk factor for autism by multiple independent research groups (Table 8.1). For instance, in a longitudinal study [3], researchers studied 15 six-month-old infants with an older sibling diagnosed with ASD (high risk, HR) and 42 infants with an older sibling without evidence of ASD and no family history of a first or second-degree relative with ASD (low risk, LR). This study revealed that the HR group exhibited significant brain overgrowth compared to the LR group, along with hyperexpansion of cortical surface area (SA) between 6 and 12 months preceding brain volume overgrowth observed between 12 and 24 months [3] (Figures 8.1A, B). Importantly, SA was identified as a predictive marker for autism diagnosis. Although this study did not confirm whether these changes were specific to autism, it demonstrated the emergence and predictive capability of early biomarkers.

Similarly, previous studies of cortical thickness (CT) and SA in ASD toddlers of the same age range have indicated comparable CT but significantly greater SA in the ASD group relative to the typically developing (TD) toddlers [6, 7]. For specific brain regions, Wolff et al. reported significantly increased SA and CT in the corpus callosum of toddlers with ASD, starting as early as 6 months [8]. A longitudinal study showed that infants with ASD had significantly greater extra-axial cerebrospinal fluid at 6–9 months, which can predict the severity of autistic symptoms at 24–36 months [9]. Head circumference (HC) has also been shown to be abnormally enlarged during early development in ASD, especially between 1 to 3 years of age [10–14], with the effect being more pronounced in males [15–17]. Cross-sectional and longitudinal studies have found that toddlers with ASD aged 2–4 years have a larger brain volume relative to typical peers, particularly in the frontal and temporal cortices [11, 18–21].

Table 8.1 Summary of studies on ASD brain volume differences

Studies	Sample (ASD/TD)	Age (years)	Findings in ASD Group
[18]	(60/52)	2–4	90% of ASD had larger brain volume
[19]	(38/39)	2–3	Enlargement of WM volumes in frontal
[10]	(48)	2–5	Increased HC between 6 to 14 months
[11]	(51/25)	0–3	Increased HC and volumes around 12 months
[12]	(16/12)	0–3	Higher growth rate in HC
[14]	(35/37)	0–2	Larger HC by 10 to 14 months
[13]	(28)	0–3	HC rapidly increased during 1 year, decelerated after
[20]	(41/44)	1.5–5	Both WM and GM were enlarged at 2.5 years
[16]	(280/609)	0–1	Increased HC from 3 to 12 months in males
[15]	(64/55)	0–2	Larger HC by age 9.5 months in males
[6]	(38/21)	2	No significant differences in CT, but an increase in SA
[9]	(33/22)	0.5–2	Larger total cerebral volumes at both 12–15 and 18–24 months
[21]	(50)	0–3	Increased volumes in global GM and WM
[7]	(112/50)	3	Greater SA and comparable CT
[17]	(400)	3–5	15% of ASD males demonstrated megalencephaly
[11]	(106/42)	0.5–2	Overgrowth of SA preceded brain volume
[22]	(24/26)	0.3–0.5	Larger cerebellar and subcortical volumes in HR infants
[23]	(58/109)	0.5–2	Faster amygdala growth between 6 and 24 months
[24]	(101)	0.3–0.5	The volumes of the left hippocampus and thalamus can predict later ASD

Gray matter (GM), white matter (WM), head circumference (HC), cortical thickness (CT), surface area (SA); HR (high risk) radial, and axial diffusivity values in the CC tracts connecting the occipital and temporal lobes [31].

Furthermore, some subcortical brain regions have frequently been implicated in ASD, with significantly larger cerebellar and subcortical volumes observed at 4–6 months and larger amygdala volumes at 12 months in patients with ASD [22, 23]. In addition, a study using the binomial logistic regression method showed that subcortical volumes (thalamus and left hippocampus) could predict later autism diagnosis [24]. These findings collectively suggest that early brain changes occur during the period in which autistic behaviors begin to emerge.

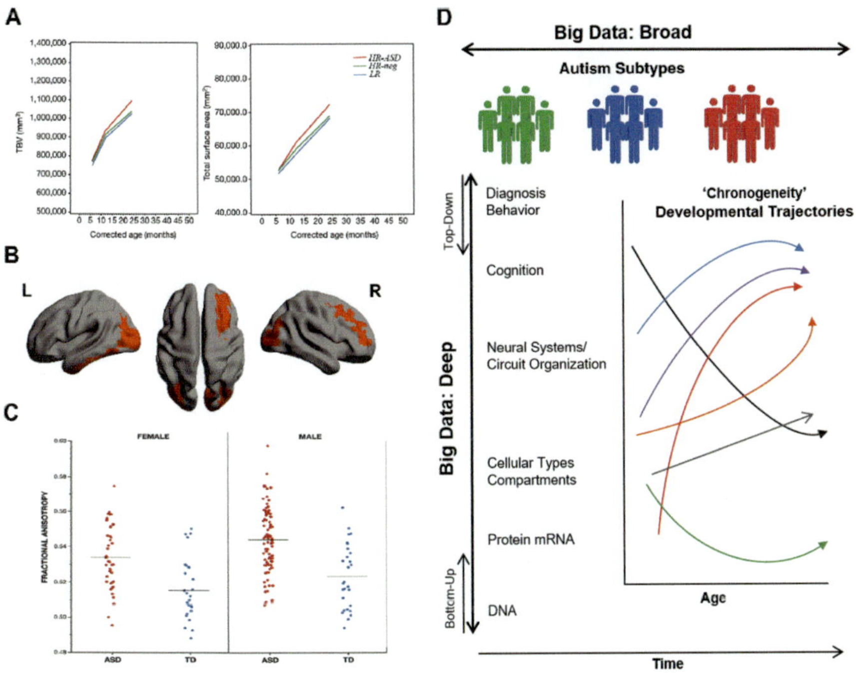

Figure 8.1 Overview of MRI-driven biomarkers and heterogeneity in autism. (A) Developmental trajectories of TBV and surface area from the HR-ASD (red), HR-neg (green), or LR (blue) groups. Adapted with permission from [3]. (B) A map of significant group differences in surface area from 6 to 12 months. The highlighted regions indicated that the HR-ASD group had significant expansion compared to the LR group. Adapted with permission from [3]. (C) Group differences in FA across individuals between the ASD and TD groups. Adapted with permission from [4]. (D) An approach towards decomposing heterogeneity might be constructing a stratified model whereby we model the subtype labels instead of one autism label and then re-examine differences on the hypothetical dependent variable of interest. The different colors are meant to represent different ASD subtypes. Adapted with permission from [92].

2.8.2.2 Diffusion MRI-based Biomarkers

In terms of microstructure, diffusion tensor imaging (DTI) has demonstrated extraordinary utility in delineating abnormal white matter (WM) development [25, 26] (Table 8.2). Findings from several longitudinal studies have reported increased fractional anisotropy (FA) in young children compared with TD controls, indicating that early atypical development of white matter pathways is associated with autistic symptoms [4, 21, 26–30] (Figure 8.1C). Moreover, Fingher et al. [31] found that young toddlers with autism exhibited larger FA and cross-sectional area in the temporal corpus callosum (CC) tract, along with abnormally low mean-Radial diffusivity (RD) and Axial diffusivity (AD) in the CC tracts connecting the occipital lobes and the temporal lobes.

Table 8.2 Review of diffusion-MRI studies in infants and toddlers with ASD

Studies	Samples (ASD/TD)	Age (years)	Findings in the ASD group
[27]	(7/18)	1.8–3.3	Increased FA in the left frontal lobe
[28]	(32/32)	3.2–3.4	Increased FA and decreased RD in CC and left cingulum
[26]	(28/64)	0.5–2	Higher FA at 6 months, lower values at 24 months
[29]	(16/41)	0.58	Longer visual orienting latencies in 7-month
[21]	(50)	0–3	Higher FA in the CC, posterior cingulate, and limbic
[30]	(61/33)	1–4	Greater FA in frontal
[32]	(68/29)	0–2.5	Larger FA and cross-sectional area of the temporal CC; Lower RD values in the CC
[32]	(116)	0.5–1	Inefficiencies at 6 months can predict 24-month ASD symptom
[33]	(32)	1.3–3	Higher FA values and number of streamlines
[4]	(127/54)	2.09–4.13	Increased FA; Increased AD in females, but decreased in males
[34]	(17/15)	0.11	A typical WM integrity in thalamic-occipital tracts in HR infants

Fractional anisotropy (FA), Radial diffusivity (RD), Axial diffusivity (AD), and corpus callosum (CC).

Additionally, WM networks in infants with ASD exhibited significantly decreased local and global efficiency in the temporal, parietal, and occipital lobes in HR infants at 24 months. This reduction in network efficiency was associated with symptom severity, suggesting a potential impact on the development of higher-level cognitive processes [32]. Another study on network connectivity patterns indicated that over-connectivity in ASD primarily involves the frontotemporal regions [33]. Furthermore, thalamocortical connectivity is disrupted at both functional and structural levels in infants at high familial risk (HR) for ASD [34]. Overall, these findings, particularly those related to early brain overgrowth around 12 months of age, are generally interpreted as reflecting an excessive number of neuron. This overabundance leads to exuberant local and short-distance cortical interactions, which impede the development of large-scale, long-distance connections between brain regions, potentially affecting the establishment of functional networks during early development [35, 36].

2.8.2.3 Functional MRI-based Biomarkers

As for the abnormal functional connectivity in infants with ASD (Table 8.3), several studies have highlighted early differences. Liu et al. found that language-related network connectivity, particularly in somatosensory regions, exhibited abnormalities in HR infants as early as 1.5 months of age [42]. Another study similarly reported atypical local functional activity in individuals with ASD [41]. In addition, Keehn et al. showed that HR infants had greater functional

Table 8.3 Review of functional-MRI studies in infants and toddlers with ASD

Studies	Samples (ASD/TD)	Age (years)	Functional Network Connectivity (FC) in ASD
[37]	(12/12)	2–3	Reduced activity in typical early language acquisition regions; Greater activation, primarily within the right and medial frontal
[38]	(29/30)	1–4	Weaker interhemispheric FC in language areas
[39]	(40/40)	1–4	Abnormally right-lateralized temporal cortex response to language
[40]	(27/37)	0.4–1	Increased FC at 3 months and decreased FC at 12 months.
[5]	(59)	0.5	FC can predict autism with greater than 96% accuracy
[41]	(20/20)	0.65–0.81	Higher ReHo; no differences in long-range connectivity.
[42]	(7/18)	0.12–0.75	Hyperconnectivity between auditory and somatosensory regions at 9 months
[43]	(24/23)	1.4–3.7	Increased FC between visual and sensorimotor networks
[34]	(24/28)	0.11	Thalamic-prefrontal underconnectivity, thalamic-occipital and thalamic-motor overconnectivity
[44]	(51/35)	1.6-3	Atypical correlations between temporal–visual FC and communication ability and between temporal–precuneus FC and expressive language ability

connectivity at 3 months but lower connectivity at 12 months compared to the TD controls [40]. Moreover, Dinstein et al. demonstrated significantly weaker interhemispheric functional connectivity in the language regions of children aged 1–4 years with ASD [38], while another study within the same age range observed increased functional connectivity between visual and sensorimotor networks in the ASD group [43]. These connectivity patterns were associated with the severity of autism symptoms. A recent study indicated that toddlers with ASD showed abnormal connectivity between visual and precuneus cortices, which are associated with communication and language function [44]. Notably, in a prospective neuroimaging study of 59 six-month-old HR infants, Emerson et al. employed a fully cross-validated machine learning algorithm to show that functional connectivity at 6 months could correctly predict 9 out of 11 infants with autism at 24 months [5]. This study also visualized positive and negative functional connections that contributed to the classification, particularly in the parietal lobe. Several studies have also reported right-lateralized abnormalities in the temporal cortex related to language processing in toddlers with autism by using task-functional stimuli, which may be linked to the failure to develop normal language in autism cohort [37, 39, 45].

When taken together, these findings suggest that atypical functional connectivity, altered by early neural activity in the first years of life, may serve as a biomarker of autism during early infancy. While MRI-based markers of autism can be detected early in life, ASD is a highly heterogeneous disorder. The effects of age, gender, and individual differences in brain growth vary, necessitating larger population studies to identify distinct autism subtypes, and each of them may associated with specific neurobiological phenotypes.

2.8.3 PARSING THE NEUROBIOLOGICAL HETEROGENEITY OF ASD

There has been growing interest in identifying subtypes of ASD [46]. These works aim to uncover homogeneous clusters to explore the biological basis of each subgroup, providing more specific insights for potential interventions. A subtyping approach incorporating multiple brain measures and employing data-driven clustering analysis may offer a more robust framework for identifying autism subtypes [47, 48]. The existence of distinct clusters in ASD is supported by findings across multiple modalities, including structural and functional MRI. Importantly, recent studies have demonstrated the effectiveness of identifying ASD subtypes in enhancing the diagnostic accuracy of ASD, underscoring the significance of neurobiological heterogeneity in understanding the etiology of ASD and advancing its precision medicine and personalized intervention.

2.8.3.1 Heterogeneity in Brain Anatomy

Recently, researchers have made efforts to dissect the neurobiological heterogeneity of ASD using brain structural MRI. These studies lie on the hypothesis that abnormal alterations in brain morphology accompany patients with ASD. By applying the traditional unsupervised clustering approaches (e.g., K-means clustering, hierarchical clustering, and spectral clustering) on structural MRI data, researchers have identified at least two neuroanatomical subtypes of ASD. For example, Liu et al. conducted semi-supervised clustering on gray and white matter volumes and classified ASD patients into two subtypes [49]. However, only using grey matter features leads to three neuroanatomical subtypes that can be commonly replicated across studies using varying samples and clustering methods. Specifically, Hong et al. reported three ASD subtypes with distinct brain structural alterations and achieved enhanced predictive performance of core ASD symptoms when models were trained separately for each subtype [50]; Chen et al. found three ASD subgroups that were significantly differed in behavioral and functional connectivity patterns [51]; by developing a novel canonical model, Shan et al. identified three ASD subtypes with distinct neuroanatomical deviation patterns from the TDs [52]. In addition to cortical structural metrics, researchers also used structural covariance between brain regions of an individual, known as brain structural co-variance network, as features for clustering analysis [53].

While these studies are important, they overlook the developmental processes of brain structure. Since ASD is a neurodevelopmental disorder characterized by age-dependent alterations in brain anatomy, age should be considered a crucial factor in clustering analysis rather than merely controlled for using computational models like the General Linear Model (GLM). A recent study by Fu et al. addressed

Table 8.4 Overview of single-model models in ASD diagnosis

Method	Samples (ASD/TD)	Advantage	Limitations	Modality	Performance
[55]	(22/22)	SVM can detect subtle and spatially distributed differences in brain networks of the ASD group	Generalizability and stability of the results	sMRI: GM, WM	Specificity of 86.0% and sensitivity of 88.0%
[56]	(19/31)	Discriminability was high using whole-brain SVM	Smaller sample and limited demographic, behavior, and genetic data	sMRI: GM, WM	Accuracy 90%
[57]	(14/28)	develop a robust technique for evaluating the volume of white matter	Small sample and coarse age range	sMRI: volume	75% under 20 years old
[58]	(82/84)	Using structural covariances in a machine-learning framework to obtain individual subject prediction	Relatively small sample size	sMRI: CT	Structural covariances among several brain regions are associated with autistic symptoms
[59]	(34/30)	Features derived from hippocampal regions also demonstrate high discriminative power	Relatively low number of subjects and limited to T1-WI MRI data only	sMRI: hippocampal texture features	Accuracy of 67.85%, sensitivity of 62.50%, specificity of 71.42%
[60]	(539/573)	Proposed a region-wise analysis of the brain using multi-scale texture features	Texture features may be more sensitive	sMRI: texture features derived from 31 brain regions	Statistically significant texture differences in the right hippocampus, left, etc.
[3]	(318/117)	SA of individuals predicted the diagnosis of later autism	Not include other relevant modalities	sMRI: SA	Positive predictive value of 81%
[61]	(149/161)	Using a deep transfer learning neural network framework for enhancing the classification	Only based on one type of feature	rs-fMRI	The highest accuracy of 70.4%

[62]	(187/183)	Proposed an Auto-ASD Network to classify	Lack generalization	fMRI	Highest accuracy of 80%.
[63]	(505/530)	A novel graph-based classification model	Not combine the fMRI and sMRI	rs-fMRI	Accuracy 76.4%
[64]	(66/66)	Using a multi-feature-based network to classify	Limited diagnostic utility of morphological features	sMRI: 7 morphological features	Accuracy 78.63%
[65]	(544/608)	Proposed a novel framework for disease diagnosis that alleviates the multisite problem	Limited by the finite computational resources	rs-fMRI	Accuracy 72.79 ± 4.62%

Structural MRI (sMRI), Functional MRI (fMRI), and rest-state FMRI (rs-fMRI) this by dividing individuals with ASD into three age groups, including children (6–11 years), adolescents (12–18 years), and young adults (18–30 years). They calculated the inter-individual similarity using four brain structural metrics and subsequently constructed a multilayer network model, with each layer representing the inter-individual similarity based on one structural metric. Using spectral clustering, they identified three subtypes of ASD for each age range, although these subtypes were not replicable across different age groups [54]. These results suggest that the clustering result of brain structure in the ASD cohort is also age-dependent, highlighting the importance of considering age when analyzing the neuroanatomical heterogeneity of ASD.

2.8.3.2 Heterogeneity in Brain Functional Connectivity

Researchers have also sought to dissect the neurobiological heterogeneity of ASD from a functional brain perspective. For example, Urchs et al. demonstrated that a simple hierarchical cluster analysis could robustly link individual brain networks to specific connectivity subtypes. They also found a moderate association between these functional connectivity subtypes and clinical diagnoses of ASD [48]. Although most fMRI studies rely on functional connectivity, which, to some extent, enhances the reliability of the findings, variations in data processing and clustering methods are also important factors affecting the results. As a result, several studies have identified 2–4 ASD subtypes using functional connectivity as features for clustering analysis [66–71]. Despite some inconsistencies in findings, these subtypes exhibit distinct patterns of functional connectivity alterations compared to the TDs and differences in corresponding clinical symptom profiles. Therefore, it cannot be definitively concluded that these ASD subgroups are incorrect; instead, more studies should focus on their reliability and biological significance. Moving forward, Buch et al. conducted clustering based on three latent dimensions of functional connectivity and revealed four ASD subgroups that were reproducible in an independent sample set [72]. They also constructed a predictive model based on the four subtypes, which could accurately predict the individual behavioral differences in patients with ASD. Their findings emphasize the potential of delineating subtypes to promote precision assessment for ASD. In addition, Zerbi et al. identified four specific patterns of network damage in an ASD mouse model, attributing pathogenetic heterogeneity as a key factor in the observed differences in connectivity patterns [73].

Other studies have constructed a normative model of functional connectivity development based on the TD cohort and estimated the deviation of functional connectivity of each individual with ASD from the typical developmental pattern before clustering analysis. This is based on the hypothesis that ASD is accompanied by abnormal developmental trajectories of the brain, such as brain overgrowth in early childhood and accelerated cortical thinning in adulthood. For example, Guo et al. calculated inter-individual deviation of functional connectivity (IDFC) from the TD group for each individual with ASD and applied K-means clustering to derive ASD subtypes [74]. Another study by Huang et al. applied support vector regression that trained on the functional connectivity of TD participants to predict the functional connectivity of patients with ASD, and the outcomes were submitted using the K-means method for subtyping analysis [70]. Li et al. move a further step to calculate the high-order similarity of individual deviation from the TDs among multiple ASD individuals, also known as a hypergraph, and then a hypergraphic community detection algorithm for clustering subgroups [75].

Although increasing studies focus on parsing the heterogeneity of autistic brains, the identified subtypes remain inconsistent across studies. Since biological heterogeneity is key to the precision diagnosis and treatment of ASD as well as the prediction of disease onset, there should be more focus placed on how to improve the interpretability and repeatability of subtypes.

2.8.4 MACHINE LEARNING-BASED DIAGNOSIS FOR ASD

Brain development is a complex and dynamic process, with disruptions potentially impacting the maturation of specific brain areas and their structure and function [76]. This is particularly relevant in the context of ASD, where neurological conditions affect the brain at multiple levels and are characterized by complex symptoms that make diagnosis challenging [77–81]. The limited understanding of ASD's biological causes and biomarkers, coupled with inconsistent diagnostic criteria [82–85], further complicates the situation. Researchers increasingly use artificial intelligence (AI) technology to address these challenges. AI's ability to identify subtle patterns is promising for studying ASD [86–89]. However, traditional unimodal analysis techniques, which focus on a single data type, may not fully capture the multidimensional nature of the pathological features in ASD, including structural, functional, and connectivity changes [90]. Multimodal modeling, which integrates data from various sources, offers a more comprehensive approach, allowing for the detection of nuanced, cross-modal patterns of abnormality. Models that rely on a single modality have limitations because they cannot fully capture the complexity and diversity of patient conditions. In contrast, multimodal models can provide richer and complementary information by integrating data from different imaging techniques and have shown great potential for improving the accuracy of diagnosis and the effectiveness of treatment [91].

2.8.4.1 Advances in the Application of Single-Modal Predictive Model in ASD Diagnosis

The current diagnosis of ASD primarily relies on behavioral assessments and clinical interviews, which, while comprehensive, do not incorporate biomarkers. This method, though effective in capturing the diversity of autism, falls short in identifying distinct biological subtypes, thereby limiting our understanding of the heterogeneity of this disorder. Recent large-scale studies analyzing data from millions of children have shed light on the need for personalized approaches. For instance, research indicates that about 30% of individuals with ASD may respond favorably to medications that target the 5-hydroxytryptaminergic system [84]. These insights underscore the necessity for individualized treatment strategies tailored to individual biochemical profiles [85]. They also lay the groundwork for developing diagnostic and therapeutic methods that utilize individual biomarkers (Figure 8.1D), potentially revolutionizing how ASD is understood and managed.

In the field of ASD diagnosis, machine learning (ML) techniques, especially support vector machines (SVM), are invaluable. These tools not only help identify ASD from control groups but also assess the severity of symptoms (Table 8.4). In the work of structural MRI data, Ecker et al. demonstrated that SVMs achieved an impressive diagnostic accuracy of about 80% in autism. This method also quantitatively measured diagnostic confidence through test margins (decision margins) [55]. Importantly, these test margins showed a positive correlation with symptom severity as measured by the Autism Diagnostic Observation Schedule (ADOS), suggesting that SVMs can effectively capture the neuroanatomical characteristics of ASD [56]. While SVMs have shown promise in classifying ASD, challenges persist, particularly in differentiating ASD from other neurodevelopmental disorders such as Attention Deficit Hyperactivity Disorder (ADHD) and Obsessive-Compulsive Disorder (OCD). Sato et al. further validated the utility of machine learning in quantifying ASD symptom severity with cortical thickness using Support Vector Regression (SVR) [58]. Chaddad et al. demonstrated the potential of hippocampal texture features as a biomarker for diagnosing and characterizing ASD with an accuracy of 67.85% [59, 60].

Additionally, Abdelrahman et al. proposed an innovative WM volume evaluation of the generated 3D mesh for potential ASD diagnosis and then conducted classification using a K Nearest Neighbor (KNN) algorithm and leave-one-out cross-validation, with an accuracy of 75% [57]. Zheng et al. constructed multi-feature-based networks using seven morphological features submitted to SVM to classify ASD groups, improving accuracy by 78.6% [64]. In order to enhance the clinical applicability of these classifiers, ongoing research focuses on improving their ability to recognize co-morbid conditions and refining their accuracy through pre-threshold analysis (PTA). Despite the success of ML, the emergence of deep learning techniques is revolutionizing the diagnostic landscape for ASD.

Deep learning (DL) has revolutionized the diagnostic process for ASD by automating the extraction of high-dimensional neuroimaging data, thereby enhancing diagnostic accuracy and differentiating ASD from other neurodevelopmental disorders. In terms of utilizing structural features, Hazlett et al. proposed a two-stage DL-SVM predictive model based on cortical SA from 6- and 12-months-old individuals to predict the diagnosis of autism in HR children at 24 months with 81% positive predictive value [3]. Using functional scans, Huang and colleagues pioneered a computational model using deep belief networks (DBNs) to analyze resting-state functional MRI data (rs-fMRI) [63]. This model, which employs graph-based feature selection and automatic hyperparameter tuning, significantly improved recognition accuracy. Its effectiveness was validated on the Autism Brain Imaging Data Exchange (ABIDE) database. Lee et al. also introduced a meta-learning framework tailored for multi-center ASD diagnosis and demonstrated the generalization ability in both seen and unseen multisite samples [65]. Eslami et al. provided an Auto-ASD-Network with a DL-SVM classify model based on fMRI, achieving more than 70% classification accuracy [62]. Li et al. developed a novel deep transfer learning neural network (DTL-NN) framework utilizing rs-fMRI to advance classification accuracy [61]. By adaptively calibrating fMRI data from various centers, the framework enabled a model capable of generalizing across unseen sites, demonstrating robust performance on the ABIDE datasets. These advancements underscore the potential of deep learning in ASD diagnosis.

However, while unimodal deep learning is promising, it may not fully capture the complexity of ASD pathophysiology. ASD's heterogeneity and multidimensionality necessitate a multifaceted approach. Researchers are increasingly exploring multimodal deep learning models that integrate diverse data sources, such as structural MRI, functional MRI, genetic data, and behavioral assessments. These models aim to provide a more comprehensive characterization of ASD, acknowledging the need for a holistic view to understand and treat this complex disorder fully.

2.8.4.2 Applications and Challenges of Multimodal Imaging in ASD Diagnosis

In the quest to better understand ASD, multimodal models are emerging as a key research focus. These sophisticated models offer a holistic view of ASD pathophysiology by integrating data from various neuroimaging techniques. Structural, functional, and diffusion MRI are employed to provide a richer diagnostic landscape. This comprehensive approach not only enhances the accuracy of ASD diagnosis but also deepens our insight into the underlying mechanisms of ASD. As shown in Table 8.5, the following review will delve into the application of multimodal models in ASD diagnosis, examining their potential to transform our diagnostic capabilities and contribute to a more nuanced understanding of ASD.

Convergence of Deep Learning and Graph Convolutional Networks

Advancements in deep learning and graph convolutional networks have significantly propelled high-dimensional brain network data analysis in ASD [93]. These techniques offer fresh insights into the structural and functional connectivity patterns in ASD brains, enhancing the precision of biomarker identification from multimodal imaging data. A notable example is Deep Learning combined with Independent Component Analysis (DL+LICA) [94], which distinguished independent components between autistic and non-autistic groups by integrating structural and functional MRI data. This study utilized sophisticated unimodal feature extraction methods, such as voxel-based morphology (VBM) and connectivity topology mapping, to deepen the understanding of brain region organization, potentially uncovering novel brain tissue phenotypes in autism.

Table 8.5 Comparison of ASD classification methods

Method	Datasets	Advantage	Limitations	Modality	Performance
[94]	EUAIMS LEAP	Improving Autism Biomarker Sensitivity	Computational limitations, small sample size	sMRI, fMRI	Identifies IC62
[95]	ADNI-2ABIDE-I	Spatiotemporal Hyperconnectivity Networks	Uninvestigated hyperedge changes	rs-fMRI	Outperforms existing methods
[96]	ABIDE I	Multimodal MRI Data for Graph Features	Future integration of more phenotypic info	sMRI, fMRI	74.7% Accuracy, 71.7% Sensitivity, 77.4% Specificity in ASD and TD Group
[97]	ABIDE	Personalized Info. with Attention Modules	Need further research on integration	sMRI, fMRI	72.08% Accuracy with AAL, 75.07% with CC200 on ABIDE
[97]	AIFB MUTAG NIH-TB portals ABIDE	Multi-Modal Graph Representation Learning	Separation of feature extraction and reasoning	sMRI, fMRI, Genomic Data, etc.	71.57% Accuracy with SVM, 71.43% with KNN on Multi-Site ASD
[98]	SNUH	Multimodal Fusion	Small sample sizes and age ranges	sMRI, DTI	Accuracy 88.8%, sensitivity 93%, specificity 83.8%
[99]	ABIDE I ABIDE II COBRE MPRC	Multimodal Fusion for Disorders classify	The fusion was conducted at the model level (not the feature level)	sMRI fMEI	Classification accuracy reached up to 83.08% for the testing data and 72.10% for the independent data
[100]	ABIDE-II	ML/ Constrained Autoregressive Model	Limited to direct structural links, impacted by complex interactions	sMRI fMRI	Classification accuracy achieved 72.34%
[101]	Own dataset	Fusion two different task fMRI	Small sample size, lack of generalizability, and data fusion complexities	Task-fMRI	Classification accuracy of 69–92.3%
[102]	ABIDE	Low-Rank Representation for Heterogeneity Reduction	Independent feature extraction and classifier training	fMRI	71.57% Accuracy with SVM, 71.43% with KNN

[104]	ABIDE ADHD-200 COBRE	Multimodal Fusion and Data Augmentation	Limited handling of missing modality	sMRI, fMRI	ASD 75.1%, ADHD 72.9%, SCZ 87.2% Accuracy
[105]	ADNI-2ABIDE-I	Multi-Template Methods for Rich Information	Potential information redundancy	rs-fMRI	Higher Accuracy
[106]	SZ/ABIDE	Convolutional Recurrent and Deep Neural Networks	Independent training of C-RNN and DNN	rs-fMRI	85.1% Accuracy with HDLFCA, 72.4% on ABIDE
[107]	HCP/ABIDE II	Functional Fiber Clustering with Riemann Framework	Further analysis needed for BOLD-Gray matter	sMRI, fMRI	84.2% Accuracy, 72.4% Sensitivity, 93.1% Specificity
[108]	ABIDE	Multi-Center Clustering for Site Heterogeneity	Nested SVD not optimal	rs-fMRI	Superior Accuracy
[109]	ABIDE	Framework Based on Graph Convolutional Networks	Need for advanced pooling methods	rs-fMRI	76.4% Accuracy, 78.6% Specificity
[110]	ABIDE	Algorithm Based on Graph Signal Processing	High sample heterogeneity	rs-fMRI	Superior Accuracy
[54]	ADNI-2/ ABIDE-I	Multi-Layer Network with Cortical Thickness and Volume	Limited Sample Size	sMRI	Superior Accuracy

Further advancements include the Spatiotemporally Weighted Multi-Hypergraph Convolutional Network (STW-MHGCN) [95], which exemplifies the power of multi-template data fusion. By constructing spatiotemporally weighted hyperconnected networks and applying deep learning models, this approach excels in ASD classification tasks, surpassing existing accuracy and area under the curve (AUC). The STW-MHGCN model enriches the study of brain diseases through multi-template data fusion, contributing to a deeper comprehension of their complexity.

Recent breakthroughs, such as the Adversarial Learning-based Node-Edge Graph Attention Network (AL-NEGAT) [96], have improved graph classification by modeling node and edge features and employing adversarial training to enhance generalization across independent datasets. The Multiview Brain Network Transformer (MBT) [97] incorporates individualized information, capturing a comprehensive range of indirect interactions in brain network connections through a higher-order attention extraction module. This not only improves diagnostic accuracy but also enriches our understanding of the neurobiological underpinnings of ASD. Additionally, Deep Learning combined with Multiplexed Graph Neural Networks (Multiplexed GNN) [98] leverages Multiplexed Graph Representation Learning to discern complex cross-modal dependencies, guiding task-specific reasoning through structured message passing. These methodologies, validated across multiple clinical databases, underscore the critical role of multimodal data fusion in enhancing brain disease analysis, emphasizing the necessity for a multidimensional approach to comprehend the complexity of disorders such as ASD fully.

Multimodal Data Fusion Techniques

Integrating multimodal data fusion and feature extraction techniques significantly advances the field of ASD diagnosis. By combining data from various imaging modalities, including structural and functional MRI, these techniques offer a more comprehensive and detailed view of brain networks. This enhanced perspective enables a more precise understanding and diagnosis of ASD. Specifically, Kim et al. applied T1-weighted MRI and DTI data of preschoolers to ML, reaching an accuracy of 88.8% [99]. In another study by Du et al., the fusion of fMRI and sMRI data to distinguish Schizophrenia and ASD with an accuracy of up to 83% [100]. Crimi et al. proposed a constrained autoregressive model with integrated functional and structural connectivity, which can effectively differentiate healthy participants and patients with ASD [101]. Chanel et al. introduced a voxel-based method based on SVM and Recursive Feature Elimination (RFE) to fusion two different task-fMRI, achieving the highest accuracy of 92.3% [102]. Combining brain anatomical and functional networks [110] offers new insights for neuropathology identification, particularly in ASD. This technique utilizes a graph signal processing framework to classify time-varying graph signals and incorporates the interaction of brain structure and function to predict ASD. Decision trees are used as the predictive model, achieving accuracy comparable to deep learning algorithms and SVMs on the ABIDE public dataset.

In addition, a prime example is the multi-site adaptive framework combined with low-rank representation (maLRR) [103], which is particularly effective for multi-center datasets like the ABIDE. This method maps data from different sites to a common latent representation space, effectively reducing heterogeneity caused by variations in data collection environments and equipment. The preprocessing involves temporal correction, motion correction, removal of interfering signals, and temporal filtering. Data normalization to the Montreal Neurological Institute (MNI) space allows for the extraction of mean time series from 116 predefined regions of interest (ROIs) based on the AAL atlas. Utilizing SVM and KNN classifiers, this approach has demonstrated improved performance over existing methods on multi-site ASD datasets [104], achieving average accuracies of 71.57% and 71.43%, respectively. In addition, a region-aware feature fusion network utilizing a multi-template and multi-graph cross-attention basis [105] offers a novel approach to brain disease diagnosis. This method integrates multi-template information into a deep learning framework, employing static and dynamic graph convolution and a two-view cross-attention mechanism to exploit functional differences in brain regions in disease manifestations. This approach achieves higher accuracy compared to existing state-of-the-art methods on the ADNI-2 and ABIDE-I datasets, and it reports other performance metrics such as sensitivity, specificity, and AUC. Parallel advancements include a hybrid deep learning framework based on the attention mechanism [106], which integrates brain connectivity and resting-state functional MRI data activity. This framework, referred to as the Hybrid Deep Learning Framework with Convolutional Attention (HDLFCA), merges a convolutional recurrent neural network (C-RNN) with a deep neural network (DNN) to improve classification accuracy and interpretability. The framework, which uses an attention module to automatically learn features in a time series and employs logistic regression for final decision-making, was validated as effective on multicenter SZ and publicly available autism datasets, outperforming 12 other models. These methodologies underscore the critical role of multimodal data fusion in enhancing the accuracy and depth of ASD diagnosis, emphasizing the necessity for a multidimensional approach to comprehend the complexity of disorders such as ASD.

Innovative Application of Specific Data Preprocessing and Analysis Methods

Diagnostic studies of ASD are being revolutionized by the use of specific data preprocessing and analysis methods that optimize the data preprocessing process and develop new techniques for extracting and utilizing neuroimaging features associated with ASD. These advancements are crucial for improving diagnostic accuracy and reliability. One innovative approach is the structured-guided functional clustering method, which clusters brain white matter fibers using a Riemannian framework [107]. This method offers a new perspective for analyzing high-dimensional, noisy, time-delayed functional sequences. It facilitates the development of a standardized white matter atlas, enhancing its flexible application across different studies. Applications on the Human

Connectome Project (HCP) and ABIDE II datasets have demonstrated the method's effectiveness in identifying ASD, with SVMs achieving the highest accuracy of 84.2% in ASD classification and a sensitivity of 72.4% and specificity of 93.1%. Further advancements include multicenter clustering and nested feature extraction (MC-NFE) method [108], which provides a new perspective for ASD detection in resting-state functional fMRI. This method significantly improves ASD detection performance by modeling inter-site heterogeneity through multicenter clustering and applying nested singular value decomposition (SVD) to extract functional connectivity features. An application on the ABIDE database has shown the superiority of this method in multicenter ASD data detection, which outperformed the existing methods.

Additionally, PLSNet [109] employs a multi-head self-attention mechanism to extract time-series features and uses positional embedding to enhance the model's perception of spatial and temporal positional information. PLSNet introduces a graph sparsification layer that effectively filters out salient brain regions associated with ASD, reducing dimensionality complexity while improving model interpretability. On the Autism Brain Imaging Data Exchange (ABIDE) public dataset, PLSNet achieved 76.4% accuracy.

2.8.5 CONCLUSIONS AND FUTURE DIRECTIONS

The application of multimodal modeling in diagnosing ASD is revolutionizing the field by integrating and analyzing data from multiple imaging modalities, such as fMRI, sMRI, and electrophysiological data like electroencephalography (EEG). This approach significantly enhances diagnostic accuracy by capturing the complex neurobiological underpinnings of ASD. By incorporating data from various sources, multimodal models provide a more nuanced understanding of the brain's structure and function, particularly valuable in ASD, a condition known for its neuroanatomical and functional heterogeneity. Using diverse MRI datasets from different clinical sites helps overcome challenges posed by variations in image acquisition parameters, making the diagnostic models more robust and generalizable. In addition, combining neuroimaging data with phenotypic information—such as age, weight, and family history—further refines classification accuracy. This integrative approach ensures that models capture a broader spectrum of ASD-related biomarkers, leading to more precise diagnoses.

Connectivity-based techniques, particularly those focused on extracting features from structural and functional neuroimaging technology, offer novel diagnostic features that contribute to developing innovative models. For instance, exploring visual and brain transformers highlights their potential to detect ASD biomarkers by analyzing specific brain regions or connectivity patterns. This suggests the possibility of developing attentional mechanisms tailored to key neural circuits involved in ASD.

Moreover, incorporating advanced techniques like transfer learning and zero-shot learning into diagnostic models holds great promise. These methods leverage pre-trained models to extract relevant features from brain MRI images, enabling better detection of subtle differences in brain structure and function associated with ASD. Other emerging research directions, such as graph theory, representation learning, migration learning, zero-shot learning, and Q-learning techniques, are also being explored, offering new insights into ASD diagnosis. These advancements not only provide new hope for early diagnosis and intervention in ASD but also pave the way for future neuroscience research. As data analysis methods and technology continue to evolve, we anticipate achieving more accurate and personalized ASD diagnoses, leading to more effective treatments and support for individuals with the disorder.

2.8.6 SEARCH STRATEGY AND SELECTION CRITERIA

We searched PubMed and Web of Science for original articles using the following search terms: "Autism Spectrum Disorders/ASD," "early childhood," "infant," "biomarkers," "magnetic resonance imaging/MRI," and "subtype" and "machine learning/deep learning/model prediction/diagnosis" alone and in combination. We also checked the references of the identified articles for any additional relevant publications. Our inclusion criteria were limited to studies written in English and published before July 2024.

REFERENCES

[1] Wetherby, A.M., J. Woods, L. Allen, J. Cleary, H. Dickinson and C. Lord. 2004. Early indicators of autism spectrum disorders in the second year of life. Journal of Autism and Developmental Disorders. 34(5): 473–493.

[2] Dawson, G., A.D. Rieder and M.H. Johnson. 2023. Prediction of autism in infants: Progress and challenges. The Lancet Neurology. 22(3): 244–254.

[3] Hazlett, H.C., H. Gu, B.C. Munsell, S.H. Kim, M. Styner, J.J. Wolff, et al. 2017. Early brain development in infants at high risk for autism spectrum disorder. Nature. 542(7641): 348–351.

[4] Andrews, D.S., J.K. Lee, M. Solomon, S.J. Rogers, D.G. Amaral and C.W. Nordahl. 2019. A diffusion-weighted imaging tract-based spatial statistics study of autism spectrum disorder in preschool-aged children. Journal of Neurodevelopmental Disorders. 11: 32.

[5] Emerson, R.W., C. Adams, T. Nishino, H.C. Hazlett, J.J. Wolff, L. Zwaigenbaum, et al. 2017. Functional neuroimaging of high-risk 6-month-old infants predicts a diagnosis of autism at 24 months of age. Science Translational Medicine. 9(393): eaag2882.

[6] Hazlett, H.C., M.D. Poe, G. Gerig, M. Styner, C. Chappell, R.G. Smith, et al. 2011. Early brain overgrowth in autism associated with an increase in cortical surface area before age 2 years. Archives of General Psychiatry. 68(5): 467–476.

[7] Ohta, H., C.W. Nordahl, A.-M. Iosif, A. Lee, S. Rogers and D.G. Amaral. 2016. Increased surface area, but not cortical thickness, in a subset of young boys with autism spectrum disorder. Autism Research. 9(2): 232–248.

[8] JWolff, J.J., G. Gerig, J.D. Lewis, T. Soda, M.A. Styner, C. Vachet, et al. 2015. Altered corpus callosum morphology associated with autism over the first 2 years of life. Brain. 138(7): 2046–2058.

[9] Shen, M.D., C.W. Nordahl, G.S. Young, S.L. Wootton-Gorges, A. Lee, S.E. Liston, et al. 2013. Early brain enlargement and elevated extra-axial fluid in infants who develop autism spectrum disorder. Brain. 136(9): 2825–2835.

[10] Courchesne, E., R. Carper and N. Akshoomoff. 2003. Evidence of brain overgrowth in the first year of life in autism. Jama. 290(3): 337–344.

[11] Hazlett, H.C., M. Poe, G. Gerig, R.G. Smith, J. Provenzale, A. Ross, et al. 2005. Magnetic resonance imaging and head circumference study of brain size in autism: birth through age 2 years. Archives of General Psychiatry. 62(12): 1366–1376.

[12] Dissanayake, C., Q.M. Bui, R. Huggins and D.Z. Loesch. 2006. Growth in stature and head circumference in high-functioning autism and Asperger disorder during the first 3 years of life. Development and Psychopathology. 18(2): 381–393.

[13] Dawson, G., J. Munson, S.J. Webb, T. Nalty, R. Abbott and K. Toth. 2007. Rate of head growth decelerates and symptoms worsen in the second year of life in autism. Biological Psychiatry. 61(4): 458–464.

[14] Mraz, K.D., J. Green, T. Dumont-Mathieu, S. Makin and D. Fein. 2007. Correlates of head circumference growth in infants later diagnosed with autism spectrum disorders. Journal of Child Neurology. 22(6): 700–713.

[15] Chawarska, K., D. Campbell, L. Chen, F. Shic, A. Klin and J. Chang. 2011. Early generalized overgrowth in boys with autism. Archives of General Psychiatry. 68(10): 1021–1031.

[16] Fukumoto, A., T. Hashimoto, K. Mori, Y. Tsuda, K. Arisawa and S. Kagami. 2011. Head circumference and body growth in autism spectrum disorders. Brain and Development. 33(7): 569–575.

[17] Amaral, D.G., D. Li, L. Libero, M. Solomon, J. Van de Water, A. Mastergeorge, et al. 2017. In pursuit of neurophenotypes: The consequences of having autism and a big brain. *In*: Autism Research. 10(5): 711–722.

[18] Courchesne, E., R. Carper and N. Akshoomoff. 2003. Evidence of brain overgrowth in the first year of life in autism. Jama. 290(3): 337–344.

[19] Carper, R.A., P. Moses, Z.D. Tigue and E. Courchesne. 2002. Cerebral lobes in autism: Early hyperplasia and abnormal age effects. Neuroimage. 16(4): 1038–1051.

[20] Schumann, C.M., C.S. Bloss, C.C. Barnes, G.M. Wideman, R.A. Carper, N. Akshoomoff, et al. 2010. Longitudinal magnetic resonance imaging study of cortical development through early childhood in autism. Journal of Neuroscience. 30(12): 4419–4427.

[21] Xiao, Z., T. Qiu, X. Ke, X. Xiao, T. Xiao, F. Liang, et al. 2014. Autism spectrum disorder as early neurodevelopmental disorder: Evidence from the brain imaging abnormalities in 2–3 years old toddlers. Journal of Autism and Developmental Disorders. 44: 1633–1640.

[22] Pote, I., S. Wang, V. Sethna, A. Blasi, E. Daly, M. Kuklisova-Murgasova, et al. 2019. Familial risk of autism alters subcortical and cerebellar brain anatomy in infants and predicts the emergence of repetitive behaviors in early childhood. Autism Research. 12(4): 614–627.

[23] Shen, M.D., M.R. Swanson, J.J. Wolff, J.T. Elison, J.B. Girault, S.H. Kim, et al. 2022. Subcortical brain development in autism and fragile X syndrome: Evidence

for dynamic, age- and disorder-specific trajectories in infancy. American Journal of Psychiatry. 179(8): 562–572.

[24] Montenegro, J.T.P., D. Seguin and E.G. Duerden. 2022. Joint attention in infants at high familial risk for autism spectrum disorder and the association with thalamic and hippocampal macrostructure. Cerebral Cortex Communications 3(3): tgac029.

[25] Gropman, A.L., B. Gertz, K. Shattuck, I.L. Kahn, R. Seltzer, L. Krivitsky, et al. 2010. Diffusion tensor imaging detects areas of abnormal white matter microstructure in patients with partial ornithine transcarbamylase deficiency. American Journal of Neuroradiology. 31(9): 1719–1723.

[26] Wolff, J.J., H. Gu, G. Gerig, J.T. Elison, M. Styner, S. Gouttard, et al. 2012. Differences in white matter fiber tract development present from 6 to 24 months in infants with autism. American Journal of Psychiatry. 169(6): 589–600.

[27] Ben Bashat, D., V. Kronfeld-Duenias, D.A. Zachor, P.M. Ekstein, T. Hendler, R. Tarrasch, et al. 2007. Accelerated maturation of white matter in young children with autism: a high b value DWI study. Neuroimage. 37(1): 40–47.

[28] Weinstein, M., L. Ben-Sira, Y. Levy, D.A. Zachor, E.B. Itzhak, M. Artzi, et al. 2011. Abnormal white matter integrity in young children with autism. Human Brain Mapping. 32(4): 534–543.

[29] Elison, J.T., S.J. Paterson, J.J. Wolff, J.S. Reznick, N.J. Sasson, H. Gu, et al. 2013. White matter microstructure and atypical visual orienting in 7-month-olds at risk for autism. American Journal of Psychiatry. 170(8): 899–908.

[30] Solso, S., R. Xu, J. Proudfoot, D.J. Hagler, Jr., K. Campbell, V. Venkatraman, et al. 2016. Diffusion tensor imaging provides evidence of possible axonal overconnectivity in frontal lobes in autism spectrum disorder toddlers. Biological Psychiatry. 79(8): 676–684.

[31] Fingher, N., I. Dinstein, M. Ben-Shachar, S. Haar, A.M. Dale, L. Eyler, et al. 2017. Toddlers later diagnosed with autism exhibit multiple structural abnormalities in temporal corpus callosum fibers. Cortex. 97: 291–305.

[32] Lewis, J.D., A.C. Evans, J.R. Pruett, Jr., K.N. Botteron, R.C. McKinstry, L. Zwaigenbaum, et al. 2017. The emergence of network inefficiencies in infants with autism spectrum disorder. Biological Psychiatry. 82(3): 176–185.

[33] Conti, E., J. Mitra, S. Calderoni, K. Pannek, K.K. Shen, A. Pagnozzi, et al. 2017. Network over-connectivity differentiates autism spectrum disorder from other developmental disorders in toddlers: A diffusion MRI study. Human Brain Mapping. 38(5): 2333–2344.

[34] Nair, A., R. Jalal, J. Liu, T. Tsang, N.M. McDonald, L. Jackson, et al. 2021. Altered thalamocortical connectivity in 6-week-old infants at high familial risk for autism spectrum disorder. Cerebral Cortex. 31(9): 4191–4205.

[35] Just, M.A., V.L. Cherkassky, T.A. Keller and N.J. Minshew. 2004. Cortical activation and synchronization during sentence comprehension in high-functioning autism: Evidence of underconnectivity. Brain. 127(8): 1811–1821.

[36] Courchesne, E., K. Pierce, C.M. Schumann, E. Redcay, J.A. Buckwalter, D.P. Kennedy, et al. 2007. Mapping early brain development in autism. Neuron. 56(2): 399–413.

[37] Redcay, E. and E. Courchesne. 2008. Deviant functional magnetic resonance imaging patterns of brain activity to speech in 2–3-year-old children with autism spectrum disorder. Biological Psychiatry. 64(7): 589–598.

[38] Dinstein, I., K. Pierce, L. Eyler, S. Solso, R. Malach, M. Behrmann, et al. 2011. Disrupted neural synchronization in toddlers with autism. Neuron. 70(6): 1218–1225.

[39] Eyler, L.T., K. Pierce and E. Courchesne. 2012. A failure of left temporal cortex to specialize for language is an early emerging and fundamental property of autism. Brain. 135(3): 949–960.

[40] Keehn, B., J. Wagner, H. Tager-Flusberg and C.A. Nelson. 2013. Functional connectivity in the first year of life in infants at risk for autism: a preliminary near-infrared spectroscopy study. Frontiers in Human Neuroscience. 7: 444.

[41] Ciarrusta, J., R. Dimitrova, D. Batalle, J. O'Muircheartaigh, L. Cordero-Grande, A. Price, et al. 2020. Emerging functional connectivity differences in newborn infants vulnerable to autism spectrum disorders. Translational Psychiatry. 10(1): 131.

[42] Liu, J., N.J. Okada, K.K. Cummings, J. Jung, G. Patterson, S.Y. Bookheimer, et al. 2020. Emerging atypicalities in functional connectivity of language-related networks in young infants at high familial risk for ASD. Developmental Cognitive Neuroscience. 45: 100814.

[43] Chen, B., A. Linke, L. Olson, C. Ibarra, S. Reynolds, R.-A. Müller, et al. 2021. Greater functional connectivity between sensory networks is related to symptom severity in toddlers with autism spectrum disorder. Journal of Child Psychology and Psychiatry. 62(2): 160–170.

[44] Xiao, Y., T.H. Wen, L. Kupis, L.T. Eyler, V. Taluja, J. Troxel, et al. 2023. Atypical functional connectivity of temporal cortex with precuneus and visual regions may be an early-age signature of ASD. Molecular Autism. 14(1): 11.

[45] Pierce, K. 2011. Early functional brain development in autism and the promise of sleep fMRI. Brain Research. 1380. 162–174.

[46] Hong, S.-J., J.T. Vogelstein, A. Gozzi, B.C. Bernhardt, B.T. Yeo, M.P. Milham, et al. 2020. Toward neurosubtypes in autism. Biological Psychiatry 88(1): 111–128.

[47] Vaidya, C.J., X. You, S. Mostofsky, F. Pereira, M.M. Berl and L. Kenworthy. 2020. Data-driven identification of subtypes of executive function across typical development, attention deficit hyperactivity disorder, and autism spectrum disorders. Journal of Child Psychology and Psychiatry. 61(1): 51–61.

[48] Urchs, S.G., A. Tam, P. Orban, C. Moreau, Y. Benhajali, H.D. Nguyen, et al. 2022. Functional connectivity subtypes associate robustly with ASD diagnosis. Elife. 11: e56257.

[49] Liu, G., L. Shi, J. Qiu and W. Lu. 2022. Two neuroanatomical subtypes of males with autism spectrum disorder revealed using semi-supervised machine learning. Molecular Autism. 13(1): 9.

[50] Hong, S.-J., S.L. Valk, A. Di Martino, M.P. Milham and B.C. Bernhardt. 2018. Multidimensional neuroanatomical subtyping of autism spectrum disorder. Cerebral Cortex. 28(10): 3578–3588.

[51] Chen, H., L.Q. Uddin, X. Guo, J. Wang, R. Wang, X. Wang, et al. 2019. Parsing brain structural heterogeneity in males with autism spectrum disorder reveals distinct clinical subtypes. Human Brain Mapping. 40(2): 628–637.

[52] Shan, X., L.Q. Uddin, J. Xiao, C. He, Z. Ling, L. Li, et al. 2022. Mapping the heterogeneous brain structural phenotype of autism spectrum disorder using the normative model. Biological Psychiatry. 91(11): 967–976.

[53] Shan, X., L.Q. Uddin, J. Xiao, C. He, Z. Ling, L. Li, et al. 2023. Exploring the heterogeneity of brain structure in autism spectrum disorder based on individual structural covariance network. Cerebral Cortex. 33(12): 7311–7321.

[54] Fu, X., Y. Wang, J. Li, H. Cai, X. Zhang, Z. Yao, et al. 2024. Decomposing Neuroanatomical Heterogeneity of Autism Spectrum Disorder Across Different Developmental Stages Using Morphological Multiplex Network Model. IEEE Transactions on Computational Social Systems. 11(5): 6557–6567.

[55] Ecker, C., V. Rocha-Rego, P. Johnston, J. Mourao-Miranda, A. Marquand, E.M. Daly, et al. 2010. Investigating the predictive value of whole-brain structural MR scans in autism: a pattern classification approach. Neuroimage 49(1): 44–56.

[56] Hoeft, F., E. Walter, A.A. Lightbody, H.C. Hazlett, C. Chang, J. Piven, et al. 2011. Neuroanatomical differences in toddler boys with fragile X syndrome and idiopathic autism. Archives of General Psychiatry. 68(3): 295– 305.

[57] Abdelrahman, M., A. Ali, A. Farag, M.F. Casanova and A. Farag. 2012. New approach for classification of autistic vs. typically developing brain using white matter volumes. 2012 Ninth Conference on Computer and Robot Vision. IEEE. 284–289.

[58] Sato, J.R., M.Q. Hoexter, P.P. de Magalhães Oliveira Jr, M.J. Brammer, D. Murphy, C. Ecker, et al. 2013. Inter-regional cortical thickness correlations are associated with autistic symptoms: a machine-learning approach. Journal of Psychiatric Research. 47(4): 453–459.

[59] Chaddad, A., C. Desrosiers, L. Hassan and C. Tanougast. 2017. Hippocampus and amygdala radiomic biomarkers for the study of autism spectrum disorder. BMC Neuroscience. 18: 1–12.

[60] Chaddad, A., C. Desrosiers and M. Toews. 2017. Multi-scale radiomic analysis of sub-cortical regions in MRI related to autism, gender and age. Scientific Reports. 7(1): 45639.

[61] Li, H., N.A. Parikh and L. He. 2018. A novel transfer learning approach to enhance deep neural network classification of brain functional connectomes. Frontiers in Neuroscience. 12: 491.

[62] Eslami, T. and F. Saeed. 2019. Auto-ASD-network: A technique based on deep learning and support vector machines for diagnosing autism spectrum disorder using fMRI data. *In*: Proceedings of the 10th ACM International Conference on Bioinformatics, Computational Biology and Health Informatics. 646–651.

[63] Huang, Z.-A., Z. Zhu, C.H. Yau and K.C. Tan. 2020. Identifying autism spectrum disorder from resting-state fMRI using deep belief network. *In*: IEEE Transactions on Neural Networks and Learning Systems. 32(7): 2847–2861.

[64] Zheng, W., T. Eilam-Stock, T. Wu, A. Spagna, C. Chen, B. Hu, et al. 2019. Multi-feature based network revealing the structural abnormalities in autism spectrum disorder. *In*: IEEE Transactions on Affective Computing. 12(3): 732–742.

[65] Lee, J., E. Kang, D.W. Heo and H.I. Suk. 2023. Site-invariant meta-modulation learning for multisite autism spectrum disorders diagnosis. *In*: IEEE Transactions on Neural Networks and Learning Systems. 35(12): 18062–18075.

[66] Feczko, E., N. Balba, O. Miranda-Dominguez, M. Cordova, S. Karalunas, L. Irwin, et al. 2018. Subtyping cognitive profiles in autism spectrum disorder using a functional random forest algorithm. Neuroimage. 172: 674–688.

[67] Kernbach, J.M., T.D. Satterthwaite, D.S. Bassett, J. Smallwood, D. Margulies, S. Krall, et al. 2018. Shared endo-phenotypes of default mode dysfunction in attention deficit/hyperactivity disorder and autism spectrum disorder. Translational Psychiatry. 8(1): 133.

[68] Easson, A.K., Z. Fatima and A.R. McIntosh. 2019. Functional connectivity-based subtypes of individuals with and without autism spectrum disorder. Network Neuroscience. 3(2): 344–362.

[69] Choi, H., K. Byeon, B.-Y. Park, J.-E. Lee, S.L. Valk, B. Bernhardt, et al. 2022. Diagnosis-informed connectivity subtyping discovers subgroups of autism with reproducible symptom profiles. NeuroImage. 256: 119212.

[70] Huang, X., Y. Ming, W. Zhao, R. Feng, Y. Zhou, L. Wu, et al. 2023. Developmental prediction modeling based on diffusion tensor imaging uncovering age-dependent heterogeneity in early childhood autistic brain. Molecular Autism. 14(1): 41.

[71] Rasero, J., A. Jimenez-Marin, I. Diez, R. Toro, M.T. Hasan and J.M. Cortes. 2023. The neurogenetics of functional connectivity alterations in autism: Insights from subtyping in 657 individuals. Biological Psychiatry. 94(10): 804–813.

[72] Buch, A.M., P.E. Vértes, J. Seidlitz, S.H. Kim, L. Grosenick and C. Liston. 2023. Molecular and network-level mechanisms explaining individual differences in autism spectrum disorder. Nature Neuroscience. 26(4): 650–663.

[73] Zerbi, V., M. Pagani, M. Markicevic, M. Matteoli, D. Pozzi, M. Fagiolini, et al. 2021. Brain mapping across 16 autism mouse models reveals a spectrum of functional connectivity subtypes. Molecular Psychiatry. 26(12): 7610–7620.

[74] Guo, X., G. Zhai, J. Liu, Y. Cao, X. Zhang, D. Cui, et al. 2022. Inter-individual heterogeneity of functional brain networks in children with autism spectrum disorder. Molecular Autism. 13(1): 52.

[75] Li, J., W. Zheng, X. Fu, Y. Zhang, S. Yang, Y. Wang, et al. 2024. Individual Deviation-Based Functional Hypergraph for Identifying Subtypes of Autism Spectrum Disorder. Brain Sciences. 14(8): 738.

[76] McPartland, J.C., B. Reichow and F.R. Volkmar. 2012. Sensitivity and specificity of proposed DSM-5 diagnostic criteria for autism spectrum disorder. Journal of the American Academy of Child and Adolescent Psychiatry. 51(4): 368–383.

[77] Matson, J.L. and M. Shoemaker. 2009. Intellectual disability and its relationship to autism spectrum disorders. Research in Developmental Disabilities. 30(6): 1107–1114.

[78] Antshel, K.M., Y. Zhang-James and S.V. Faraone. 2013. The comorbidity of ADHD and autism spectrum disorder. Expert Review of Neurotherapeutics. 13(10): 1117–1128.

[79] Lombardo, M.V., T. Pramparo, V. Gazestani, V. Warrier, R.A. Bethlehem, C.C. Barnes, et al. 2018. Large-scale associations between the leukocyte transcriptome and BOLD responses to speech differ in autism early language outcome subtypes. Nature Neuroscience. 21(12): 1680–1688.

[80] Zaboski, B.A. and E.A. Storch. 2018. Comorbid autism spectrum disorder and anxiety disorders: A brief review. Future Neurology. 13(1): 31–37.

[81] Tang, S., N. Sun, D.L. Floris, X. Zhang, A. Di Martino and B.T. Thomas Yeo. 2020. Reconciling dimensional and categorical models of autism heterogeneity: A brain connectomics and behavioral study. Biological Psychiatry. 87(12): 1071–1082.

[82] Lord, C., M. Rutter, S. Goode, J. Heemsbergen, H. Jordan, L. Mawhood, et al. 1989. Austism diagnostic observation schedule: A standardized observation of communicative and social behavior. Journal of Autism and Developmental Disorders. 19(2): 185–212.

[83] Lord, C., M. Rutter and A. Le Couteur. 1994. Autism Diagnostic Interview-Revised: A revised version of a diagnostic interview for caregivers of individuals with possible pervasive developmental disorders. Journal of Autism and Developmental Disorders. 24(5): 659–685.

[84] Hranilovic, D., Z. Bujas-Petkovic, R. Vragovic, T. Vuk, K. Hock and B. Jernej. 2007. Hyperserotonemia in adults with autistic disorder. Journal of Autism and Developmental Disorders. 37: 1934–1940.

[85] Ecker, C., W. Spooren and D. Murphy. 2013. Developing new pharmacotherapies for autism. Journal of Internal Medicine. 274(4): 308–320.

[86] Plitt, M., K.A. Barnes, G.L. Wallace, L. Kenworthy and A. Martin 2015. Resting-state functional connectivity predicts longitudinal change in autistic traits and adaptive functioning in autism. Proceedings of the National Academy of Sciences. 112(4): E6699–E6706.

[87] Rohr, C.S., S. Kamal and S. Bray. 2020. Building functional connectivity neuromarkers of behavioral self-regulation across children with and without autism spectrum disorder. Developmental Cognitive Neuroscience. 41: 100747.

[88] Xiao, J., H. Chen, X. Shan, C. He, Y. Li, X. Guo, et al. 2021. Linked social—Communication dimensions and connectivity in functional brain networks in autism spectrum disorder. Cerebral Cortex. 31(8): 3899–3910.

[89] Ilioska, I., M. Oldehinkel, A. Llera, S. Chopra, T. Looden, R. Chauvin, et al. 2023. Connectome-wide mega-analysis reveals robust patterns of atypical functional connectivity in autism. Biological Psychiatry. 94(1): 29–39.

[90] Vaswani, A., N. Shazeer, N. Parmar, J. Uszkoreit, L. Jones, A.N. Gomez, et al. 2017. Attention is all you need. *In*: 31st Conference on Neural Information Processing Systems (NIPS 2017), Long Beach, CA, USA. pp. 1–11.

[91] Ahmed, M.R., Y. Zhang, Y. Liu and H. Liao. 2020. Single volume image generator and deep learning-based ASD classification. IEEE Journal of Biomedical and Health Informatics. 24(11): 3044–3054.

[92] Lombardo, M.V., M.-C. Lai and S. Baron-Cohen. 2019. Big data approaches to decomposing heterogeneity across the autism spectrum. Molecular Psychiatry. 24(10): 1435–1450.

[93] Horien, C., D.L. Floris, A.S. Greene, S. Noble, M. Rolison, L. Tejavibulya, et al. 2022. Functional connectome–based predictive modeling in autism. Biological Psychiatry. 92(8): 626–642.

[94] Oblong, L.M., A. Llera, T. Mei, K. Haak, C. Isakoglou, D.L. Floris, et al. 2023. Linking functional and structural brain organisation with behaviour in autism: A multimodal EU-AIMS Longitudinal European Autism Project (LEAP) study. Molecular Autism. 14(1): 32.

[95] Liu, Z., L. Tong, L. Chen, Z. Jiang, F. Zhou, Q. Zhang, et al. 2023. Deep learning based brain tumor segmentation: A survey. Complex and Intelligent Systems. 9(1): 1001–1026.

[96] Chen, Y., J. Yan, M. Jiang, T. Zhang, Z. Zhao, W. Zhao, et al. 2022. Adversarial learning based node-edge graph attention networks for autism spectrum disorder identification. IEEE Transactions on Neural Networks and Learning Systems. 35(6): 7275–7286.

[97] Dong, Q., H. Cai, Z. Li, J. Liu and B. Hu. 2024. A multiview brain network transformer fusing individualized information for autism spectrum disorder diagnosis. IEEE Journal of Biomedical and Health Informatics. 28(8): 4854–4865.

[98] D'Souza, N.S., H. Wang, A. Giovannini, A. Foncubierta-Rodriguez, K.L. Beck, O. Boyko, et al. 2024. Fusing modalities by multiplexed graph neural networks for outcome prediction from medical data and beyond. Medical Image Analysis. 93: 103064.

[99] Kim, J.I., S. Bang, J.-J. Yang, H. Kwon, S. Jang, S. Roh, et al. 2022. Classification of preschoolers with low-functioning autism spectrum disorder using multimodal MRI data. Journal of Autism and Developmental Disorders. 1–13.

[100] Du, Y., X. He, P. Kochunov, G. Pearlson, L.E. Hong, T.G.M. van Erp, et al. 2022. A new multimodality fusion classification approach to explore the uniqueness of schizophrenia and autism spectrum disorder. Human Brain Mapping. 43(12): 3887–3903.

[101] Crimi, A., L. Dodero, V. Murino and D. Sona. 2017. Case-control discrimination through effective brain connectivity. *In*: 2017 IEEE 14th International Symposium on Biomedical Imaging (ISBI 2017). IEEE. 970–973.

[102] Chanel, G., S. Pichon, L. Conty, S. Berthoz, C. Chevallier and J. Grèzes. 2016. Classification of autistic individuals and controls using cross-task characterization of fMRI activity. *In*: NeuroImage: Clinical. 10: 78– 88.

[103] Wang, M., D. Zhang, J. Huang, P.-T. Yap, D. Shen and M. Liu. 2020. Identifying autism spectrum disorder with Multi-Site fMRI via low-rank domain adaptation. IEEE Transactions on Medical Imaging. 39(3): 644–655.

[104] Liu, R., Z.-A. Huang, Y. Hu, Z. Zhu, K.-C. Wong, K.C. Tan, et al. 2022. Attention-like multimodality fusion with data augmentation for diagnosis of mental disorders using MRI. IEEE Transactions on Neural Networks and Learning Systems. 35(6): 7627–7641.

[105] Ma, Y., W. Cui, J. Liu, Y. Guo, H. Chen and Y. Li 2023. A multi-graph cross-attention based region-aware feature fusion network using multi-template for brain disorder diagnosis. IEEE Transactions on Medical Imaging. 43(3): 1045–1059.

[106] Zhao, M., W. Yan, N. Luo, D. Zhi, Z. Fu, Y. Du, et al. 2022. An attention-based hybrid deep learning framework integrating brain connectivity and activity of resting-state functional MRI data. Medical Image Analysis. 78: 102413.

[107] Zhao, Y., Z. Yang, Z. Ding and J. Su. 2023. A riemannian framework for structurally curated functional clustering of brain white matter fibers. IEEE Transactions on Medical Imaging. 42(8): 2414–2424.

[108] Wang, N., D. Yao, L. Ma and M. Liu 2022. Multi-site clustering and nested feature extraction for identifying autism spectrum disorder with resting-state fMRI. Medical Image Analysis. 75: 102279.

[109] Wang, Y., H. Long, Q. Zhou, T. Bo and J. Zheng 2023. Plsnet: Position-aware GCN-based autism spectrum disorder diagnosis via FC learning and ROIs sifting. Computers in Biology and Medicine. 163: 107184.

[110] Itani, S. and D. Thanou. 2021. Combining anatomical and functional networks for neuropathology identification: A case study on autism spectrum disorder. Medical Image Analysis. 69: 101986.

Chapter **2.9**

Multi-Structure Segmentation for STN-DBS Surgery via Contrastive Learning

Congyu Tian[1], Manxi Lin[2], Doudou Zhang[3], Jialun Pei[4] and Weixin Si[1*]

[1]Shenzhen Institutes of Advanced Technology, Chinese Academy of Sciences

[2]Department of Applied Mathematics and Computer Science, Technical University of Denmark

[3]Department of Neurosurgery, Shenzhen Second People's Hospital

[4]Department of Computer Science and Engineering, The Chinese University of Hong Kong

2.9.1 INTRODUCTION

Parkinson's disease (PD), the second most common neurodegenerative disorder after Alzheimer's disease, causes motor and non-motor symptoms that significantly impact patients' quality of life. Deep brain stimulation (DBS) of the subthalamic nucleus (STN) is a well-established and effective neurosurgical treatment for alleviating motor symptoms in PD. Accurate localization and segmentation of key brain structures, i.e., STN, red nucleus, brain sulci, gyri, and ventricles, are crucial for effective pre-operative planning of STN-DBS. Traditionally, the localization and segmentation of these structures have relied solely on the manual manipulation of surgeons. Locating the STN, in particular, depends on direct delineation on

*For Correspondence: siweixin@suat-sz.edu.cn

DOI: 10.1201/9781003518754-14

T2-weighted MRI or indirect segmentation based on brain atlases. This process is often supplemented with intraoperative microelectrode recordings to refine the target location since STN is such a small anatomical size. Unfortunately, these traditional methods are time-consuming and heavily dependent on the expertise of surgeons, limiting their clinical applications.

Recent advances in machine learning for medical imaging analysis provide opportunities to enhance the accuracy and efficiency of STN-DBS surgeries. Deep learning techniques, especially convolutional neural networks (CNNs), have shown great promise in medical image segmentation, enabling the precise delineation of complex anatomical structures. Besides, these automated segmentation architectures based on deep learning can substantially cut down on time and workforce requirements, thereby improving overall surgical efficiency.

Although a series of methods based on the U-Net architecture have shown superior performance in numerous medical image segmentation tasks, the complexity of brain multi-structure segmentation makes a direct application of these networks less than optimal. On the one fold, recognizing tiny structures in the task (e.g., STN and red nucleus) and irregular structures (brain sulci, gyri, etc.) are difficult for most existing segmentation models. On the other fold, the variability in the location and shape of individual structures poses another challenge to these segmentation networks.

To overcome these issues, we propose a hierarchical attention U-Net framework based on contrastive learning. First, we introduce a coarse-to-fine workflow, complemented by hierarchical attention, to improve the recognition of tiny structures. Second, we employ contrastive learning strategies to enhance the discrimination of different structures. Additionally, we incorporate an ensemble module to boost segmentation results further. Experimental results demonstrate that our framework achieves competitive improvements in overall segmentation performance compared to existing methods.

2.9.2 RELATED WORKS

The application of deep learning in medical image segmentation has revolutionized the field, providing tools that can accurately and efficiently segment complex anatomical structures. U-Net, a convolutional network architecture designed for biomedical image segmentation, has been widely adopted owing to its ability to combine low-level and high-level features through skip connections in its encoder-decoder architecture. However, vanilla U-Net often struggles with recognizing small structures and distinguishing those with complex boundaries.

In recent years, a significant amount of work based on U-Net has been proposed to address these issues. Isensee et al. [1] proposed an adaptive medical image segmentation framework, namely nnU-Net, which is a simple U-Net architecture together with a robust training scheme. Fu et al. [2] developed HMRNet, which fuses multi-scale features with an additional high-resolution branch that maintains contextual information. Similarly, Zhang et al. [3] proposed HMNet, utilizing multi-resolution branches adapting different brain tumor shapes and sizes. Liu et al. [4] introduced FMMsWC, a triple-path U-Net for segmenting ventricles. Ottom et al. [5] proposed ZNet to segment 2D brain tumors in MR images. Additionally, some researchers have attempted multi-stage approaches for multi-structure segmentation of the brain. Baxter and Jannin [6] introduced a two-stage separable learning workflow for STN segmentation, including a localization stage and a segmentation stage.

Tomassini et al. [7] introduced a two-stage 3D U-Net for brain extraction and multi-structure segmentation. Some other works have sought to improve segmentation performance by introducing more modalities. Yue et al. [8] presented ACFNet for brain tumor segmentation, incorporating adaptive feature fusion and prediction inconsistency guidance. Wang et al. [9] developed SDPN, integrating local and global features with a multi-spectrum attention module, significantly improving segmentation performance for lesions with variable locations. Zhu et al. [10] proposed a brain tumor segmentation method by fusing semantic and edge features in multi-modal MRI to achieve accurate segmentation. Zhang et al. [11] proposed a novel multi-modal medical transformer (mmFormer) for incomplete multi-modal learning of brain tumor segmentation. Yang et al. [12] developed F^2Net, which can fuse arbitrary numbers of multi-modal images and integrate the multi-modal features into the shared network to get complementary segmentation results.

Many works introduce transformers, a recently popular network backbone, for medical image segmentation. Kiya et al. [13] introduced the Vision Transformer (ViT) framework for brain tumor segmentation. Jiang et al. [14] introduced the Swin Transformer for brain architecture segmentation, utilizing a window attention mechanism that is more applicable to brain segmentation tasks. Yu et al. [15] proposed UNesT, a hierarchical transformer design for local communication among spatially adjacent patches. Lin et al. [16] combined clinical knowledge with a hybrid CNN-Transformer model to leverage multi-modality image features for brain tumor segmentation. Yuan et al. [17] proposed CTC-Net, which features a CNN encoder for capturing spatial contextual information and a Transformer encoder for modeling long-range dependencies.

Although a large number of works have made improvements to brain segmentation tasks, most of them are only designed for the binary segmentation task of simple structures (e.g., tumors), which is not realistic for most brain structure segmentation scenarios.

As a result, these models often struggle with different anatomical structures of complex shapes and varying sizes. We consider the solution for the multi-class brain segmentation task with contrastive learning, a coarse-to-fine workflow, and ensemble learning.

2.9.3 METHOD

This chapter introduces a novel brain multi-structure segmentation framework for STN-DBS surgery via contrastive learning, as illustrated in Figure 9.1. The network works in a coarse-to-fine cascade flow. First, a vanilla U-Net provides preliminary segmentation results of key brain structures. Based on these results, we perform region-of-interest (ROI) detection. The cropped ROIs are then fed into our improved feature extraction network and two segmentation heads, which produce the segmentation results for different groups of structures. We further introduce ensemble learning to enhance the performance. We train the vanilla U-Net for ROI detection and the feature extraction network sequentially. The feature extraction network is first pre-trained with contrastive learning and then fine-tuned to the segmentation task.

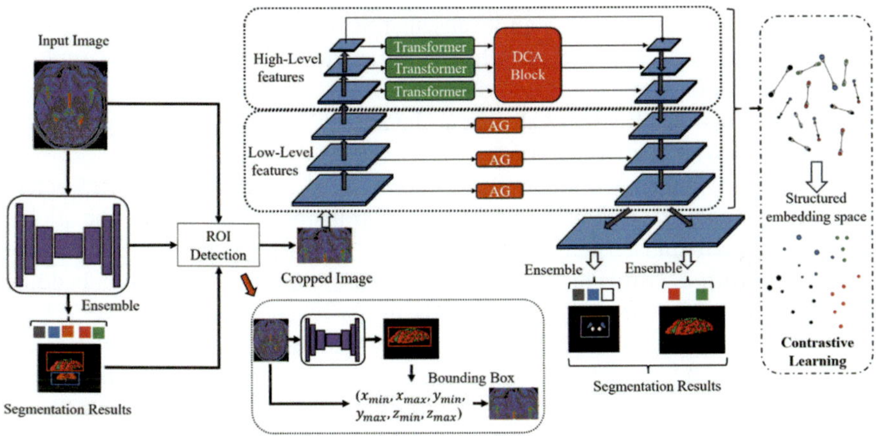

Figure 9.1 Diagram of our proposed framework. The input image will first be segmented by a vanilla U-Net for ROI detection. Subsequently, the cropped ROIs will be fed into a shared hierarchical attention U-Net pre-trained by contrastive learning to extract features. Finally, two segmentation heads with ensemble learning will be employed to achieve more precise segmentation for each structure.

2.9.3.1 Coarse-to-Fine Workflow and Multi-Head Segmentation

The sulci and gyri structures usually have complex shapes with co-occurrence. Compared to other structures, they are more isolated in location. , We treat them separately for better segmentation from other structures, i.e., STNs, red nuclei, and ventricles. Intuitively, zooming into the regions of interest (ROIs) improves the segmentation precision, especially for tiny structures. To this end, we introduce a two-stage workflow for coarse-to-fine segmentation, which localizes the ROIs at the first stage and performs accurate segmentation at the second stage.

In the first stage, we train a simple U-Net to conduct rough segmentation on the structures, on which we extract the bounding boxes of "sulci and gyri," as well as "other structures." These bounding boxes are used to describe the ROIs in the input image and serve as input for the following stage. In the second stage, the two cropped images are converted into corresponding feature maps by a shared feature extraction network (Section 2.9.3.2) respectively. We employ two segmentation heads consisting of 3 convolutional layers, one for brain sulci and gyri and the other for STNs, red nucleus, and ventricles. The extracted feature maps are passed to the corresponding segmentation heads to obtain segmentation results.

2.9.3.2 Hierarchical Attention U-Net

We propose a hierarchical attention U-Net as the feature extraction network, illustrated in Figure 1. Our U-Net includes six convolutional layers in the encoder and decoder, respectively. According to existing works, in the first few layers of U-Net, e.g., the first three convolutional layers, the network learns low-level features from the images, such as the texture information of anatomical structures. In the following layers, with the increase of the layer depth, the features become more and more abstract, with high-level semantic meanings. Considering the level of features, we employ different attention strategies to enhance the features of different layers for skip connection. For the low-level features from the first three layers, we adapt the attention gates from the Attention U-Net, where the features are enhanced with spatial attention.

We further exploit the global dependencies in the high-level features before the skip connection. Specifically, we use a transformer to model the global context. In each transformer layer, we replace the original positional encoding embedding with a learnable embedding PE, representing each token embedding T as $T = T^* + PE$, where T^* is the vanilla image token embedding, like ViT. In addition, we enhance the high-level features by introducing a dual cross-attention (DCA) module [18] to interact with the features from different layers. The module first fuses tokens of different sizes at the same location across multiple layers to capture the long-distance dependencies between different layers. The fused tokens are then passed through the channel cross-attention module and the spatial cross-attention module to fuse the tokens in the channel and spatial domains, respectively. The channel cross-attention (CCA) operation can be denoted as:

$$CCA(Q_i, K, V) = Softmax\left(\frac{Q_i K^T}{\sqrt{d}}\right)V, \tag{1}$$

where Q_i represents the linear mapping of each token T_i, d is the channel dimension, and K, V are the linear mappings of T_c obtained by normalizing and concatenating all tokens along the channel dimension. We denoted the output of each token from CCA as T_i^c, and their channel concatenation as T_c. Similarly, the spatial cross-attention (SCA) operation can be written as:

$$SCA\left(\bar{Q}, \bar{K}, \overline{V_i}\right) = Softmax\left(\frac{\bar{Q}\bar{K}^T}{\sqrt{d}}\right)\overline{V_i}, \tag{2}$$

where $\overline{V_i}$ represents the linear mapping of each token T_i^c, and $\bar{Q}$, $\bar{K}$ are the linear mappings of T_c. This dual cross-attention mechanism ensures that both channel and spatial dependencies between different layers are effectively captured and integrated, enhancing the overall segmentation performance.

2.9.3.3 Contrastive Pre-Training

We employ contrastive learning to enhance the separability of different structure features in the latent space. We adopt the pixel-to-pixel contrastive learning approach to pre-train our hierarchical attention U-Net. We split each image into patches. During training, the network is optimized by minimizing the distance between each patch and its positive samples, i.e., patches with the same structure, while maximizing the distance between it and its negative samples in the embedding space. For each patch, the loss function is computed as follows:

$$L = -\log \frac{\exp(S^p)}{\exp(S^p) + \exp(S^n)} \tag{3}$$

where S^p represents the score of positive samples obtained by computing the average similarity between the query patch feature and the positive patch features in the same batch, and S^n is calculated in a similar way for negative samples. This contrastive learning strategy enhances the network to differentiate between various brain structures.

2.9.3.4 Ensemble Learning

Ensemble methods are widely used inference strategies in machine learning, commonly consisting of three types: bagging, boosting, and stacking. In our framework, we employ a bagging strategy. We train all networks using five-fold cross-validation to obtain five different models and then aggregate the predictions from these models to obtain the final prediction result. This approach allows us to enhance the robustness and accuracy of our predictions by leveraging the diverse outputs from multiple models.

2.9.4 EXPERIMENTS

We perform a series of comparative and ablation experiments to validate the effectiveness of our method. This section presents the choice of experimental methods, the relevant parameter settings, and the experimental dataset. In addition, we illustrate and analyze the experimental results of the comparison and ablation studies. We build our codebase upon the official implementation of nnU-Net. All other baselines are implemented with the MONAI [19] framework. Experiments were performed on an NVIDIA RTX A6000 GPU and implemented with Python 3.9, PyTorch 2.0.0, and MONAI 1.4. For a fair comparison, we used the AdamW optimizer with a learning rate of le-3 to train all the models for 100 epochs with a batch size of 2; we chose the cosine annealing learning rate scheduler to adjust the learning rate. In this stage, we used RandFlip and RandRotate in MONAI for data augmentation. For contrastive learning, we utilized SGD as an optimizer and a cosine annealing learning rate scheduler to train the model for 100 epochs with a learning rate of le-2; the weight decay and momentum of the SGD optimizer were le-5 and 0.99, the batch size was set to 4, the patch size used in this stage was (96, 96, 96) and the dimension of the projected features was 512.

2.9.4.1 Dataset

All our experiments were performed on a private dataset consisting of 98 patients with PD who had undergone STN-DBS surgery (age range: 30–72 years; mean disease duration: 6.9 years). The raw MRI data contains T1-weighted and T2-weighted imaging. T1 images have a better illustration of the anatomical structures, while T2 is better in presenting tissue lesions. The 3-T MRI T1-weighted and T2-weighted images were obtained using a 64-channel head coil on a 3-T MRI system (Prisma, Siemens). All ground truth labels in the data were annotated by two radiologists with over six years of experience in neuroradiology. The labeled structures include sulci, gyri, red nucleus, ventricles, and the subthalamic nucleus. We utilize 80 of these cases as a training set and the remaining 18 cases as a test set, performing 5-fold cross-validation on the training set. In the preprocessing stage, we pad all the 3D volumes to the size of 256 × 256 × 256.

2.9.4.2 Model Performance

We compare our model performance with serval state-of-the-art methods, including U-Net, nnU-Net, and Attention U-Net. nnU-Net is one of the most widely used medical image segmentation frameworks. Attention U-Net employs the gated attention mechanism.

The sample-average dice similarity coefficient (DSC) of all methods for segmentation on the test set is shown in Table 9.1. According to the results, our model outperforms all the other methods in 3 out of the 5 anatomical structures, especially in the challenging segmentation of sulci and gyri. We attribute this to our coarse-to-fine workflow and contrastive learning. Specifically, the introduced ROI detection allows the network to focus on the ROIs, improving the segmentation accuracy. Our proposed contrastive learning significantly enhances the learned features, discriminating different structures. On the segmentation of the red nucleus and cerebral ventricles, our method is still competitive to most of the baselines, with dice scores of 84.33 and 94.17.

Table 9.1 Segmentation performance of different methods in the brain segmentation task. "DSC" in the table means the average dice score over all the samples in the test set

Methods	**DSC (%)**				
	Cerebral Sulci	**Cerebral Gyri**	**Red Nucleus**	**Cerebral Ventricles**	**Subthalamic Nucleus**
U-Net [20]	29.33	66.22	77.98	90.01	61.95
nnU-Net [1]	33.70	75.44	82.41	93.02	72.98
Attention U-Net [21]	30.98	67.72	78.13	92.31	66.50
Our method	**35.25**	**78.56**	**84.33**	**94.17**	**75.62**

2.9.4.3 Ablation Study

We conducted a series of ablation experiments to validate the effectiveness of our contributions. The experiment results of the ablation study for multi-structure segmentation on the test set are shown in Table 9.2. We evaluated the model performance with the sample-average dice score. Our approach includes a series of improvements over U-Net. As a consequence, we use U-Net as the baseline for ablation experiments.

We can see that after introducing our proposed hierarchical attention mechanism, the dice scores of each structure are significantly improved, especially for the segmentation of the STNs and the red nucleus. This indicates that the hierarchical attention mechanism we introduced effectively helps the network focus on small structures that U-Net cannot recognize clearly.

After embedding the ROI detection strategy, the dice scores for brain sulci and gyri exhibit a substantial improvement, whereas the enhancement is less noticeable for other structures. This can be attributed to the two-step approach of performing a coarse segmentation to identify ROIs, followed by a detailed segmentation of these specific regions. For sulci and gyri structures, which are relatively independently located, this approach allows the network to concentrate on segmenting these two types of structures, minimizing interference from other structural features when establishing long-distance dependencies.

The results with the ensemble indicate that using the ensemble method can slightly enhance segmentation performance, as evidenced by the various indicators being improved by nearly 1% in dice. Additionally, we incorporated contrastive learning into the hierarchical attention U-Net network to evaluate its optimization capabilities. The findings reveal that the network with contrastive learning improves segmentation across all types, with the most significant gains observed in sulci and gyri. The findings reveal that the network with contrastive learning improves segmentation across all types, with the most significant gains observed in sulci and gyri. As the most prominent and challenging to distinguish in the dataset, these structures benefit greatly from the introduced pixel contrastive learning approach.

2.9.5 DISCUSSION

Accurate segmentation of multiple brain structures is essential for surgeons planning STN-DBS surgery. Compared to previous deep learning-based methods, our approach introduces contrastive learning for multi-class structure segmentation, specifically tailored to the characteristics of the target brain structures. The proposed method significantly outperforms current well-known methods in most structures, providing physicians with more accurate and valuable location information, especially for STNs and gyri.

Although our method does not achieve the highest segmentation metrics for the red nucleus and ventricles, its performance is sufficient to meet the needs of most STN-DBS surgical scenarios. Comparative experiments reveal that the difference is slight, while our method's segmentation performance for red nuclei and ventricles is not the best. In contrast, our method shows significant improvement in segmenting other structures. This is because our proposed hierarchical attention U-Net can adjust the model's attention at different levels and perform multilayer

Table 9.2 Experiment results of ablation study

	Modules				DSC (%)				
	Hierarchical Attention	**ROI Detection**	**Ensemble**	**Contrastive Learning**	**Cerebral Sulci**	**Cerebral Gyri**	**Red Nucleus**	**Cerebral Ventricles**	**Subthalamic Nucleus**
Baseline					29.33	66.22	77.98	90.01	61.95
	✓				33.78	76.83	83.66	93.35	74.12
U-Net	✓	✓			34.67	77.74	83.85	93.27	74.30
	✓		✓		34.35	77.17	83.24	93.79	75.36
	✓			✓	34.80	78.24	83.89	94.11	75.54
Our method	✓	✓	✓	✓	**35.25**	**78.56**	**84.33**	**94.17**	**75.62**

fusion on high-level features, allowing effective handling of multi-structures with various shapes and sizes. Additionally, ablation experiments reveal that the proposed ROI detection mechanism enables independent processing of sulci and gyri, yielding better segmentation results due to their complex and interrelated shapes. Finally, incorporating contrastive learning significantly enhances our method's sensitivity to different structures, thus effectively improving overall performance in brain multi-structure segmentation.

2.9.6 CONCLUSION

In this chapter, we introduce a fully automated brain multi-structure segmentation framework that aids surgeons by providing localization and shape information for pre-operative planning of STN-DBS. Experimental results indicate that our method achieves DSCs of 35.25%, 78.56%, 84.33%, 94.17%, and 75.62% for the sulcus, gyrus, red nucleus, ventricles, and subthalamic nucleus, respectively, outperforming current state-of-the-art methods in overall performance. The hierarchical attention mechanism and dual cross-attention in our approach facilitate efficient feature extraction from different structures. Furthermore, the inclusion of ROI detection and ensemble learning enhances segmentation accuracy. Besides, we also leverage contrastive learning to better distinguish between various structures. Nonetheless, there is potential for improved brain sulci segmentation, evidenced by a DSC of 35.25%. Future efforts will focus on integrating foundational models to enhance further the segmentation accuracy of all structures, particularly the sulci, aiming for automated high-precision segmentation necessary for STN-DBS surgery.

REFERENCES

[1] Fabian Isensee, Paul F. Jaeger, Simon Kohl, Jens Petersen and Klaus H. Maier-Hein. 2021. nnU-Net: A self-configuring method for deep learning-based biomedical image segmentation. Nature Methods. 18(2): 203–211.

[2] Hao Fu, Guotai Wang, Wenhui Lei, Wei Xu, Qianfei Zhao, Shichuan Zhang, et al. 2022. HMRNet: High and multi-resolution network with bidirectional feature calibration for brain structure segmentation in radiotherapy. IEEE Journal of Biomedical and Health Informatics. 26(9): 4519–4529.

[3] Ruifeng Zhang, Shasha Jia, Mohammed Jajere Adamu, Weizhi Nie, Qiang Li and Ting Wu. 2023. HMNet: Hierarchical multi-scale brain tumor segmentation network. Journal of Clinical Medicine. 12(2): 538.

[4] Jinping Liu, Mengke Li, Subo Gong, Ardashir Mohammadzadeh and Guanyi Yang. 2023. Toward right ventricle segmentation in cardiac MRIs via feature multiplexing and multiscale weighted convolution. IEEE Journal of Biomedical and Health Informatics. 27(6): 2922–2931.

[5] Mohammad Ashraf Ottom, Hanif Abdul Rahman and Ivo D. Dinov. 2022. Znet: deep learning approach for 2D MRI brain tumor segmentation. IEEE Journal of Translational Engineering in Health and Medicine. 10: 1–8.

[6] John S.H. Baxter and Pierre Jannin. 2022. Combining simple interactivity and machine learning: A separable deep learning approach to subthalamic nucleus localization and segmentation in MRI for deep brain stimulation surgical planning. Journal of Medical Imaging. 9(4): 045001–045001.

[7] Selene Tomassini, Haidar Anbar, Agnese Sbrollini, M.H.D. Jafar Mortada, Laura Burattini and Micaela Morettini. 2023. A Double-Stage 3D U-Net for On-Cloud Brain Extraction and Multi-Structure Segmentation from 7T MR Volumes. Information 14(5): 282.

[8] Guanghui Yue, Guibin Zhuo, Tianwei Zhou, Weide Liu, Tianfu Wang and Qiuping Jiang. 2023. Adaptive cross-feature fusion network with inconsistency guidance for multi-modal brain tumor segmentation. IEEE Journal of Biomedical and Health Informatics.

[9] Jing Wang, Shuyi Li, Luyue Yu, Aixi Qu, Qing Wang, Ju Liu, et al. 2023. SDPN: A slight dual-path network with local-global attention guided for medical image segmentation. IEEE Journal of Biomedical and Health Informatics. 27(6): 2956–2967.

[10] Zhiqin Zhu, Xianyu He, Guanqiu Qi, Yuanyuan Li, Baisen Cong and Yu Liu. 2023. Brain tumor segmentation based on the fusion of deep semantics and edge information in multimodal MRI. Information Fusion 91: 376–387.

[11] Yao Zhang, Nanjun He, Jiawei Yang, Yuexiang Li, Dong Wei, Yawen Huang, et al. 2022. mmformer: Multimodal medical transformer for incomplete multi-modal learning of brain tumor segmentation. *In*: International Conference on Medical Image Computing and Computer-Assisted Intervention. Springer. 107–117.

[12] Hengyi Yang, Tao Zhou, Yi Zhou, Yizhe Zhang and Huazhu Fu. 2023. Flexible fusion network for multi-modal brain tumor segmentation. IEEE Journal of Biomedical and Health Informatics. 27(7): 3349–3359.

[13] Hitoshi Kiya, Teru Nagamori, Shoko Imaizumi and Sayaka Shiota. 2022. Privacy-preserving semantic segmentation using vision transformer. Journal of Imaging. 8(9): 233.

[14] Yun Jiang, Yuan Zhang, Xin Lin, Jinkun Dong, Tongtong Cheng and Jing Liang. 2022. SwinBTS: A method for 3D multimodal brain tumor segmentation using Swin transformer. Brain Sciences. 12(6): 797.

[15] Xin Yu, Qi Yang, Yinchi Zhou, Leon Y. Cai, Riqiang Gao, Ho Hin Lee, et al. 2023. Unest: local spatial representation learning with hierarchical transformer for efficient medical segmentation. Medical Image Analysis. 90: 102939.

[16] Jianwei Lin, Jiatai Lin, Cheng Lu, Hao Chen, Huan Lin, Bingchao Zhao, et al. 2023. CKD-TransBTS: Clinical knowledge-driven hybrid transformer with modality-correlated cross-attention for brain tumor segmentation. IEEE Transactions on Medical Imaging. 42(8): 2451–2461.

[17] Feiniu Yuan, Zhengxiao Zhang and Zhijun Fang. 2023. An effective CNN and Transformer complementary network for medical image segmentation. Pattern Recognition. 136: 109228.

[18] Gorkem Can Ates, Prasoon Mohan and Emrah Celik. 2023. Dual cross-attention for medical image segmentation. Engineering Applications of Artificial Intelligence 126: 107139.

[19] Jianwei Lin, Jiatai Lin, Cheng Lu, Hao Chen, Huan Lin, Bingchao Zhao, et al. 2022. Monai: An open-source framework for deep learning in healthcare. arXiv preprint arXiv:2211.02701.

[20] Olaf Ronneberger, Philipp Fischer and Thomas Brox. 2015. U-net: Convolutional networks for biomedical image segmentation. *In*: Medical image computing and computer-assisted intervention–MICCAI 2015: 18th international conference, Munich, Germany. Proceedings, Part III 18. Springer. 234–241.

[21] Ali Hatamizadeh, Yucheng Tang, Vishwesh Nath, Dong Yang, Andriy Myronenko, Bennett Landman, et al. 2022. Unetr: Transformers for 3D medical image segmentation. *In*: Proceedings of the IEEE/CVF Winter Conference on Applications of Computer Vision. 574–584.

Chapter 2.10

Alzheimer's Disease Diagnosis Methods Based on Biomedical Data

Jin Liu*, Xu Tian and Mengshen He
The School of Computer Science and Engineering,
Central South University, Changsha 410083, China

2.10.1 INTRODUCTION

Alzheimer's disease (AD) is an irreversible neurodegenerative disorder that progressively leads to comprehensive deterioration in memory, cognition, and motor abilities. AD is the leading cause of dementia, accounting for 70% of cases worldwide. It is projected that by 2050, the prevalence of dementia will triple. The neurodegenerative process in AD is believed to start 20 years or more before the onset of clinical symptoms. Genomic data, from healthy individuals (since genetic information, such as genotypes, remains constant) provide some of the earliest indications of differences between patients. As the disease progresses, certain AD-related genes become differentially expressed, leading to amyloid plaque deposition, tau protein abnormalities, and progressive damage to neurons and brain microstructures. After years of structural and functional degeneration, individuals experience noticeable symptoms, such as memory loss and language difficulties caused by damage to specific brain regions. These issues eventually impair the ability to perform daily activities, leading to severe conditions like amnesia, aphasia, and agnosia, and ultimately result in death. Given that there

*For Correspondence: liujin06@csu.edu.cn

DOI: 10.1201/9781003518754-15

is currently no cure for AD, accurate, objective, and timely diagnosis is crucial. According to [1], the progression of AD can be categorized into the following three stages:

- **Preclinical AD:** At this stage, molecular changes in the brain begin, detectable through blood tests and cerebrospinal fluid (CSF) analysis, despite the absence of noticeable clinical symptoms. This phase can start up to 20 years before any symptoms appear.
- **Mild Cognitive Impairment (MCI):** Patients or their family members notice cognitive difficulties, temporary memory loss, and related symptoms. Although individuals in this stage can still carry out daily activities, they often require some assistance and support. Notably, 10–15% of patients in this stage progress to AD yearly. Based on the progression, MCI can be further divided into progressive MCI (pMCI) and stable MCI (sMCI). This is a critical phase for intervention aimed at delaying neurodegeneration.
- **AD-Related Dementia:** Patients exhibit clear clinical symptoms, including significant changes in memory, cognition, language, and motor functions. At this stage, individuals progressively lose the ability to live independently, relying on family members or professional caregivers for daily support.

Biomedical data for diagnosing AD are available at various stages of the disease. However, due to the diversity in clinical presentations, subjectivity in evaluations by patients and physicians during clinical assessments and the unknown patterns of association among different biomarkers in molecular omics data and brain imaging data, effectively utilizing a broad spectrum of biomedical data for AD diagnosis—particularly in the early stages—remains a significant challenge. Given the recent advancements in artificial intelligence, specifically in machine learning (ML) and deep learning (DL), computer-aided diagnosis of AD has become increasingly essential to enhance diagnosis based on biomedical data. Furthermore, the availability of large-scale datasets, particularly the Alzheimer's Disease Neuroimaging Imaging Initiative (ADNI) dataset, has also driven the development of ML and DL-based computational models for AD diagnosis.

In recent years, a growing number of ML- and DL-based methods have been developed for AD diagnosis. Molecular omics data, including genomics, transcriptomics, and proteomics, are among the earliest biomedical indicators that reflect AD progression. Given the high dimensionality of these data, low-parameter models, such as statistical approaches and traditional machine learning techniques, are often used for diagnosing AD through molecular omics data. Molecular changes affect brain structure and function, eventually developing into observable manifestations in brain imaging data related to AD. Based on clinical diagnostic experience with AD, manually extracted structural and functional brain features were initially employed to assess AD progression using brain imaging data. With advancements in end-to-end models in the field of computer vision, an increasing number of AD diagnostic methods have moved away from predefined brain region segmentation and feature extraction. Instead, deep learning models such as Convolutional Neural Networks (CNNs), Recurrent Neural Networks (RNNs), and Transformers have become the primary frameworks. Unlike brain imaging data, patients' spontaneous behaviors represent a more holistic manifestation of AD-related symptoms and are among the most intuitive and easily evaluated indicators of AD. With the progress in foundational models from natural image and natural language analysis, spontaneous behavioral data—such as gait, speech, and language—have garnered increasing attention from researchers, playing a significant role in community monitoring and daily care for AD patients.

Molecular omics, brain imaging, and spontaneous behavior data are closely related to AD diagnosis and represent key categories of biomedical data. Therefore, in the following sections, we will provide a comprehensive review of AD diagnostic methods based on these three different levels of biomedical data. Specifically, Sections 2.10.2, 2.10.3, and 2.10.4 will cover methods grounded in molecular omics, brain imaging, and spontaneous behavior data, respectively. In Section 2.10.5, we will discuss diagnostic approaches that integrate multi-level biomedical data. Subsequently, Section 2.10.6 will present a comparison and discussion of the advantages and limitations of the current methods, along with an overview of relevant datasets, codes, and tool resources. Finally, in Section 2.10.7, we will summarize the current AD diagnostic methods based on biomedical data and identify future research directions and potential areas for further development.

2.10.2 Molecular Omics Data-based Methods

Molecular omics technologies provide a comprehensive view of the systemic pathophysiology of AD, encompassing genomics, transcriptomics, proteomics, and metabolomics. Innovations in these areas have emerged as powerful tools for studying early biomarkers of AD [2]. Genomics, in particular, quantifies and characterizes all genes and mutations in patients, identifying risk genes associated with AD and enhancing our understanding of the fundamental causes behind AD onset and progression. Transcriptomics plays a key role in investigating the regulatory mechanisms of AD risk genes and their associations with complex traits, helping to identify transcriptional programs and molecular processes linked to specific phenotypes. Proteomics focuses on the final products of gene expression—proteins—including protein levels, post-translational modifications, and protein-protein interactions, thereby identifying proteins and related genes involved in AD pathology. Metabolomics, which examines the full set of metabolites within a cell at a given moment, reflects the overall activity and environmental state of the cell and can reveal ongoing pathological processes in AD. Thus, molecular omics data provide a microscopic perspective on cellular processes in AD, enabling the identification of biomarkers associated with the early progression of the disease.

2.10.2.1 Single-Omics Methods

Genomics, the study of an organism's complete genetic material, has been widely used to investigate specific genetic variations related to disease, treatment, and prognosis [3]. Genome-wide association studies (GWAS) aim to identify associations between common genetic variations and phenotypes in a population where deoxyribonucleic acid is genotyped in the form of single nucleotide polymorphisms (SNPs) [4]. To diagnose AD from genomic data, Alatrany et al. [5] used random forest models to select SNPs associated with AD and developed an ensemble model comprising a multi-layer perceptron (MLP) and a CNN for AD diagnosis. The experimental results validated the effectiveness of their feature selection strategy and the ensemble model in diagnosing AD. Subsequently, Alatrany et al. [6] further enhanced the feature selection process by developing a hybrid method based on association testing, principal component analysis (PCA), and the Boruta algorithm to identify the most promising AD predictors. These selected features were then forwarded to a wide, deep neural network model for AD diagnosis. The experimental results confirmed the effectiveness of this feature selection approach. Purely data-driven feature selection methods that do not consider AD-specific associations often result in suboptimal performance. Jo et al. [7] proposed a novel three-step deep learning approach for identifying phenotypically relevant SNPs and developing an accurate AD diagnosis model to address this. In this approach, the entire genome was divided into optimally sized non-overlapping segments, from which deep features were extracted using a CNN. Phenotype impact scores were then calculated to identify SNP segments associated with AD. Finally, the identified SNPs were used to train a CNN to develop the AD diagnosis model. In addition to data-driven approaches for SNP and gene selection, some studies have explored specific gene pathways, such as ferroptosis. Wang et al. [8] investigated the association between ferroptosis-related genes and AD. They collected three AD gene expression datasets from the GEO database, identified AD-related module genes, and overlapped them with ferroptosis-related genes to determine hub genes (including JUN, SLC2A1, TFRC, ALB, and NFE2L2). Logistic regression was then used to distinguish AD patients from controls. The experimental results demonstrated that ferroptosis-related genes could be used to diagnose AD ($p < 0.05$), achieving an AUC of 0.643 for the diagnostic model.

Besides genes such as APOE, APP, PSEN1, and PSEN2, over 500 other genes have been identified over the years. However, their relationship with AD remains unclear. In order to address this issue, AD research has expanded to downstream omics fields, from genomics to transcriptomics, proteomics, and metabolomics. While genomics provides a static view of specific diseases, other molecular omics are dynamic and influenced by environmental changes [9]. Plasma biomarkers related to AD, such as amyloid and tau pathologies, have experienced rapid development in recent years. Stevenson et al. [10] attempted to define AD using an integrated set of plasma biomarkers rather than clinical assessments. They used these biomarkers to diagnose AD, achieving an AUC of 0.81. Their experimental results showed that plasma biomarkers accurately reflect the biochemically defined risk of AD and help distinguish it from other types of dementia. The combination of phosphorylated tau protein (P-tau) and other biomarkers collected from plasma may provide an accurate prediction of the risk of AD progression. Palmqvist et al. [11] showed that using P-tau alone could achieve an AUC of 0.83 for predicting AD progression within four years. When P-tau, demographic information, and cognitive scale data were integrated through a logistic regression model, the AUC increased to 0.91. Ablation studies of different feature types revealed that P-tau played the most significant role in predicting AD progression, surpassing demographic and cognitive scale features.

Considering the unknown risk genes associated with AD, Sun et al. [12] employed a fully data-driven approach to identify AD-related risk genes from gene expression data. They initially identified 120 differentially expressed genes (DEGs) through statistical tests, then used random forest (RF) to select six key genes (including KLF15, MAFF, ITPKB, SST, DDIT4, and NRXN3). Finally, they constructed an MLP based on these key genes for AD diagnosis. The lowest AUC of their model was 0.810, indicating that they successfully identified genetic biomarkers associated with AD and developed a novel AD diagnostic model.

Yu et al. [13] also directly selected DEGs from raw data rather than relying on previously reported risk genes. They screened DEGs from five gene expression datasets, identified hub genes using Cytoscape, and applied least absolute shrinkage and selection operator (LASSO) logistic regression to identify potential diagnostic biomarkers. Their experimental results showed that 16 hub genes became dysregulated as AD progressed, and the diagnostic model based on these genes achieved an AUC of 0.985. Given the advancements in bioinformatics data collection technologies, such as high-throughput methods, Mahendran et al. [14] developed a predictive model based on deep belief networks, utilizing methylation and gene expression microarray data to diagnose AD. To address the high-dimensional low sample size issue in raw data, they implemented a two-stage data-driven feature selection process: initially identifying DEGs and differentially methylated positions, followed by narrowing down candidate genes through an ensemble-based feature selection method. The experimental results demonstrated the effectiveness of the two-stage gene selection process and the deep belief network-based predictive model.

2.10.2.2 Multi-Omics Methods

From genomics to transcriptomics and proteomics, the mechanisms by which genetic factors lead to the onset and progression of AD remain unclear. Wingo et al. [15] integrated AD-related GWAS results with the human brain proteome to conduct proteome-wide association studies (PWAS) for AD, followed by Mendelian randomization and colocalization analyses. Their study identified 11 genes consistent with a causal role in AD, independent of APOE, providing new insights into the mechanisms of AD pathogenesis. The association between the genome and proteome is specific to different stages of AD progression. Altmann et al. [16] explored the roles of different loci during multiple stages of AD progression based on a Cox proportional hazards regression model. Their analysis revealed stage-dependent effects of genetic risk for AD, particularly for late-onset AD. Considering the deeply hidden information behind high-dimensional genetic data, Abbas et al. [17] developed a deep learning (DL)-based method to integrate

DNA methylation data and gene expression data for AD diagnosis. They used an autoencoder to extract minimal continuous feature representations from raw genetic data, which were then integrated with multiple machine-learning models for AD diagnosis. Wang et al. [18] further integrated three molecular omics data types, including mRNA expression data, DNA methylation data, and microRNA expression data, for AD diagnosis. They constructed a graph neural network (GNN) to extract deep representations of different molecular omics data while considering population relationships, followed by tensor fusion to integrate multi-omics representations for AD diagnosis. Similarly, Gong et al. [19] proposed a novel multi-omics integration method called the Multi-omics Attention Deep Learning Network for biomedical data classification. First, they used three fully connected layers and a self-attention mechanism to extract features from each molecular omics type and constructed patient relationships based on a graph structure. Then, they applied the feature vectors learned from self-attention to generate class labels and used a Multi-Omics Correlation Discovery Network to learn cross-omics correlations in the label space. Finally, an MLP with softmax was used to diagnose AD.

Despite significant advances in AD-related molecular omics research, multiple challenges remain. Although GWAS has identified more than 70 genes or genetic loci associated with AD risk, most of the data come from non-Hispanic white individuals in Europe and North America. This disparity has led to genetic information bias, limiting the understanding of AD in other racial groups and hindering the development of personalized treatment approaches. Moreover, the estimated heritability of AD remains lower than expected, likely due to insufficient research on rare variants and a lack of comprehensive multi-omics data. Identifying rare variants poses several challenges, including limited sample sizes and technical difficulties. While rare autosomal dominant forms of AD manifest in middle age, the more common forms occur in old age, with pathological heterogeneity being the norm. This complicates understanding disease progression mechanisms, necessitating more multi-omics data and interdisciplinary collaborative research to uncover its complexity. To fill the gaps in current knowledge, expanding genomic sequencing and analysis in underrepresented regions globally, incorporating blood-based biomarkers, and improving biomarkers are essential for a comprehensive understanding of the genetic architecture of AD and the variability of dementia worldwide.

2.10.3 BRAIN IMAGING DATA-BASED METHODS

The molecular progression in AD patients gradually affects brain structure and function, leading to neurodegeneration. The accumulation of extracellular protein fragments known as amyloid-beta (referred to as amyloid plaques) and abnormal forms of tau protein inside neurons (referred to as tau tangles) are the most prominent AD-related pathological changes in the brain. Additionally, reduced metabolism and brain atrophy are characteristic neurodegenerative processes associated with AD due to the gradual damage to neurons and the decreased metabolic capacity of cells in specific brain regions. For example, hippocampal astrocytes have emerged as an independent risk factor for dementia progression, and hippocampal neurodegeneration may be more directly related to cognitive and clinical decline than other pathological features. Thus, AD is associated with pathological amyloid deposition, structural brain atrophy, and altered brain metabolism. Structural magnetic resonance imaging (sMRI) is used to detect brain atrophy, while functional imaging modalities such as positron emission tomography (PET) and functional MRI (fMRI) can detect hypometabolism and brain dysfunction.

2.10.3.1 Single-Modal Methods

Structural magnetic resonance imaging (sMRI) is an outstanding imaging technique that can produce high-resolution anatomical images of the brain. It can precisely differentiate between gray and white matter, clearly depicting changes such as the widening and deepening of sulci and ventricles during the progression of dementia [20]. Additionally, sMRI allows imaging of the brain in any direction, enabling precise measurements of key regions such as the hippocampus and amygdala, which are crucial indicators for assessing brain atrophy. Structural changes in areas like the medial temporal lobe, hippocampus, and olfactory cortex can be used to detect MCI, as these regions exhibit significant neurofibrillary tangles and amyloid plaques in the early stages of the disease, aiding early diagnosis. Hippocampal neurodegeneration may be more directly associated with cognitive and clinical decline compared to other pathological features, which has prompted researchers to use hippocampal volume rather than whole-brain imaging to predict the conversion of MCI to stable MCI or dementia. Sathiyamoorthi et al. [21] preprocessed collected sMRI scans and extracted morphological measurements of AD-relevant regions of interest, using an MLP for AD diagnosis based on these features. They first applied a 2D adaptive bilateral filter for image restoration on the raw sMRI and used adaptive histogram adjustment (AHA) for image enhancement to improve sMRI contrast information. Then, they segmented AD regions of interest using an adaptive mean shift corrected expectation-maximization algorithm and calculated various features using a second-order 2D gray-level co-occurrence matrix. Finally, an MLP-based classifier was used for AD diagnosis based on the selected features. Experimental results demonstrated that the proposed steps effectively enhanced model accuracy and efficiency. Bron et al. [22] also used sMRI for AD diagnosis. Unlike other studies, they compared different preprocessing methods, including minimal preprocessing and preprocessing into specific gray matter maps, and different diagnostic algorithms such as support vector machines (SVM) and CNN. Their experimental results revealed performance differences due to pre-processing methods and variations in the regions of interest (ROIs) focused on by different diagnostic models, highlighting the complexity of AD-related brain regions and the potential advantages of ensemble models.

Deep learning models can more flexibly focus on AD-related brain regions than machine learning models. Fan et al. [23] proposed a U-Net model for

AD diagnosis using sMRI. In their method, multi scale brain imaging features were fused and combined with deep supervision, effectively utilizing AD-related imaging features at various scales. Their method was validated on the ADNI datasets, demonstrating that multi-scale feature extraction and deep supervision can significantly improve model performance. Additionally, they used a 3D Grad-CAM method to visualize the regions that the model focused on for AD diagnosis, finding that the model paid more attention to features in the ventricles, hippocampus, and certain cortical areas known to be affected by AD. Mehmood et al. [24] employed a transfer learning approach to prevent overfitting small AD datasets, adapting a VGG model pre-trained on natural images to the AD diagnosis task. Experimental results showed that their model outperformed state-of-the-art models in test accuracy. Considering the local brain atrophy caused by AD, sMRI scans may show only a few regions with significant structural changes that are highly correlated with AD pathology. Zhu et al. [25] proposed a dual-attention multi-instance deep learning network. Specifically, this network consisted of three main components: a patch network with spatial attention blocks to extract discriminative features from each sMRI patch, an attention-based multi-instance learning pooling operation to generate a global weighted representation, and an attention-aware global classifier to further learn overall features and make AD-related diagnostic decisions. Experimental results indicated that the model could identify class-discriminative pathological locations and achieve better classification performance in terms of both accuracy and generalizability. The receptive field of CNNs is local rather than global, which makes it challenging for CNNs to capture global brain information. Fan et al. [26] proposed a brain-inspired global-local information fusion network for AD diagnosis. This network used CNNs to capture morphological features of local brain regions and used a graph convolutional network (GCN) to establish long-distance relationships between different spatial locations, thereby inheriting the advantages of both CNNs and GCNs, resulting in improved performance. Han et al. [27] developed a novel multi-template meta-data regularization network for AD diagnosis to exploit the impact of metadata on AD diagnosis. Specifically, they considered the confounding effects of the correlation between metadata and AD and designed weakly supervised metadata learning and mutual information minimization modules to learn metadata and disentangle it from class-related representations, explaining the metadata regularization in disease diagnosis. Experimental results validated the importance of considering metadata in AD diagnostic models. In addition to integrating more information for AD diagnosis, another common approach to enhance model performance is to include subjects from more medical centers, thereby increasing the sample size. Lei et al. [28] proposed a Transformer-based multi-site federated domain adaptation framework. This framework not only extracted correlations between multi-atlas regions of interest, capturing rich brain information but also integrated sMRI data from different sites while eliminating data heterogeneity.

PET is a functional imaging technique that measures brain metabolism and specific pathological biomarkers by injecting radioactive tracers. It is particularly useful for directly detecting amyloid-beta and tau protein deposits, which are closely associated with AD pathology. PET can be performed for amyloid-beta using specific radioligands such as ^{18}F-Florbetapir and ^{18}F-Flutemetamol. These tracers bind to amyloid-beta accumulated in the brain, with excessive amyloid-beta accumulation being one of the hallmark pathological features of AD. Park et al. [29] developed an ML-based framework for AD staging diagnosis using ^{18}F-Flortaucipir PET. In this framework, they extracted the standardized uptake value ratio (SUVR) from PET and combined it with clinical variables such as age, gender, education level, and Mini-Mental State Examination (MMSE) scores. AD diagnosis was performed using logistic regression, SVM, extreme gradient boosting (XGBoost), and MLP models. Experimental results showed that the AUC for each diagnostic model using tau SUVR features was higher than clinical variables alone, especially for SUVR features in the entorhinal cortex and amygdala, demonstrating the effectiveness of SUVR as an imaging feature. Accumulation of amyloid-beta (Aβ) is also one of the most common neurobiological biomarkers for AD. Ding et al. [30] investigated whether radiomic features from Aβ PET could serve as AD predictors and provide a neurobiological basis. In their study, they proposed radiomic features for Aβ PET imaging of each brain region, including intensity features (primarily reflecting grayscale distribution) and texture features (primarily reflecting grayscale homogeneity). An SVM model was used for AD diagnosis. Experimental results showed that the radiomic features extracted from Aβ PET could effectively be used for AD diagnosis and were significantly correlated with clinical indicators such as APOE genotype, polygenic risk score, and cognitive scores. To explore the impact of different feature extraction methods, Zhou et al. [31] developed a novel deep learning radiomics (DLR) model based on ^{18}F-FDG PET images. They compared DLR features with ROI radiomic features and SUVR features, validating the advantages of deep learning in radiomic feature extraction. Deep learning models are more flexible in extracting imaging features from PET. Kishore et al. [32] constructed an end-to-end deep learning method based on a pre-trained VGG model for AD diagnosis using PET, while Thakur et al. [33] developed an AD diagnostic model based on ResNet. To effectively integrate 3D spatial information from PET, Duan et al. [34] proposed a broad-based network model (BLADNet) for MCI diagnosis using PET. This method employed a novel broad neural network to enhance PET features extracted by a 2D CNN. Since BLADNet can search for information in a broad space by adding new BLS blocks without retraining the entire network, it improved the accuracy of AD classification. Considering the limited sample size and high acquisition cost of PET, Baydargil et al. [35] employed an adversarial training approach, incorporating a generative adversarial network (GAN) into the diagnostic model to further enhance its performance in AD diagnosis. To reduce PET acquisition costs through imaging acceleration, Zhao et al. [36] proposed an image denoising method called Monte Carlo Denoising Network for accelerated PET images. They selected PET images with normal scan times and reduced scan times to generate the necessary training data. Objective metrics and subjective evaluations by radiologists validated the effectiveness of the PET image denoising method, showing that it could reduce PET scan times from a normal level of 20 to 5 minutes while maintaining acceptable image quality for correctly diagnosing amyloid-beta levels.

fMRI can detect functional connectivity network (FCN) abnormalities in the brains of AD and MCI patients, particularly impairments in the default mode network. FCN of brain networks refers to the synchrony between regions detected from low-frequency fluctuations in blood oxygen level-dependent (BOLD) sequences. The DMN is the most commonly studied brain network in fMRI research and is involved in memory consolidation tasks. Consistent evidence shows that FCN within the DMN is reduced in AD patients compared to healthy controls, particularly between the posterior and anterior cortical areas, such as the posterior cingulate cortex and medial prefrontal cortex. Khatri et al. [37] investigated functional brain networks at a resting-state frequency range of 0.01–0.027, primarily including the DMN. They applied graph theory to compute nodal features (degree, path length, and centrality) and used feature selection methods to reduce the dimensionality of the raw network features, training SVM and RF classifiers based on the highly significant feature vectors. Experimental results validated the impact of AD on the DMN. Zamani et al. [38] incorporated raw FCN measures and graph-theoretical measures into their analysis framework. They input the features into multiple evolutionary algorithms and statistical methods to select a feature subset and used an MLP with two hidden layers to diagnose AD. Integrating fMRI as an FCN overlooks the fine-grained dynamic changes within brain networks. Sun et al. [39] conducted a longitudinal study on brain networks for AD diagnosis. They extracted fMRI data from individual subjects at different follow-ups and developed a deep learning method based on a residual CNN and a multi-layer long short-term memory (LSTM) network to diagnose and longitudinally predict AD effectively. FC represents an undirected network of spontaneous associations between brain regions. However, correlation does not necessarily imply causation. Using fMRI, Biswas et al. [40] constructed causal functional connectivity (C-FCN), providing a directed network representing causal relationships between brain regions. Their study used the time-aware Peter-Clark algorithm to infer causal functional connectivity across the brain. They compared the C-FCN results in the AD diagnosis task with other related methods in the literature and conducted exploratory analysis on differences in C-FCN edge strength between the AD and cognitively normal groups. FCN characterizes first-order relationships between brain regions, ignoring higher-order interactions, which limits its application in AD diagnosis. Lei et al. [41] developed a new framework to leverage higher-order dynamic interactions between brain regions for AD diagnosis. Specifically, they used a sliding window method to generate a series of fMRI sub-sequences and used these subsequences to construct a series of dynamic FCNs. They then constructed a high-order FCN based on the topological similarity between each pair of FCNs. Next, they extracted network features from the high-order FCN, selected features using the least absolute shrinkage and selection operator (LASSO), and performed AD diagnosis using an SVM. Experimental results showed that by considering both the dynamic and higher-order properties of brain networks, the proposed method achieved promising results in AD diagnosis and successfully identified biomarkers associated with the disease.

FCN naturally has a graph structure, and graph neural networks (GNNs) are widely used for AD diagnosis based on FCN. Qin et al. [42] extended the excellent CNN framework to GCN-based brain network analysis and proposed a U-shaped hierarchical GCN framework (U-GCN), which includes downsampling, upsampling, and skip connection operators for graph data. Experimental results validated the effectiveness of this framework. Considering the hierarchical characteristics of brain and population networks, Zhang et al. [43] constructed a local-to-global graph neural network (LG-GNN) to address this issue. A local ROI-GNN was used to learn feature embeddings of the brain, and then a global subject-level GNN was established. Experimental results showed that LG-GNN achieved state-of-the-art performance in various evaluation metrics for AD diagnosis. Zhou et al. [44] also recognized the local characteristics of GCN operations and proposed a method for coupling global representation learning with local sequential features, enhancing FCN representation learning using convolution operations and a self-attention mechanism to extract topological information from local to global FCN. Experiments on AD and attention deficit hyperactivity disorder (ADHD) demonstrated the superiority of this method. FCN construction is influenced by prior knowledge, such as atlases. Gan et al. [45] proposed a multi-atlas integrated FCN analysis framework to reduce the impact of atlas selection and subject heterogeneity. They proposed a multi-graph fusion method to explore shared and complementary information between two FCNs, producing highly discriminative fMRI data representations for AD diagnosis. Their method was validated on various dementia and psychiatric conditions, including AD. Experimental results showed that the proposed framework achieved optimal diagnostic performance by selecting reasonable brain regions for classification tasks compared to state-of-the-art FCN analysis methods. Ma et al. [46] not only considered the limitations of using a single atlas but also considered the complementary information between static and dynamic brain networks and functional differences between different brain regions. To address these limitations, they proposed a regional-aware feature fusion network based on multi-graph cross-attention, where the multi graph cross-attention network was used to explore deep features contained in multi-template data and the regional-aware feature fusion network was used to consider the potential relationships between static and dynamic features of different brain regions, further improving the discriminative power of features. FCN reflects the pairwise relationships between brain regions. Zhang et al. [47] constructed a diffusion kernel attention network based on a transformer to address the challenge of higher-order brain connectivity. Specifically, they used kernel attention to replace the original dot-product attention module in the transformer and further explored the diffusion process of attention to include broader interactions between indirectly connected brain regions. Extensive experimental studies on the ADNI dataset showed that the proposed method outperformed competing methods. Hyper-connectivity networks (HCNs) are also a common approach to reveal higher-order interactions between multiple brain regions. Liu et al. [48] proposed a spatiotemporal-weighted HCN to capture high-order spatiotemporal characteristics of more comprehensive brain activity and developed a multi-atlas deep fusion model to extract and fuse deep interaction information between different templates. Experimental results showed that the proposed method outperformed state-of-the-art methods for AD diagnosis, and the abnormal spatiotemporal hyper-edges it identified were important for analyzing brain abnormalities in AD. Despite advances in FCN analysis methods, they still lack interpretability. Xu et al. [49] proposed a contrastive dual-attention block and an interpretable graph pooling method to apply GNNs to brain networks. Their case studies confirmed that the patterns extracted by their method matched domain knowledge in the neuroscience literature, with the potential to enhance understanding of brain networks and AD.

2.10.3.2 Multi-Modal Methods

Multi-modal fusion can integrate information from modalities in different stages. According to the stage of fusion, multi-modal fusion can be divided into early fusion, late fusion, and hybrid fusion [50]. Early fusion fuses multi-modal data in the raw data space [51, 52]. Late fusion constructs models for different modalities and fuses their predicted values [53, 54]. Hybrid fusion first extracts mid-level features from each modality and then integrates them into a single compact representation [55, 56].

Early fusion attempts to combine two modalities into a new one. For brain imaging data, the most common approach is the fusion of sMRI and PET. Kong et al. [57] proposed an image fusion method that combines sMRI and PET of AD patients, then used a 3D CNN to evaluate the effectiveness of the image fusion method for AD diagnosis. Experimental results showed that the proposed model achieved better results in terms of accuracy, sensitivity, and specificity. Dwivedi et al. [58] also fused sMRI and PET using wavelet transformation for AD diagnosis. To fuse information from different modalities, Zhang et al. [51] extracted important image features from multiple input images and used several fusion rules, such as element-wise maximum, minimum, and average, to fuse features from multiple images. In addition to obtaining important information from individual modalities, it is also necessary to estimate the importance of different modalities. Zhao et al. [52] further divided features into low-frequency and high-frequency domains and adopted different fusion strategies for different domains. For medical images, Li et al. [59] constructed an edge enhancement module and a global refinement module to enhance the visual effect of the proposed fusion network. They added semantic guidance to facilitate the training of the fusion network. Directly fusing images from different modalities may not be an ideal choice for AD diagnostic models. On the one hand, although early fusion creates a new modality, it may lead to the loss of diagnostic-related information since it typically follows a two-stage fusion-diagnosis model, where the first stage is not guided by AD diagnosis. On the other hand, image fusion struggles to handle heterogeneous multi-modal data, such as sMRI and fMRI, where the former is 3D, and the latter is 4D.

Late fusion constructs separate models for each modality and combines the predictions of these models using ensemble learning. The advantage of late fusion is that it allows for designing classifiers specific to each modality and combines heterogeneous base learners into a single model. Shukla et al. [60] extracted features from sMRI and PET and constructed an ensemble classifier to integrate the diagnostic results from different modalities. Junaid et al. [54] used different classifiers in the diagnosis and demonstrated that different classifiers could accurately diagnose different subjects. Additionally, Liu et al. [53] used a graph learning network to construct diagnostic models for different modalities. Considering the role of each modality in diagnosis, they used a two-step integration strategy to fuse the predictions of all models. Qiu et al. [61] constructed a two-stage model for AD diagnosis using sMRI along with clinical information such as age, gender, and scale scores. In this method, the sMRI diagnostic results were combined with other clinical information and used for cognitive classification and risk prediction in the second stage. Although it is straightforward to design a separate model for each modality in late fusion, it is time-consuming, expensive, and lacks cross-modal joint learning.

Hybrid fusion allows one to model relationships between different modalities, leverage cross-modal collaboration, and find better task-relevant representations. Tu et al. [62] proposed a novel multi-modal feature transformation and fusion model for AD diagnosis. They used feature transformation to avoid feature dimensional differences between different modalities and further mined significant features for AD diagnosis. They designed an ANN-based framework to fuse the transformed features with neuroimaging features extracted by CNN for AD diagnosis. Du et al. [56] proposed a novel sparse multi-task mixed-effects longitudinal method that modeled the association between different modalities. Their study showed that correlations indeed exist between different modalities. There are complex correlations between modalities, especially for specific brain regions. To perform multi-modal fusion in the feature space, Wang et al. [63] constructed different graphs based on various modalities and used a hypergraph regularization term to merge inter-modal and cross-modal information. Similarly, Zheng et al. [64] proposed a multi-modal graph learning method. This method used modality-aware representation learning to aggregate features from each modality by leveraging modality correlations and complementarities. Additionally, it captured the underlying graph structure through an effective adaptive graph learning approach, revealing intrinsic relationships between samples effectively improving model performance at both the modality and sample levels. Considering the heterogeneity and complementarity of multi-modal data, Lei et al. [65] proposed a new framework for AD diagnosis that integrates genetic, imaging, proteomic, and clinical data. This framework integrates multi-modal features into a graph structure and uses a feature induction learning module to learn feature representations of different modalities in the same feature space. It performs multi-modal fusion based on a hierarchical graph composed of nodes from different modalities, thereby mitigating the impact of feature heterogeneity.

To overcome overfitting caused by an increase in modality numbers, Ning et al. [66] proposed a relation-induced multi-modal shared representation learning method for AD diagnosis. This method obtained multi-modal shared representations by learning a bidirectional mapping between the original space and shared space. In this shared space, a relation regularizer was used to encourage learning the inherent latent associations of multi-modal data. Experimental results on two independent AD datasets showed that the proposed method outperformed several state-of-the-art methods. Considering the discriminative information between samples under multi-modal data, Zhu et al. [67] proposed a deep multi-modal discriminative and Explainable Network method. This method aligns samples in a discriminative common space and provides a new approach to identifying important brain regions (ROIs) for AD diagnosis. It used generalized canonical correlation analysis as a correlation constraint to generate a discriminative common space and employed knowledge distillation to capture the influence of brain regions on AD classification, achieving better performance and interpretability. Qiu et al. [68] proposed a novel multi-modal diagnostic network based on multi-fusion and disease-induced learning to alleviate inherent differences between multi-modal images, enhancing MCI diagnosis by effectively fusing multi-modal data. Specifically, this method enhanced feature representations from a global, local, and latent learning perspective to effectively alleviate modality heterogeneity and used disease-induced region-aware learning to identify AD-related brain regions, thereby effectively enhancing the interpretability of the model.

Multi-modal fusion provides an irreplaceable opportunity to leverage complementary cross-modal information between different brain imaging data. However, most deep models, such as convolutional neural networks and their numerous extensions, can only operate on regular Euclidean data (e.g., voxels in 3D sMRI), neglecting the natural graph structure of brain networks. Zhang et al. [69] developed a graph-based deep neural network. The topology of the brain network was initialized using DTI and iteratively updated by incorporating functional information from fMRI. Using multi-modal brain networks effectively improved the model's ability to distinguish between MCI and healthy individuals. Yang et al. [70] integrated functional and structural connectivity data from the brain, specifically fMRI and diffusion tensor imaging (DTI), for AD diagnosis. Their study proposed a cross-modal graph neural network that used dynamic graph learning and mutual learning to capture inter-modal dependencies, carefully coupling inter-modal representations into a combined space to infer inter-modal relationships. Experiments on neurodegenerative diseases like AD and Parkinson's disease (PD) demonstrated the superiority of this diagnostic method, with good diagnostic performance and localization of multi-modal connectomic biomarkers. Using multi-modal data also poses challenges for brain network analysis, such as high-dimensional data and interpretability. Zhou et al. [71] proposed a multi-modal sparse interpretable GCN framework for diagnosing AD and its precursor stage MCI. This method learned sparse region importance probabilities to identify regions of interest and connection importance probabilities to reveal disease-specific brain network connections. Experimental results showed that sparse ROIs could effectively enhance AD diagnosis, and the identified abnormalities were significantly related to AD clinical symptoms. Song et al. [72] also introduced a dual-modal fusion brain connectivity network combining fMRI and DTI and proposed three mechanisms to improve AD diagnosis performance within the current GCN.

First, they considered the relationship between structure and function by introducing a DTI intensity penalty term to construct a functional connectivity network. Second, they constructed a multi-center population graph to account for the influence of data sources, gender, acquisition devices, and disease status. Third, they proposed a complex attention mechanism to perform feature pooling based on feature statistics. Experimental results on multiple AD datasets showed that this method outperformed other related algorithms. Considering both intra-region features and inter-region connectivity, Liu et al. [73] integrated anatomical and morphological information from sMRI with complementary information from fMRI. In this study, they developed an enhanced multi-modal graph convolutional network for AD diagnosis based on the fusion of brain region structural and functional graphs.

Multi-modal brain imaging data has promoted the improvement of AD diagnostic model performance, but there are still obstacles and limitations to multi-modal methods in real-world scenarios, such as modality imbalance and missing modalities. To address the issue of modality imbalance, Han et al. [74] proposed a new Doubly Supervised Transfer Classifier (DSTC) algorithm based on transfer learning, which utilizes supervised knowledge transfer between modalities using shared labels and block-diagonal low-rank constraints. For the problem of incomplete modalities in AD diagnosis, Chen et al. [75] proposed a disentangle-then-distill framework. They designed a disentanglement module to decompose images into modality-shared and modality-specific representations, followed by a distillation module. In cross-modal distillation, they created a lateral inter-modal transfer unit to interpolate the representations of missing modalities. Experimental results showed that this method achieved superior AD and MCI diagnosis performance. Based on the association between brain imaging data and genetic data, Wang et al. [76] proposed a deep multi-modal disentangled correlation analysis network. This method decomposed each modality's information into shared and specific components, establishing a nonlinear relationship between imaging and genetic data, and simultaneously synthesized modality mask vectors to integrate genetic and imaging data for disease diagnosis. Since the nonlinear mapping between modalities was constructed, the shared genetic representation could be used to estimate missing multi-modal data. Similarly, Ko et al. [77] developed a multi-modal learning method based on adversarial generative networks. This method extracted feature vectors from genetic data and mapped them to feature vectors of imaging data. It also implemented a dot-product fusion method for genetic and imaging features and used the fused multi-modal features for downstream AD diagnosis tasks. Unlike imputation of representations, Liu et al. [78] developed a multi-task model that simultaneously synthesized missing modality data and performed AD diagnosis. This model is a Joint Neuroimage Synthesis and Representation Learning (JSRL) framework that contains two components: a generative adversarial network for synthesizing missing images and a classification network for AD diagnosis. These two components were incorporated into a joint learning framework by sharing the same features. In multi-modal AD diagnosis tasks based on sMRI and PET, this model achieved leading performance in both cross-modal synthesis and AD diagnosis tasks.

2.10.4 LIMITATIONS AND FUTURE WORKS

Despite significant advancements in Alzheimer's disease (AD) diagnosis using biomedical data, several limitations persist, hindering its widespread clinical application. One of the major challenges lies in the availability and diversity of data. Current research primarily relies on large-scale public datasets such as ADNI, which predominantly consist of North American and European populations. This leads to a lack of generalizability in diagnostic models when applied to underrepresented ethnic groups. Moreover, many datasets lack longitudinal data, making it difficult to model disease progression and accurately predict future cognitive decline. Additionally, missing data remains a critical issue in multi-modal approaches, as obtaining comprehensive genomic, imaging, and behavioral data from each patient is often impractical due to high acquisition costs, patient compliance issues, and technical constraints.

Another significant limitation is the heterogeneity of AD biomarkers and disease progression. AD is a complex and multifactorial disorder, with variations in genetic, molecular, structural, and functional biomarkers across individuals. Current diagnostic models often focus on classifying patients into predefined categories (e.g., AD vs. CN, MCI vs. AD), yet they fail to capture the full spectrum of disease subtypes and individualized risk factors. Furthermore, the relationships between different modalities, such as molecular omics and neuroimaging features, remain poorly understood, limiting the interpretability and biological relevance of multi-modal fusion models. As a result, while AI-driven models have achieved promising classification performance, their ability to provide clinically meaningful insights remains constrained.

Integrating multi-modal data poses additional challenges, as each modality presents distinct data structures, resolutions, and noise characteristics. Existing fusion strategies—early, late, and hybrid fusion—each have inherent drawbacks. Early fusion may lead to information loss due to differences in data representation across modalities, while late fusion, which treats each modality independently before aggregating predictions, often fails to capture meaningful cross-modal interactions. Hybrid fusion methods, although promising, introduce increased computational complexity and a higher risk of overfitting, particularly when training deep learning models on limited sample sizes. The alignment of multi-modal data remains a critical issue, as variations in spatial and temporal resolutions between imaging and molecular data can hinder effective integration.

Interpretability remains another major barrier to clinical adoption. Most deep learning models, particularly convolutional neural networks (CNNs) and transformers, function as black-box systems, making it difficult for clinicians to understand how decisions are made. While visualization techniques such as Grad-CAM and SHAP enhance explainability, they often provide only post-hoc interpretations rather than intrinsic model transparency. Clinicians require models that not only yield high accuracy but also offer interpretable and actionable insights into disease mechanisms. Trust in automated diagnostic tools remains limited without clear explanations of how AI models derive their conclusions. Furthermore, computational feasibility and clinical integration present practical constraints. Many state-of-the-art deep learning models require substantial computational resources, which may not be readily available in all clinical settings, particularly in resource-limited healthcare environments. The high cost of acquiring high-quality biomedical data, such as PET imaging and multi-omics sequencing, further limits the scalability of these methods. Additionally, most AI-based diagnostic models are developed and evaluated in controlled research environments but are rarely tested in real-world clinical workflows. Seamless integration into electronic health record (EHR) systems, real-time inference capabilities, and regulatory approval processes remain critical hurdles before AI-driven AD diagnostics can be deployed on a large scale.

In order to address these limitations, future research should prioritize the development of more diverse and representative datasets, incorporating underrepresented populations and expanding longitudinal data collection efforts. Advanced data augmentation and self-supervised learning techniques could help mitigate the impact of missing data while improving model robustness. Additionally, improving multi-modal fusion strategies by leveraging graph neural networks (GNNs), hypergraph learning, and causal inference methods may enable more effective integration of heterogeneous biomedical data, facilitating a deeper understanding of disease mechanisms. Enhancing model interpretability through explainable AI (XAI) techniques, such as attention mechanisms, knowledge distillation, and hybrid AI approaches that combine deep learning with domain knowledge, will be crucial for gaining clinical trust.

Furthermore, optimizing computational efficiency and enabling real-time clinical deployment should be a key focus. Lightweight deep learning architectures, federated learning for secure multi-institutional collaboration, and cloud-based diagnostic frameworks could enhance the accessibility of AI-driven AD diagnosis. Additionally, integrating AI with personalized medicine approaches, incorporating lifestyle and environmental factors alongside genetic and imaging data, could pave the way for individualized risk assessments and targeted interventions. By addressing these challenges, future research can move towards more accurate, interpretable, and clinically applicable AI-driven AD diagnosis and progression prediction solutions.

2.10.5 CONCLUSION

Alzheimer's disease (AD) remains a major global health challenge, necessitating accurate, objective, and early diagnosis to enable timely interventions. With the rapid advancement of biomedical data acquisition technologies, molecular omics, brain imaging, and behavioral data have become crucial sources for AD diagnosis. Machine learning and deep learning approaches have significantly improved the ability to extract valuable insights from this data, facilitating automated and data-driven diagnostic frameworks. This survey comprehensively reviewed recent research on AD diagnosis, focusing on single-modal and multi-modal methodologies and their respective strengths and limitations.

Despite the substantial progress in AI-assisted AD diagnosis, several challenges remain. Data heterogeneity, limited generalizability, and the difficulty of integrating multi-modal information continue to hinder the robustness and clinical applicability of current models. Additionally, the lack of explainability in deep learning models reduces their acceptance among clinicians, while the computational cost and high data acquisition expenses present further barriers to large-scale implementation. Addressing these challenges requires the development of more diverse and representative datasets, advanced multi-modal fusion strategies, and interpretable AI models that can offer meaningful insights into disease progression. Furthermore, optimizing computational efficiency and integrating AI-driven diagnostics into real-world clinical workflows will be critical to bridging the gap between research advancements and practical applications.

Future research should emphasize interdisciplinary collaboration between computer science, neuroscience, and clinical medicine to refine AI-driven diagnostic models. The field can move toward more precise, interpretable, and scalable AD diagnostic solutions by incorporating emerging technologies such as federated learning, causal inference, and personalized medicine. Ultimately, synergistically leveraging AI and biomedical data has the potential to revolutionize AD diagnosis and provide new opportunities for early intervention and improved patient outcomes.

REFERENCES

[1] M. Khojaste-Sarakhsi, Seyedhamidreza Shahabi Haghighi, S.M.T. Fatemi Ghomi and Elena Marchiori. 2022. Deep learning for Alzheimer's disease diagnosis: A survey. Artificial Intelligence in Medicine. 130: 102332.

[2] Philip Scheltens, Bart De Strooper, Miia Kivipelto, Henne Holstege, Gael Chételat, Charlotte E. Teunissen, et al. 2021. Alzheimer's disease. The Lancet. 397(10284): 1577– 1590.

[3] Shea J. Andrews, Alan E. Renton, Brian Fulton-Howard, Anna Podlesny-Drabiniok, Edoardo Marcora and Alison M. Goate. 2023. The complex genetic architecture of Alzheimer's disease: Novel insights and future directions. EBioMedicine. 90.

[4] Valentina Escott-Price and John Hardy. 2022. Genome-wide association studies for Alzheimer's disease: Bigger is not always better. Brain Communications. 4(3): fcac125.

[5] A. Alatrany, A. Hussain, J. Mustafina and D. Al-Jumeily. 2021. A novel hybrid machine learning approach using deep learning for the prediction of Alzheimer disease using genome data. *In*: Intelligent Computing Theories and Application: 17th International Conference, ICIC 2021, Shenzhen, China. Proceedings, Part III 17. Springer. 253–266.

[6] Abbas Saad Alatrany, Wasiq Khan, Abir Hussain, Dhiya Al-Jumeily and Alzheimer's Disease Neuroimaging Initiative. 2023. Wide and deep learning based approaches

for classification of Alzheimer's disease using genome-wide association studies. PLOS One. 18(5): e0283712.

[7] Taeho Jo, Kwangsik Nho, Paula Bice and Andrew J. Saykin and the Alzheimer's Disease Neuroimaging Initiative. 2022. Deep learning-based identification of genetic variants: application to Alzheimer's disease classification. Briefings in Bioinformatics. 23(2): bbac022.

[8] Ying Wang, Guohua Chen and Wei Shao. 2022. Identification of ferroptosis-related genes in Alzheimer's disease based on bioinformatic analysis. Frontiers in Neuroscience. 16: 823741.

[9] Christiane Reitz, Margaret A. Pericak-Vance, Tatiana Foroud and Richard Mayeux. 2023. A global view of the genetic basis of Alzheimer disease. Nature Reviews Neurology. 19(5): 261–277.

[10] Joshua Stevenson-Hoare, Amanda Heslegrave, Ganna Leonenko, Dina Fathalla, Eftychia Bellou, Lauren Luckcuck, et al. 2023. Plasma biomarkers and genetics in the diagnosis and prediction of Alzheimer's disease. Brain. 146(2): 690–699.

[11] Sebastian Palmqvist, Pontus Tideman, Nicholas Cullen, Henrik Zetterberg, Kaj Blennow, The Alzheimer's Disease Neuroimaging Initiative, et al. 2021. Prediction of future Alzheimer's disease dementia using plasma phospho-tau combined with other accessible measures. Nature Medicine. 27(6): 1034–1042.

[12] Dazhong Sun, Haojun Peng and Zhibing Wu. 2022. Establishment and analysis of a combined diagnostic model of Alzheimer's disease with random forest and artificial neural network. Frontiers in Aging Neuroscience. 14: 921906.

[13] Wuhan Yu, Weihua Yu, Yan Yang and Yang Lü. 2021. Exploring the key genes and identification of potential diagnosis biomarkers in Alzheimer's disease using bioinformatics analysis. Frontiers in Aging Neuroscience. 13: 602781.

[14] Nivedhitha Mahendran and Durai Raj Vincent PM. 2023. Deep belief network-based approach for detecting Alzheimer's disease using the multi-omics data. Computational and Structural Biotechnology Journal. 21: 1651–1660.

[15] Aliza P. Wingo, Yue Liu, Ekaterina S. Gerasimov, Jake Gockley, B.A. Logsdon, Duc M. Duong, et al. 2021. Integrating human brain proteomes with genome-wide association data implicates new proteins in Alzheimer's disease pathogenesis. Nature Genetics. 53(2): 143–146.

[16] Andre Altmann, Leon M. Aksman, Neil P. Oxtoby, Alexandra L. Young, ADNI, Daniel C. Alexander, et al. 2024. Towards cascading genetic risk in Alzheimer's disease. Brain. 147(8): 2680–2690.

[17] Zeeshan Abbas, Hilal Tayara and Kil To Chong. 2022. Alzheimer's disease prediction based on continuous feature representation using multi-omics data integration. Chemometrics and Intelligent Laboratory Systems. 223: 104536.

[18] Tongxin Wang, Wei Shao, Zhi Huang, Haixu Tang, Jie Zhang, Zhengming Ding, et al. 2021. MOGONET integrates multi-omics data using graph convolutional networks allowing patient classification and biomarker identification. Nature Communications. 12(1): 3445.

[19] Ping Gong, Lei Cheng, Zhiyuan Zhang, Ao Meng, Enshuo Li, Jie Chen, et al. 2023. Multi-omics integration method based on attention deep learning network for biomedical data classification. Computer Methods and Programs in Biomedicine. 231: 107377.

[20] Zhaomin Yao, Hongyu Wang, Wencheng Yan, Zheling Wang, Wenwen Zhang, Zhiguo Wang, et al. 2023. Artificial intelligence-based diagnosis of Alzheimer's disease with brain MRI images. European Journal of Radiology. 165: 110934.

[21] V. Sathiyamoorthi, A. K. Ilavarasi, K. Murugeswari, S. T. Ahmed, B. A. Devi and M. Kalipindi. 2021. A deep convolutional neural network based computer aided diagnosis system for the prediction of Alzheimer's disease in MRI images. Measurement. 171: 108838.

[22] Esther E. Bron, Stefan Klein, J.M. Papma, Lize C. Jiskoot, Vikram Venkatraghavan, Jara Linders, et al. 2021. Cross-cohort generalizability of deep and conventional machine learning for MRI-based diagnosis and prediction of Alzheimer's disease. NeuroImage: Clinical. 31: 102712.

[23] Zhonghao Fan, Johann Li, Liang Zhang, Guangming Zhu, Ping Li, Xiaoyuan Lu, et al. 2021. U-net based analysis of MRI for Alzheimer's disease diagnosis. Neural Computing and Applications. 33: 13587–13599.

[24] Atif Mehmood, Shuyuan Yang, Zhixi Feng, Min Wang, Al Smadi Ahmad, Rizwan Khan, et al. 2021. A transfer learning approach for early diagnosis of Alzheimer's disease on MRI images. Neuroscience. 460: 43–52.

[25] Wenyong Zhu, Liang Sun, Jiashuang Huang, Liangxiu Han and Daoqiang Zhang. 2021. Dual attention multi-instance deep learning for Alzheimer's disease diagnosis with structural MRI. IEEE Transactions on Medical Imaging. 40(9): 2354–2366.

[26] Chen-Chen Fan, Hongjun Yang, Liang Peng, Xiao-Hu Zhou, Zhen-Liang Ni, Zeng-Guang Hou, et al. 2022. BGL-Net: A brain-inspired global-local information fusion network for Alzheimer's disease based on sMRI. IEEE Transactions on Cognitive and Developmental Systems. 15(3): 1161–1169.

[27] Kangfu Han, Gang Li, Zhiwen Fang and Feng Yang. 2023. Multi-template meta-information regularized network for Alzheimer's disease diagnosis using structural MRI. IEEE Transactions on Medical Imaging. 43(5): 1664–1676.

[28] Baiying Lei, Yun Zhu, Enmin Liang, Peng Yang, Shaobin Chen, Houyou Hu, et al. 2023. Federated domain adaptation via transformer for multi-site alzheimer's disease diagnosis. IEEE Transactions on Medical Imaging. 42(12): 3651–3664.

[29] Sang Won Park, Na Young Yeo, Jinsu Lee, Suk-Hee Lee, Junghyun Byun, Dong Young Park, et al. 2023. Machine learning application for classification of Alzheimer's disease stages using ^{18}F-flortaucipir positron emission tomography. BioMedical Engineering Online. 22(1): 40.

[30] Yanhui Ding, Kun Zhao, Tongtong Che, Du Kai, Shuyu Liu and Yong Liu. 2021. Quantitative radiomic features as new biomarkers for Alzheimer's disease: An amyloid PET study. Cerebral Cortex. 31(8): 3950–3961.

[31] Ping Zhou, Rong Zeng, Lun Yu, Yabo Feng, Chuxin Chen, Fang Li, et al. 2021. Deep-learning radiomics for discrimination conversion of Alzheimer's disease in patients with mild cognitive impairment: A study based on ^{18}F-FDG PET imaging. Frontiers in Aging Neuroscience. 13: 764872.

[32] Nand Kishore and Neelam Goel. 2023. Deep learning based diagnosis of Alzheimer's disease using FDG-PET images. Neuroscience Letters. 817: 137530.

[33] Mahima Thakur and U. Snekhalatha. 2022. Multi-stage classification of Alzheimer's disease from ^{18}F-FDG-PET images using deep learning techniques. Physical and Engineering Sciences in Medicine. 45(4): 1301–1315.

[34] Junwei Duan, Yang Liu, Huanhua Wu, Jing Wang, Long Chen, C. L. Philip Chen, et al. 2023. Broad learning for early diagnosis of Alzheimer's disease using FDG-PET of the brain. Frontiers in Neuroscience. 17: 1137567.

[35] Husnu Baris Baydargil, Jang-Sik Park and Do-Young Kang. 2021. Anomaly analysis of Alzheimer's disease in PET images using an unsupervised adversarial deep learning model. Applied Sciences. 11(5): 2187.

[36] Zhao Peng, Ming Ni, Hongming Shan, Yu Lu, Yongzhe Li, Yifan Zhang, et al. 2021. Feasibility evaluation of PET scan-time reduction for diagnosing amyloid-β levels in Alzheimer's disease patients using a deep-learning-based denoising algorithm. Computers in Biology and Medicine. 138: 104919.

[37] Uttam Khatri and Goo-Rak Kwon. 2022. Alzheimer's disease diagnosis and biomarker analysis using resting-state functional MRI functional brain network with multi-measures features and hippocampal subfield and amygdala volume of structural MRI. Frontiers in Aging Neuroscience. 14: 818871.

[38] Jafar Zamani, Ali Sadr and Amir-Homayoun Javadi. 2022. Classification of early-MCI patients from healthy controls using evolutionary optimization of graph measures of resting-state fMRI, for the Alzheimer's disease neuroimaging initiative. PLoS One. 17(6): e0267608.

[39] Haijing Sun, Anna Wang and Shanshan He. 2022. Temporal and spatial analysis of Alzheimer's disease based on an improved convolutional neural network and a resting-state fMRI brain functional network. International Journal of Environmental Research and Public Health. 19(8): 4508.

[40] Rahul Biswas and SuryaNarayana Sripada. 2023. Causal functional connectivity in Alzheimer's disease computed from time series fMRI data. Frontiers in Computational Neuroscience. 17: 1251301.

[41] Baiying Lei, Shuangzhi Yu, Xin Zhao, Alejandro F. Frangi, Ee-Leng Tan, Ahmed Elazab, et al. 2021. Diagnosis of early Alzheimer's disease based on dynamic high order networks. Brain Imaging and Behavior. 15: 276–287.

[42] Zhiwei Qin, Zhao Liu and Ping Zhu. 2022. Aiding Alzheimer's disease diagnosis using graph convolutional networks based on rs-fMRI Data. *In*: 2022 15th International Congress on Image and Signal Processing, BioMedical Engineering and Informatics (CISP-BMEI). IEEE. 1–7.

[43] Hao Zhang, Ran Song, Liping Wang, Lin Zhang, Dawei Wang, Cong Wang, et al. 2022. Classification of brain disorders in rs-fMRI via local-to-global graph neural networks. IEEE Transactions on Medical Imaging. 42(2): 444–455.

[44] Jie Zhou, Biao Jie, Zhengdong Wang, Zhixiang Zhang, Tongchun Du, Weixin Bian, et al. 2024. LCGNet: Local sequential feature coupling global representation learning for functional connectivity network analysis with fMRI. IEEE Transactions on Medical Imaging. 43(12): 4319–4330.

[45] Jiangzhang Gan, Zi-Wen Peng, Xiaofeng Zhu, Rongyao Hu, Junbo Ma and Guorong Wu. 2021. Brain functional connectivity analysis based on multi-graph fusion. Medical Image Analysis. 71: 102057.

[46] Yulan Ma, Weigang Cui, Jingyu Liu, Yuzhu Guo, Huiling Chen, Yang Li, et al. 2023. A multi-graph cross-attention based region-aware feature fusion network using multi-template for brain disorder diagnosis. IEEE Transactions on Medical Imaging. 43(3): 1045–1059.

[47] Jianjia Zhang, Luping Zhou, Lei Wang, Mengting Liu and Dinggang Shen. 2022. Diffusion kernel attention network for brain disorder classification. IEEE Transactions on Medical Imaging. 41(10): 2814–2827.

[48] Zhihua Liu, Lei Tong, Long Chen, Zheheng Jiang, Feixiang Zhou, Qianni Zhang, et al. 2023. Deep learning based brain tumor segmentation: A survey. Complex and Intelligent Systems. 9(1): 1001–1026.

[49] Jiaxing Xu, Qingtian Bian, Xinhang Li, Aihu Zhang, Yiping Ke, Miao Qiao, et al. 2024. Contrastive graph pooling for explainable classification of brain networks. IEEE Transactions on Medical Imaging. 43(9): 3292–3305.

[50] Ankita Gandhi, Kinjal Adhvaryu, Soujanya Poria, Erik Cambria and Amir Hussain. 2023. Multimodal sentiment analysis: A systematic review of history, datasets, multimodal fusion methods, applications, challenges and future directions. *In*: Information Fusion. 91: 424–444.

[51] Yu Zhang, Yu Liu, Peng Sun, Han Yan, Xiaolin Zhao and Li Zhang. 2020. IFCNN: A general image fusion framework based on convolutional neural network. Information Fusion. 54: 99–118.

[52] Zixiang Zhao, Haowen Bai, Jiangshe Zhang, Yulun Zhang, Shuang Xu, Zudi Lin, et al. 2023. Cddfuse: Correlation-driven dual-branch feature decomposition for multi-modality image fusion. *In*: Proceedings of the IEEE/CVF Conference on Computer Vision and Pattern Recognition. 5906–5916.

[53] Jin Liu, Hao Du, Rui Guo, Harrison X. Bai, Hulin Kuang and Jianxin Wang. 2022. Mmgk: Multimodality multiview graph representations and knowledge embedding for mild cognitive impairment diagnosis. IEEE Transactions on Computational Social Systems. 11(1): 389–398.

[54] Muhammad Junaid, Sajid Ali, Fatma Eid, Shaker El-Sappagh and Tamer Abuhmed. 2023. Explainable machine learning models based on multimodal time-series data for the early detection of Parkinson's disease. Computer Methods and Programs in Biomedicine. 234: 107495.

[55] Xia-an Bi, Sheng Luo, Siyu Jiang, Yu Wang, Zhao-Xu Xing and Luyun Xu. 2023. Explainable and programmable hypergraph convolutional network for imaging genetics data fusion. Information Fusion. 100: 101950.

[56] Lei Du, Ying Zhao, Jianting Zhang, Muheng Shang, Jin Zhang, Junwei Han, et al. 2023. Identification of genetic risk factors based on disease progression derived from longitudinal brain imaging phenotypes. IEEE Transactions on Medical Imaging. 43(3): 928–939.

[57] Zhaokai Kong, Mengyi Zhang, Wenjun Zhu, Yang Yi, Tian Wang, B. Zhang, et al. 2022. Multi-modal data Alzheimer's disease detection based on 3D convolution. Biomedical Signal Processing and Control. 75: 103565.

[58] Shubham Dwivedi, Tripti Goel, M. Tanveer, R. Murugan and Rahul Sharma. 2022. Multimodal fusion-based deep learning network for effective diagnosis of Alzheimer's disease. IEEE MultiMedia. 29(2): 45–55.

[59] Jiawei Li, Jinyuan Liu, Shihua Zhou, Qiang Zhang and Nikola Kasabov. 2023. GeSeNet: A general semantic-guided network with couple mask ensemble for medical image fusion. IEEE Transactions on Neural Networks and Learning Systems. 35(11): 16248–16261.

[60] Amar Shukla, Rajeev Tiwari and Shamik Tiwari. 2023. Alzheimer's disease detection from fused PET and MRI modalities using an ensemble classifier. Machine Learning and Knowledge Extraction. 5(2): 512–538.

[61] Shangran Qiu, Matthew I. Miller, Prajakta S. Joshi, Joyce C. Lee, Chonghua Xue, Yunruo Ni, et al. 2022. Multimodal deep learning for Alzheimer's disease dementia assessment. Nature Communications. 13(1): 3404.

[62] Yue Tu, Shukuan Lin, Jianzhong Qiao, Yilin Zhuang and Peng Zhang. 2022. Alzheimer's disease diagnosis via multimodal feature fusion. Computers in Biology and Medicine. 148: 105901.

[63] Meiling Wang, Wei Shao, Shuo Huang and Daoqiang Zhang. 2023. Hypergraph-regularized multimodal learning by graph diffusion for imaging genetics based Alzheimer's Disease diagnosis. Medical Image Analysis. 89: 102883.

[64] Shuai Zheng, Zhenfeng Zhu, Zhizhe Liu, Zhenyu Guo, Yang Liu, Yuchen Yang, et al. 2022. Multi-modal graph learning for disease prediction. IEEE Transactions on Medical Imaging. 41(9): 2207–2216.

[65] Baiying Lei, Yafeng Li, Wanyi Fu, Peng Yang, Shaobin Chen, Tianfu Wang, et al. 2024. Alzheimer's disease diagnosis from multi-modal data via feature inductive learning and dual multilevel graph neural network. Medical Image Analysis. 103213.

[66] Zhenyuan Ning, Qing Xiao, Qianjin Feng, Wufan Chen and Yu Zhang. 2021. Relation-induced multi-modal shared representation learning for Alzheimer's disease diagnosis. IEEE Transactions on Medical Imaging. 40(6): 1632–1645.

[67] Qi Zhu, Bingliang Xu, Jiashuang Huang, Heyang Wang, Ruting Xu, Wei Shao, et al. 2022. Deep multi-modal discriminative and interpretability network for Alzheimer's disease diagnosis. IEEE Transactions on Medical Imaging. 42(5): 1472–1483.

[68] Zifeng Qiu, Peng Yang, Chunlun Xiao, Shuqiang Wang, Xiaohua Xiao, Jing Qin, et al. 2024. 3D Multimodal fusion network with disease-induced joint learning for early Alzheimer's Disease Diagnosis. IEEE Transactions on Medical Imaging. 43(9): 3161–3175.

[69] Lu Zhang, Li Wang, Jean Gao, Shannon L. Risacher, Jingwen Yan, Gang Li, et al. 2021. Deep fusion of brain structure-function in mild cognitive impairment. Medical Image Analysis. 72: 102082.

[70] Yanwu Yang, Chenfei Ye, Xutao Guo, Tao Wu, Yang Xiang, Ting Ma, et al. 2023. Mapping multi-modal brain connectome for brain disorder diagnosis via cross-modal mutual learning. IEEE Transactions on Medical Imaging. 43(1): 108–121.

[71] Houliang Zhou, Lifang He, Brian Y. Chen, Li Shen and Yu Zhang. 2024. Multi-modal diagnosis of Alzheimer's Disease using interpretable graph convolutional networks. *In*: 2023 IEEE International Conference on Bioinformatics and Biomedicine (BIBM), Istanbul, Turkiye, 2023, pp. 1004–1007.

[72] Xuegang Song, Feng Zhou, Alejandro F. Frangi, Jiuwen Cao, Xiaohua Xiao, Yi Lei, et al. 2022. Multicenter and multichannel pooling GCN for early AD diagnosis based on dual-modality fused brain network. IEEE Transactions on Medical Imaging. 42(2): 354–367.

[73] Liangliang Liu, Yu-Ping Wang, Yi Wang, Pei Zhang and Shufeng Xiong. 2022. An enhanced multi-modal brain graph network for classifying neuropsychiatric disorders. Medical Image Analysis. 81: 102550.

[74] Xiangmin Han, Xiaoyan Fei, Jun Wang, Tao Zhou, Shihui Ying, Jun Shi, et al. 2022. Doubly supervised transfer classifier for computer-aided diagnosis with imbalanced modalities. IEEE Transactions on Medical Imaging. 41(8): 2009–2020.

[75] Yuanyuan Chen, Yongsheng Pan, Yong Xia and Yixuan Yuan. 2023. Disentangle first, then distill: A unified framework for missing modality imputation and

Alzheimer's disease diagnosis. IEEE Transactions on Medical Imaging. 42(12): 3566–3578.

[76] Tao Wang, Xiumei Chen, Jiawei Zhang, Qianjin Feng and Meiyan Huang. 2023. Deep multimodality-disentangled association analysis network for imaging genetics in neurodegenerative diseases. Medical Image Analysis. 88: 102842.

[77] Wonjun Ko, Wonsik Jung, Eunjin Jeon and Heung-Il Suk. 2022. A deep generative–discriminative learning for multimodal representation in imaging genetics. IEEE Transactions on Medical Imaging. 41(9): 2348–2359.

[78] Yunbi Liu, Ling Yue, Shifu Xiao, Wei Yang, Dinggang Shen and Mingxia Liu. 2022. Assessing clinical progression from subjective cognitive decline to mild cognitive impairment with incomplete multi-modal neuroimages. Medical Image Analysis. 75: 102266.

Chapter **2.11**

Applications of Hypergraph Learning for Brain Disorder Diagnosis with Neuroimaging: A Survey

Mengshen He, Jianxin Wang and Jin Liu*
The School of Computer Science and Engineering, Central South University, Changsha 410083, China

2.11.1 INTRODUCTION

Brain disorders significantly impact patients' quality of life, markedly increasing the risk of complications and mortality while imposing a substantial burden on healthcare systems. Traditional diagnostic approaches for brain disorders mainly rely on clinical diagnostic criteria, medical history collection, and physicians' subjective judgment and experience. However, several factors can lead to misdiagnosis, including the diverse clinical presentations of the same disease, symptom overlap and genetic similarities across different disorders, and the considerable heterogeneity in disease progression among patients. Furthermore, traditional methods lack objective biological evidence, making it difficult to provide accurate biomarkers or to deeply investigate pathological mechanisms, which limits our understanding of brain disorders and the development of effective treatments. Thus, developing objective and accurate diagnostic methods is essential for improving the diagnosis and treatment of brain disorders.

*For Correspondence: liujin06@csu.edu.cn

DOI: 10.1201/9781003518754-16

Neuroimaging techniques have provided clinicians and researchers with methods to examine structural and functional changes in brain disorders [1–4]. Commonly used modalities include structural magnetic resonance imaging (sMRI/T1w) [5], diffusion tensor imaging (DTI) [6], and functional magnetic resonance imaging (fMRI) [7, 8].

The high dimensionality and complex spatial-temporal relationships inherent in neuroimaging data pose significant challenges for traditional analysis methods. In recent years, graph learning approaches, particularly graph neural networks (GNNs) [9–22], have emerged as powerful tools for neuroimaging analysis. Graph learning can naturally capture the brain's inherent network structure and functional connectivity patterns by modeling the brain as a network where brain regions are vertices, and their connections are edges. However, recent studies [23] have revealed a critical limitation of this approach: the brain is an inherently complex system where multiple regions simultaneously interact to support various cognitive functions, characterized by abundant higher-order connections. While conventional GNNs excel at modeling pairwise relationships between brain regions, they are fundamentally limited to these second-order interactions. This limitation prevents them from capturing the crucial higher-order relationships that are essential for understanding the brain's complex network structures and the intricate mechanisms underlying brain disorders.

Researchers have introduced hypergraph learning [24, 25] to overcome these limitations, where hyperedges can connect multiple vertices simultaneously, representing complex associations between brain regions. This advancement has led to the development of hypergraph brain networks (HBNs) and hypergraph neural networks (HGNNs), which can effectively capture higher-order relationships among multiple regions of interest (ROIs) and identify complex patterns between subjects. Recent studies have demonstrated that these hypergraph-based approaches significantly outperform traditional graph methods in both diagnostic accuracy and biomarker identification for brain disorders [26–30]. This breakthrough not only enhances our understanding of individual differences in brain disorders but also provides more reliable biological evidence through improved classification performance.

Nevertheless, hypergraph-based methods in neuroimaging analysis research have not yet been fully developed or widely applied despite their significant potential for advancement. To further develop this field, this paper presents a comprehensive review of the application of hypergraph learning in neuroimaging analysis of brain disorders, discussing existing challenges and future research directions.

The remainder of this survey is organized as follows: Section 2.11.2 comprehensively introduces the fundamental concepts and mathematical definitions of hypergraphs. Section 2.11.3 presents a systematic review of hypergraph learning methods and algorithms. Section 2.11.4 elaborates on the practical applications of hypergraph learning in brain disorder diagnosis, focusing on various neurological and psychiatric conditions. Section 2.11.5 introduces relevant datasets and computational tools that support hypergraph-based neuroimaging analysis. Finally, Section 2.11.6 concludes the survey by summarizing current challenges and exploring promising future research directions in this emerging field.

2.11.2 HYPERGRAPH DEFINITION

In graph theory, a traditional graph consists of vertices and edges connecting these vertices. However, simple binary edges are insufficient to fully capture the multivariate relationships between elements in certain complex relationships and structures. In order to address this limitation, the concept of a hypergraph was introduced [24]. A hypergraph is a generalized graph structure that allows edges (referred to as hyperedges in hypergraph) to connect two or more vertices, thereby better representing multivariate relationships. A hypergraph is an extension of the traditional mathematical structure of graph theory. In a standard graph, edges only connect two vertices, whereas in a hypergraph, hyperedges can connect more than two vertices, allowing hypergraphs to represent more complex relationships.

A **hypergraph** G is defined as $G = (V, E, W)$, where V is a vertex set, E is a hyperedge set and each hyperedge is assigned with a weight by W. The hypergraph G can also be represented by an incidence matrix H of size $|V| \times |E|$, where each entry is defined as:

$$h(v, e) = \begin{cases} 1, & \text{if } v \in e \\ 0, & \text{if } v \notin e \end{cases} \tag{1}$$

where $v \in \mathcal{V}$ and $e \in \mathcal{E}$.

To further elaborate on the components of the hypergraph structure, we define its funda- mental elements as follows:

Vertex: A vertex is a fundamental element of a hypergraph, and all vertices together form the vertex set V. Vertices are typically denoted by the letter v, with the vertex set represented as $V = \{v_1, v_2, \ldots, v_n\}$.

Hyperedge: A hyperedge is a collection of one or more vertices, and all such hyperedges together form the set E. Each hyperedge e is a subset of the vertex set, $e \subseteq V$. The weight matrix $W = \mathrm{diag}(\{w(e_i)\}_{i=1}^{|E|}) \in \mathbb{R}^{|E| \times |E|}$ is a diagonal matrix where each diagonal element $w(e_i)$ represents the weight assigned to hyperedge e_i for $1 \leq i \leq |E|$.

2.11.2.1 Vertex Definition

In neuroimaging analysis, two primary approaches exist for vertex definition in hypergraphs. The first approach defines vertices as ROIs based on established anatomical or functional criteria, where hyperedges encode higher-order relationships among multiple ROIs through various neurobiological dimensions (functional connectivity, structural connectivity, or pathological associations). This ROI-based method captures complex multi-vertex interactions within brain networks, enabling sophisticated analyses of network topology and neural information flow. The second approach defines vertices as individual subjects, where hyper-edges represent multivariate interrelationships among subjects through clinical phenotypes, genetic architectures, or neurocognitive profiles. This subject-level framework facilitates the analysis of population-level patterns, which is crucial for understanding disease transmission dynamics and phenotypic variations across populations.

Brain ROI-based hypergraph vertex definition typically relies on brain atlases, with three primary ROI delineation approaches. The first approach utilizes structural priors, such as the Automated Anatomical Labelling atlas (AAL) [31], Harvard-Oxford atlas (HO) [32], and Brainnetome atlases [33], which is particularly effective for analyzing structural connectivity patterns. The second approach employs functional brain atlases, including the Craddock atlas [34], AICHA atlas [35], and Schaefer atlases [36], providing functionally homogeneous ROI divisions for studying functional connectivity. The third approach adopts data-driven methods such as Independent Component Analysis (ICA) [37, 38], Sparse Dictionary Learning (SDL) [39, 40], and deep learning methods [41–43], which extract ROIs directly from neuroimaging data to capture individual variability and novel connectivity patterns.

For ROI-based hypergraphs, vertex feature extraction is crucial in hypergraph construction. The first approach employs original time series as vertex features, preserving neural activity dynamics with high dimensionality and noise susceptibility challenges. The second approach derives features by processing raw time series through various methods. Among these, functional connectivity (FC) matrices, calculated using correlation coefficients (e.g., Pearson or Spearman), are commonly used to capture synchronous activities between brain regions. Other processing methods include frequency domain features, complexity measures (e.g., entropy, fractal dimension), and temporal statistics (e.g., mean, variance, kurtosis). Additionally, advanced feature extraction techniques such as manifold learning, deep learning, and other dimensionality reduction methods can be employed to obtain more sophisticated representations of brain activity patterns.

In the context of brain disorder research, subject-level hypergraph construction represents another effective approach, where individual subjects serve as vertices. In this framework, hyperedges connect subjects who exhibit similar functional connectivity patterns. Unlike traditional hypergraph brain network models that only represent connections between brain regions within a single individual, this approach effectively captures complex inter-subject relationships, revealing high-order patterns across individuals. The extraction of vertex features in subject-level hypergraphs encompasses multiple information domains. Clinical features include demographic variables (age and gender), disease chronology, symptom severity metrics, and therapeutic interventions. Genetic and molecular features comprise gene expression profiles, SNPs, and protein expression patterns. Behavioral and cognitive features are derived from standardized psychological instruments and cognitive assessments. Additionally, imaging features such as gray matter volume, cortical thickness, and white matter integrity indices are utilized to analyze inter-individual anatomical variation.

2.11.2.2 Hyperedge Definition

In brain disorder analysis, hyperedges can be constructed through three primary approaches: distance-based methods, representation-based methods, and other specialized construction methods. Each approach captures distinct aspects of higher-order relationships in brain networks, thereby offering unique perspectives for subsequent analysis.

Among these approaches, distance-based hypergraph construction methods, particularly the K-nearest neighbors (KNN) approach, have gained widespread adoption [44–47]. The KNN-based method constructs hypergraphs by leveraging similarities between data points to capture local structural patterns. This approach systematically identifies the K most similar neighbors for each vertex based on their feature similarities and combines these vertices to form hyperedges. The construction process follows these steps: First, an appropriate similarity measure function is selected to evaluate the similarity between vertices $\mathbf{x}_i$ and $\mathbf{x}_j$. Common similarity measures include Euclidean distance, cosine similarity, and Pearson correlation coefficient. Taking Euclidean distance as an example:

$$d(x_i, x_j) = \left\| x_i - x_j \right\|_2 = \sqrt{\sum_{k=1}^{n} (x_{ik} - x_{jk})^2} \tag{2}$$

where x_i, $x_j \in \mathbb{R}^n$ are feature vectors of vertices, $\mathbf{x}_{ik}$ and $\mathbf{x}_{jk}$ represent the k-th dimension of vectors $\mathbf{x}_i$ and $\mathbf{x}_j$, respectively.

For each vertex $\mathbf{x}_i$, the K nearest vertices are selected as its neighbors based on the chosen similarity measure, forming the neighbor set $\mathcal{N}_i$. Using Euclidean distance as the measure:

$$\mathcal{N}_i = \text{arg top } K_{x_j \in \mathcal{V}, j \neq i}(-d(x_i, x_j)) \tag{3}$$

where $\mathcal{V}$ is the set of vertices, and arg top K denotes selecting the K vertices that minimize the distance.

Each vertex $\mathbf{x}_i$ is combined with its neighbor set $\mathcal{N}_i$ to form a hyperedge e_i:

$$e_i = \{x_i\} \cup \mathcal{N}_i \tag{4}$$

The KNN-based hypergraph construction methods effectively utilize the similarity information between vertices to generate hypergraphs that reflect the local structure of the data. In representation-based hyperedge construction methods [48–51], data can be analyzed through linear representations in the feature space. We will now explain how hypergraphs are constructed using sparse representations. The sparse representation-based hypergraph construction method uses concepts from sparse coding and compressed sensing to capture higher-order relationships among vertices. Each vertex is represented as a linear combination of other vertices while keeping this combination sparse. The method solves a sparse optimization problem for each vertex to find a set of sparse coefficients. These coefficients allow the vertex to be rebuilt linearly using a small number of other vertices. The vertices with non-zero sparse coefficients then form a hyperedge. Sparse representation aims to efficiently represent data using a limited number of basis elements. In the context of hypergraph construction, consider N vertices, where each vertex $\mathbf{x}_i$ can be expressed as a linear combination of other vertices:

$$x_i = \sum_{j \neq i} c_{ij} x_j \tag{5}$$

where c_{ij} denotes the sparse coefficient, representing the contribution of vertex $\mathbf{x}_j$ in the representation of vertex $\mathbf{x}_i$. The requirement of sparsity implies that most of the coefficients c_{ij} should be zero, retaining only a few non-zero coefficients.

To ensure the sparsity of the representation, the sparse coefficients $\mathbf{c}_i = [c_{i1}, c_{i2}, \ldots, c_{iN}]^T$ are typically determined by solving the following optimization problem:

$$\min_{c_i} \|x_i - Xc_i\|_2^2 + \lambda \|c_i\|_1 \tag{6}$$

where $X = [x_1, x_2, \ldots, x_N]$ is the vertex feature matrix. λ is the regularization parameter, which balances the reconstruction error and the sparsity of the solution. $\|c_i\|_1$ represents the ℓ_1 norm of $\mathbf{c}_i$, promoting a sparse solution.

This optimization problem can be efficiently solved using methods such as Lasso regression to obtain the sparse coefficients $\mathbf{c}_i$. Once the sparse coefficients $\mathbf{c}_i$ are obtained, hyperedges can be constructed through the following steps:

1. **Non-zero Coefficient Selection:** Identify all vertices $\mathbf{x}_j$ for which $c_{ij} = 0$ as the neighbors of vertex $\mathbf{x}_i$:

$$\mathcal{N}_i = \{x_j \mid c_{ij} \neq 0\} \tag{7}$$

2. **Hyperedge Formation**: Combine vertex $\mathbf{x}_i$ with its neighbor set $\mathcal{N}_i$ to form a hyper-edge e_i:

$$e_i = \{x_i\} \cup \mathcal{N}_i \tag{8}$$

3. **Hyperedge Deduplication**: In order to avoid redundant hyperedges, a deduplication process is applied to ensure that each hyperedge is unique within the hypergraph.

The hypergraph construction method based on sparse representation effectively uncovers higher-order relationships among vertices through sparse coding, resulting in hypergraphs that reflect the intrinsic structure of the data.

Beyond distance-based and representation-based hypergraph construction methods, knowledge-based approaches are also widely used [52–58]. Domain-specific information can take various forms. In biological networks, hypergraphs can be built using known biological pathways and protein interaction data. In neuroscience, hyperedges can be created based on anatomical connections or functional module patterns. Furthermore, multimodal information can be used to group objects with properties similar to vertices on a hyperedge.

2.11.3 HYPERGRAPH LEARNING

After constructing the hypergraph, hypergraph learning becomes essential. Traditional hypergraph learning methods rely on spectral and optimization theories. These methods utilize spectral techniques to construct hypergraph Laplacian operators and perform eigendecomposition, which helps map hypergraph structures to the frequency domain and reveal complex data relationships. The learning process is viewed as information flows across the hypergraph structure to minimize label differences between strongly connected vertices.

The foundation of hypergraph learning theory was established by [59], who formulated it as information flow on hypergraph structures. Their work focused on reducing label differences between strongly connected vertices through transductive inference. This theoretical framework was subsequently applied to various domains: Huang [60] utilized it for video object segmentation, while [61] applied it to model image relationships and ranking. Research then progressed towards improving hypergraph structures through hyperedge weight learning. [62] introduced L2 regularization for optimal weight learning. Researchers [63] investigated hyperedge correlations, proposing that related hyperedges should have similar weights. For multi-modal data, [64] developed multi-hypergraph structures to weigh different modal sub-hypergraphs. While these methods possess strong mathematical foundations, they face challenges with large-scale data due to high computational costs and limited feature representation capabilities. These limitations motivated the development of hypergraph neural networks.

Hypergraph neural networks are an emerging technology that aims to synergize the powerful modeling capabilities of hypergraphs with the representational capabilities of neural networks. This is achieved through specially designed hypergraph convolution operators that learn structural-semantic representations. Existing hypergraph neural networks can be broadly classified into two categories: spectral methods and spatial methods.

2.11.3.1 Spectral-based Hypergraph Neural Networks

Spectral-based hypergraph convolutional methods are rooted in hypergraph spectral theory. These methods define convolution operations in the frequency domain to capture complex high-order relationships in hypergraph structures. Like spectral convolutions in traditional graph neural networks, they use eigenvalue decomposition of the hypergraph Laplacian operator to transform signals from the time domain to the frequency domain. This helps handle higher-order connections that occur when hyperedges link multiple vertices.

For example, in the Hypergraph Neural Networks (HGNN) proposed by [45], the spectral convolution on hypergraphs works as follows: given a hypergraph $G = (\mathcal{V}, \mathcal{E}, \Delta)$ with N vertices, the hypergraph Laplacian Δ is an $N \times N$ positive semi-definite matrix. The eigen decomposition $\Delta = \Phi\Lambda\Phi^T$ can be employed to obtain the orthonormal eigenvectors $\Phi = [\phi_1, \ldots, \phi_N]$ and a diagonal matrix $\Lambda = \text{diag}(\lambda_1, \ldots, \lambda_N)$ containing the corresponding non-negative eigenvalues. The Fourier transform for a signal $x = (x_1, \ldots, x_N)$ on the hypergraph is defined as $\hat{\mathbf{x}} = \Phi^T x$, where the eigenvectors are regarded as the Fourier basis, and the eigenvalues are interpreted as frequencies. The spectral convolution of a signal $\mathbf{x}$ and a filter $\mathbf{g}$ can be defined as:

$$g \star x = \Phi\left((g^T) \odot (\Phi^T x)\right) = \Phi g(\Lambda)\Phi^T x, \tag{9}$$

where $\odot$ denotes the element-wise Hadamard product and $g(\Lambda) = \text{diag}(g(\lambda_1), \ldots, g(\lambda_N))$ is a function of the eigenvalues.

Based on this spectral convolution formulation, for a hypergraph signal $\mathbf{X}^t$ at layer t, the hypergraph convolution layer can be formulated as:

$$X^{t+1} = \sigma(D_v^{-1/2} HWD_e^{-1} H^T D_v^{-1/2} X^t \Theta), \tag{10}$$

where Θ is the learnable filter parameter, and σ is a non-linear activation function. The result $\mathbf{X}^{t+1}$ is the output of the convolution layer, which can be used for further learning.

There are still some other methods that use spectral convolution on hypergraphs. Bai et al. introduced the Hypergraph Convolution and Hypergraph Attention Networks [57], which utilize a spectral convolution operator similar to that in HGNN but incorporate an attention mechanism to adaptively learn the importance of vertices within hyperedges. Researchers [65] proposed HyperGCN, a graph convolutional network based on hypergraph spectral theory. HyperGCN first unfolds the hypergraph into a regular graph using specific rules and then performs standard graph convolutional operations on the resulting graph.

2.11.3.2 Spatial-based Hypergraph Neural Networks

Spatial-based methods differ from spectral-based methods in obtaining new representations of central vertices by aggregating representations from neighboring vertices. Spatial hypergraph convolutional methods define convolution operations directly in the spatial domain of hypergraphs, updating vertex representations by aggregating local neighborhood information. This approach includes the following key steps. First, for each vertex, its set of neighboring vertices is defined, including directly connected vertices and vertices indirectly connected through hyperedges. An aggregation function is then designed to perform weighted summation or averaging of the information from neighboring vertices. Finally, the aggregated neighborhood information is combined with the vertex's own features to update its representation.

In General hypergraph neural networks (HGNN+) proposed by [52], each vertex in the hypergraph updates itself by aggregating neighbor vertex messages based on the path between the central vertex and its neighborhood vertices. This path in a hypergraph, called a **hyperpath**, between two distinct vertices v_1 and v_k is defined as a sequence:

$$P(v_1, v_k) = (v_1, e_1, v_2, e_2, \ldots, v_{k-1}, e_k, v_k), \tag{11}$$

where vertices v_j and v_{j+1} belong to the same vertex subset indicated by a hyperedge e_j. Each pair of adjacent vertices in a hyperpath is separated by a hyperedge. The message in the hypergraph between two vertices is propagated through related hyperedges, utilizing the higher-order relationships modeled by hyperedges, compared to simple graphs.

For message propagation from vertex to hyperedge and from hyperedge to vertex using hyperpaths, we define the Inter-neighbor Relation over the vertex set $\mathcal{V}$ and hyperedge set $\mathcal{E}$:

$$N = \{(v, e) \mid H(v, e) = 1, v \in \mathcal{V}, e \in \mathcal{E}\}, \tag{12}$$

where H is the incidence matrix of the hypergraph $G = (\mathcal{V}, \mathcal{E}, W)$.

Definition 1: Vertex Inter-neighbor Set of a Hyperedge For a hyperedge $e \in \mathcal{E}$, the vertex inter-neighbor set $N_v(e)$ is defined as:

$$N_v(e) = \{v \mid v \in N_e, v \in \mathcal{V}, e \in \mathcal{E}\} \tag{13}$$

Definition 2: Hyperedge Inter-neighbor Set of a Vertex For a vertex $v \in \mathcal{V}$, the hyperedge inter-neighbor set $N_e(v)$ is defined as:

$$N_e(v) = \{e \mid v \in N_v, v \in \mathcal{V}, e \in \mathcal{E}\} \tag{14}$$

Following Definitions 1 and 2, we introduce the message-passing of neighbor vertex message aggregation via hyperpaths for one spatial hypergraph convolution layer.

Given a vertex $\alpha \in \mathcal{V}$ of the hypergraph $G = (\mathcal{V}, \mathcal{E}, W)$, we aim to aggregate messages from its hyperedge inter-neighbor set $N_e(\alpha)$. To obtain these hyperedge messages for each hyperedge $\beta \in N_e(\alpha)$, we aggregate messages from the vertex inter-neighbor set $N_v(\beta)$.

The hypergraph convolution layer can be defined by specifying the message-update functions, including the vertex message function $M_v^t(\cdot)$, hyperedge update function $U_e^t(\cdot)$, hyperedge message function $M_e^t(\cdot)$, and vertex update function $U_v^t(\cdot)$, as follows:

$$M_v^t(x_\alpha^t) = \frac{x_\alpha^t}{|N_v(\beta)|} \tag{15}$$

$$U_e^t(w_\beta, m_\beta^t) = w_\beta \cdot m_\beta^t \tag{16}$$

$$M_e^t(x_\alpha^t, y_\beta^t) = \frac{y_\beta^t}{|N_e(\alpha)|} \tag{17}$$

$$U_v^t(x_\alpha^t, m_\alpha^{t+1}) = \sigma(m_\alpha^{t+1} \cdot \Theta^t) \tag{18}$$

Where $\Theta^t \in \mathbb{R}^{C_t \times C_{t+1}}$ is a trainable parameter of layer t, and $\sigma(\cdot)$ is a non-linear activation function such as ReLU. Note that $x_\alpha^t/|N_v(\beta)|$ and $y_\beta^t/|N_v(\alpha)|$ are normalized vertex and hyperedge features, which help in stabilizing convergence and preventing overfitting. Let X^t be the input vertex feature set at layer t, and from Definitions 1 and 2, the incidence matrix $H^T \in \{0, 1\}^{M \times N}$ can control the hyperedge inter-neighbor set of each vertex feature. Thus, the matrix version of *HGNN Conv+* is written as:

$$X^{t+1} = \sigma(D_v^{-1} H W D_e^{-1} H^T X^t \Theta^t), \tag{19}$$

where D_v and D_e are the degree matrices for the vertices and hyperedges, respectively, and W is the hyperedge weight matrix.

There are still some other methods that use spatial convolution on hypergraphs [66]. proposed HyperSAGE, which achieves efficient convolution on hypergraphs by performing message passing in the spatial domain. [67] introduced the All Set method, which unifies set functions on hypergraphs, further enriching the research on spatial hypergraph convolutions.

Researchers [68] proposed the Dynamic Hypergraph Neural Networks (DHGNN), a model specifically designed for dynamic hypergraphs. This method employs the k-nearest neighbors (k-NN) algorithm to generate basic hyperedges and expands the set of adjacent hyperedges through clustering algorithms, such as k-means clustering. Through this dynamic hypergraph construction approach, both local and global relationships can be extracted.

2.11.4 APPLICATIONS IN BRIAN DISORDER DIAGNOSIS

Brain disorders represent significant challenges in modern healthcare, profoundly impacting individuals across different age groups and life stages. Among the most challenging neurological and psychiatric conditions, Alzheimer's disease (AD), as the most common neurodegenerative disorder in elderly populations, represents age-related cognitive deterioration with characteristic structural and functional brain alterations. Autism spectrum disorder (ASD), a widely recognized neurodevelopmental condition affecting children worldwide, exemplifies disorders characterized by distinctive social-communication deficits and repetitive behaviors. Attention deficit hyperactivity disorder (ADHD), predominantly manifesting in school-age children, represents disorders affecting attention and executive function during critical developmental periods. These disorders are particularly suitable for hypergraph-based analysis as they involve complex pathological patterns across multiple brain regions and networks, often presenting with heterogeneous symptoms and varying degrees of severity. In the following sections, we focus on applying hypergraph learning methods in neuroimaging-based diagnosis of these disorders, demonstrating how these advanced computational approaches can extract and utilize higher-order relationships from brain imaging data for improved diagnostic accuracy. The general framework for brain disorder diagnosis based on hypergraph learning is illustrated in Figure 11.1, which consists of four main stages: neuroimaging pre-processing to ensure data quality, hypergraph construction to model high-order relationships among samples, hypergraph learning to extract discriminative features, and classification for brain disorder diagnosis.

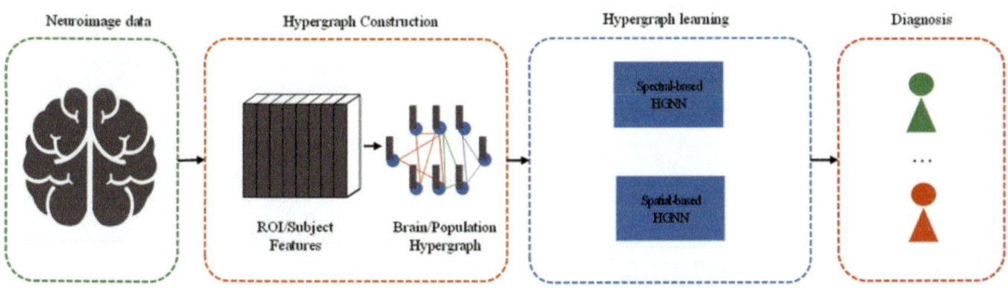

Figure 11.1 The general framework for brain disorder diagnosis based on hypergraph learning (HGCN: Hypergraph Convolutional Network).

2.11.4.1 Alzheimer's Disease

AD, the most prevalent neurodegenerative disorder affecting approximately 44 million people worldwide [69], is characterized by progressive cognitive decline and memory impairment. Its pathological signatures include the accumulation of β-amyloid plaques, the formation of neurofibrillary tangles, and extensive neuronal degeneration, particularly in brain regions crucial for memory function [70]. These neuropathological alterations manifest primarily as structural abnormalities, notably hippocampal atrophy, and cortical thinning, which can be detected through structural neuroimaging techniques such as T1w MRI. Moreover, complementary neuroimaging modalities, including functional MRI and PET imaging, can capture functional and metabolic alterations, collectively providing powerful tools for early diagnosis and disease progression monitoring.

Table 11.1 summarizes representative studies utilizing hypergraph-based methods for AD diagnosis, providing substantial experimental evidence for the superiority of hypergraph learning in AD diagnostic applications.

Table 11.1 Diagnosis of AD based on hypergraph learning

Method	Modality	Number	Acc (%)
[71]	T1w	AD: 41, MCI: 36	AD/MCI: 73.69
[72]	fMRI	MCI: 45, NC: 46	NC/MCI: 82.49
[73]	fMRI	AD: 623, NC: 591	AD/NC: 99.09
[74]	fMRI	MCI: 100, NC: 192	NC/MCI: 74.14
[75]	fMRI	AD: 107, MCI: 107, NC: 107	AD/NC: 97.2, MCI/NC: 87.2, AD/MCI: 85.3
[76]	T1w	AD: 223, MCI: 125, NC: 170	AD/NC: 91.08, MCI/NC: 76.10, AD/MCI: 84.07
[77]	fMRI	EMCI: 51, NC: 72	NC/EMCI: 82.87
[78]	fMRI, DTI	MCI: 10, NC: 17	NC/MCI: 96.3
[79]	fMRI, DTI	AD: 50, EMCI: 69, LMCI: 25, NC: 75	AD/NC: 93.02, AD/EMCI: 90.24, AD/LMCI: 72.00, EMCI/NC: 80.00, LMCI/NC: 91.17
[80]	fMRI, DTI, T1w	AD: 63, EMCI: 82, LMCI: 76, NC: 78	EMCI/NC: 87.50, LMCI/NC: 91.56, AD/NC: 95.57
[81]	fMRI, DTI, T1w	AD: 64, EMCI: 82, LMCI: 76, NC: 178	EMCI/NC: 87.50, LMCI/NC: 92.20, AD/NC: 96.47

Unimodal Neuroimaging

In unimodal AD diagnosis, researchers analyze single imaging modalities (T1w or fMRI) through hypergraph learning to assess brain alterations and facilitate disease diagnosis. Researchers [28, 82] constructed hypergraph brain networks from resting-state fMRI time series using sparse representation techniques and employed a manifold regularization-based multi-task feature selection method to jointly select the most discriminative features. Researchers also [72] proposed a method for constructing dynamic functional brain networks through hypergraph MR (HMR), extending the MR approach to enhance biological significance. Moreover, [71] constructed hypergraph brain networks based on the nearest neighbor algorithm and designed a Hypergraph Convolutional Autoencoder (HCAE) framework to capture many-to-many relationships between brain regions. They [73] introduced a construction method for dynamic, hyperbrain networks and proposed an evolving hypergraph convolutional network, incorporating attention mechanisms to enhance representational learning capabilities. Lastly, [76] utilized the K- Nearest Neighbors (KNN) method to construct hypergraphs for each time point of sMRI data, representing relationships among subjects, and subsequently fused the hypergraphs based on the importance of each time point's data to obtain the final hypergraph. Hypergraph convolution was then applied to learn higher-order information among objects while performing feature dimensionality reduction.

Multimodal Neuroimaging

In multimodal AD diagnosis, the disease manifests through structural changes (e.g., hippocampal atrophy), functional disruptions, and clinical symptoms (e.g., cognitive decline). Multimodal analysis combines different imaging types (T1w, fMRI) to assess brain alterations comprehensively. Hypergraph learning fuses cross-modal features effectively, enabling better characterization of inter-regional interactions and improving diagnostic accuracy. Researchers [78] construct a multimodal hyperconnected network by considering information from diffusion tensor imaging and resting-state functional MRI data simultaneously. Subsequently, different types of network features are extracted from the hyperconnected network, and the most discriminative features are jointly selected using a manifold regularized multi-task feature selection method; [83] embed diffusion tensor imaging information from the structural brain network into a functional brain network constructed based on functional magnetic resonance data using Laplacian graphs to build a hyper-order functional connectivity. By utilizing sparse representation methods, a brain network containing both functional and structural features is obtained and projected into a kernel space for classification through multi-task learning. Researchers [84] proposed a hypergraph p-Laplacian regularized multi-task feature selection (HpMTFS) method for AD classification. Specifically, feature selection for each modality is treated as a separate task, and the shared features of the multimodal data are jointly extracted using a group sparse regularizer.

Recent studies have integrated hypergraph neural networks with multimodal imaging for brain disease analysis, demonstrating improved performance. Lastly, [80] proposed a novel Multi-modal Representation Learning and Adversarial Hypergraph Fusion (MRL-AHF) framework aimed at diagnosing AD using complete tri-modal images. They [81] introduced a prior knowledge-guided adversarial representation learning and hypergraph-aware network (PGARLHPN) to predict abnormal brain connectivity using tri-modal medical images. Researchers [85] proposed a brain network-specific hypergraph neural network (BrainHGNN) to identify neurological event propagation patterns in AD. The BrainHGNN approach constructs hypergraphs using ROI identity encoding and random walk-based sampling strategies, preserving the unique identities of brain regions while characterizing the intrinsic properties of brain network organization.

2.11.4.2 Autism Spectrum Disorder

ASD is classified as a neurodevelopmental psychiatric disorder in the Diagnostic and Statistical Manual of Mental Disorders (DSM-5) [86]. Distinct from purely neurological conditions, ASD's classification as a psychiatric disorder reflects its complex manifestation across multiple domains—behavioral, cognitive, and social functioning—rather than being limited to neurological symptoms alone. In contrast to AD's progressive deterioration pattern, ASD emerges during early developmental stages and exhibits significant heterogeneity in both its clinical presentation and severity across individuals [87].

Table 11.2 summarizes representative studies utilizing hypergraph learning methods for ASD diagnosis. In ASD diagnostic practice, as the disorder primarily manifests through abnormal changes in social interaction, behavioral patterns, and cognitive functions, researchers commonly employ fMRI to capture dynamic changes in brain functional connectivity patterns. Extensive experimental evidence demonstrates that hypergraph learning methods exhibit significant advantages in processing these complex functional connectivity patterns, comprehensively characterizing higher-order relationships among brain regions and delivering more accurate ASD diagnostic results.

Table 11.2 Diagnosis of ASD based on hypergraph learning

Method	Modality	Number	Acc (%)
[88]	fMRI	ASD: 44, NC: 53	ASD/NC: 66.10
[89]	fMRI	ASD: 45, NC: 47	ASD/NC: 87.65
[90]	T1w	ASD: 155, NC: 186	ASD/NC: 76.70
[91]	fMRI	ASD: 245, NC: 272	ASD/NC: 69.00
[92]	fMRI	ASD: 527, NC: 569	ASD/NC: 70.90
[93]	fMRI	ASD: 45, NC: 47	ASD/NC: 80.31
[30]	fMRI	ASD: 539, NC: 573	ASD/NC: 76.60
[94]	fMRI	ASD: 384, NC: 428	ASD/NC: 75.34
[95]	fMRI	ASD: 167, NC: 188	ASD/NC: 78.54
[96]	fMRI	ASD: 91, NC: 76	ASD/NC: 75.63
[29]	fMRI	ASD: 528, NC: 586	ASD/NC: 73.60
[97]	fMRI	ASD: 206, NC: 243	ASD/NC: 73.52
[98]	fMRI, DTI	ASD: 33, NC: 20	ASD/NC: 79.90

Unimodal Neuroimaging

In unimodal ASD diagnosis, researchers mainly use fMRI data through hypergraph learning to study brain connectivity patterns, as functional alterations closely relate to ASD's behavioral symptoms. This approach enables the analysis of complex multi-regional brain interactions. Researchers [88, 89] utilized hypergraph learning methods to explore subnetworks that significantly differentiate between two clinical cohorts, aiming to construct biomarkers. They [99] constructed hypergraphs by thoroughly examining all possible subnetworks across all subjects. The objective function of hypergraph learning aims to jointly optimize the weights of all hyperedges. Furthermore, they [93] developed a method to construct higher-order functional connectivity networks (FCNs) via hypergraphs. They first build low-order FCNs from rs-fMRI data, then identify each region's closely related networks as "good friends." By computing correlations from averaged time series of these "good friends," they generate higher-order hypergraph FCNs that capture multi-regional interactions. With the advancement of deep learning and hypergraph neural networks, [90] constructed a multi-view hypergraph neural network (HGNN) using multi-kernel unsupervised learning, where each network captures a specific view of the brain connectome to effectively differentiate between ASD and normal control (NC) subjects.

The researchers [30] introduced a spatiotemporal weighted higher-order convolutional network (STW-HCN) to capture the higher-order spatiotemporal characteristics of brain activity more comprehensively and proposed a novel multi-template deep fusion model, the spatiotemporal weighted multi-hypergraph convolutional network (STW-MHGCN), to integrate multiple templates of STW-HCN and extract deep relational information between different templates. They [94] introduced HyperGALE, which constructs hypergraphs by combining learned hyperedges with a gated attention mechanism. This approach significantly enhances the model's ability to interpret complex brain imaging data, providing deeper insights into the characterization of biomarkers for ASD. [95] proposed CcSi-MHAHGEL to integrate multiple brain atlases from multi-site fMRI data. They model brain networks as hypergraphs for each atlas and develop a multi-view hyperedge-aware HGCN with adaptive hyperedge weights to extract FCN embeddings.

Multimodal Neuroimaging

Multimodal ASD diagnosis considers both brain abnormalities and behavioral symptoms. While structural changes exist, ASD primarily manifests through functional impairments in social interaction, repetitive behaviors, and communication. Functional neuroimaging, particularly fMRI-derived measures (e.g., Pearson correlation, partial correlations, and dynamic connectivity), proves valuable in studying brain networks when combined with behavioral and clinical assessments. The researchers [96] proposed a multimodal dynamic hypergraph learning framework for diagnosing autism in children, which integrates static functional connectivity (sFC) and dynamic functional connectivity (dFC). After extracting features from each subject's sFC and dFC, they constructed two hypergraphs to represent the complex correlations between different subjects under static and dynamic modes, respectively. To further adjust inappropriate or erroneous connections, they employed multimodal dynamic hypergraph learning to jointly learn data correlations and predict subject labels. Researchers [29] proposed a Hypercomplex Graph Neural Network (HC-GNN) that models multimodal networks as hypercomplex tensor graphs. In their approach, HC-GNN is conceptualized as a dynamic spatial graph where carefully learned inter-modal associations are represented as adjacency matrices. HC-GNN enriches deep coupling of multimodal representations through cross-embedding and cross-aggregation, utilizing hypercomplex operations for inter-modal crossing.

Researchers [98] introduced transformer models into hypergraph-based multimodal brain disease diagnosis, integrating multiple information from fMRI and DTI to enhance diagnostic accuracy. The transformer refines structural embeddings by incorporating higher-order relationships derived from functional networks, thereby improving brain disease diagnosis. They [97] proposed a deep learning framework called FedHNN (Federated Learning with Hypergraph Neural Networks) that integrates multimodal feature fusion and hypergraph neural networks to address privacy protection concerns and enhance ASD diagnosis. The framework employs federated learning strategies where local models train independently in a distributed manner without data sharing, enabling rapid expansion of medical datasets for robust and scalable prediction models. To improve privacy protection performance, they enhanced the multimodal fusion hypergraph model through a hypergrap fusion strategy that captures inter-modal complementarity and correlations, making it suitable for ASD diagnostic tasks.

2.11.4.3 Attention Deficit Hyperactivity Disorder

ADHD is a neurodevelopmental condition marked by inattention, hyperactivity, and impulsivity. The disorder manifests through disrupted attention and executive function networks. Functional neuroimaging, particularly fMRI analysis, reveals altered connectivity patterns in ADHD patients, especially when integrated with behavioral and cognitive assessments. Researchers [100] applied a Bayesian change point model (BCCPM) for dynamic assessments of the brain, constructing hypergraphs to represent brain functional connectivity networks using sparse models. They [101] proposed a multi-stage graph learning framework consisting of (1) a pre-training stage using self-supervised graph learning for insufficient fMRI data supervision and (2) a fine-tuning stage employing supervised graph learning for brain disease diagnosis. They [92] proposed a hypergraph attention network for classifying functional brain networks (FC-HAT), which dynamically updates the hypergraph and its node embeddings during the training process. Researchers [102] developed HyperBrain, an unsupervised anomaly detection framework for temporal hypergraph brain networks. The method models fMRI time series as temporal hypergraphs to capture dynamic higher-order interactions and employs a customized temporal walk (BrainWalk) with neural encodings to detect abnormal brain region co-activations.

Researchers [103] proposed the Hierarchical Hyperedge Graph Transformer network (HH-GraphFormer), which builds hierarchical interactions of the brain and generates hyperedge graphs to detail relationships at various scales. Based on hyperedges formed from the doubly stochastic matrices of self-attention maps of the transformer, multiple sub-graphs are constructed to depict diverse inter-ROI dependencies. Furthermore, a cluster-based aggregation module is presented to aggregate the topological properties of multiple sub-graphs by gathering sub-graph embeddings.

Table 11.3 summarizes representative studies utilizing hypergraph-based methods for ADHD diagnosis, providing substantial experimental evidence for the superiority of hypergraph learning in ADHD diagnostic applications.

Table 11.3 Diagnosis of ADHD based on hypergraph learning

Method	Modality	Number	Acc (%)
[89]	fMRI	ADHD: 118, NC: 98	ADHD/NC: 65.08
[100]	fMRI	ADHD: 23, NC: 45	ADHD/NC: 97.59
[92]	fMRI	All: 850	ADHD/NC: 69.20
[28]	fMRI, T1w	ADHD: 118, NC: 98	ADHD/NC: 82.90
[29]	fMRI, EEG	ADHD: 150, NC: 105	ADHD/NC: 81.60
[104]	fMRI	ADHD: 118, NC: 98	ADHD/NC: 86.70
[105]	fMRI	ADHD: 218, NC: 222	ADHD/NC: 65.30
[102]	fMRI	ADHD: 50, NC: 50	ADHD/NC: 92.33 (AUC)
[103]	fMRI	ADHD: 261, NC: 311	ADHD/NC: 65.90 (AUC)

2.11.4.4 Discussion

In the domain of brain disorder research, hypergraph learning has emerged as a powerful analytical framework, significantly advancing disease diagnosis through both unimodal and multimodal approaches. While unimodal analysis has established hypergraph-based network features as valuable diagnostic biomarkers for disorders such as AD and ASD, multimodal applications have further enhanced diagnostic accuracy by integrating complementary characteristics across diverse neuroimaging modalities. Notably, existing studies have demonstrated promising diagnostic performance through hypergraph-based methods, underscoring the exceptional capability of hypergraphs in capturing higher-order functional interactions in the brain. Beyond its primary applications in AD, ASD, and ADHD, hypergraph learning has demonstrated remarkable efficacy in analyzing various neurological and psychiatric conditions, including depression, schizophrenia, and Parkinson's disease [106–112], through its unique capability to model complex brain networks and capture their higher-order relationships.

With rapid technological advancement, the joint analysis of multimodal multi-omics data has been extensively applied in brain disorder research, yielding particularly significant breakthroughs in genomics [113–123]. Researchers have innovatively leveraged hypergraph learning methods in multi-omics analysis of brain disorders, achieving groundbreaking results through the integration of multidimensional data and systematic investigation of disease mechanisms. These hypergraph-based multi-omics analytical approaches not only effectively capture complex interactions across different omics levels but also provide novel insights into the molecular mechanisms underlying diseases. Given the inherent complexity and hierarchical nature of biological systems, hypergraph learning-based multi-omics integration demonstrates tremendous potential and is emerging as a crucial direction in future brain disorder research.

2.11.5 DATASETS AND TOOLS

In hypergraph, learning-based neuroimaging analysis for brain disorder diagnosis, datasets, and analytical tools play fundamental roles in advancing research and facilitating reproducibility. This chapter presents a comprehensive overview of resources commonly utilized in this field, encompassing both neuroimaging datasets and analytical tools. Specifically, we systematically compile and discuss widely used brain imaging datasets that significantly contribute to disorder diagnosis research. Additionally, we introduce essential analytical tools, including specialized neuroimaging processing platforms and hypergraph learning frameworks, which form the technical foundation for brain disorder analysis. These resources collectively enable researchers to effectively conduct hypergraph-based studies on brain disorders by capturing complex higher-order relationships in neuroimaging data.

2.11.5.1 Datasets

In the study of brain disorders, the quality and diversity of datasets significantly influence the analysis results. Commonly used datasets include the Alzheimer's Disease Neuroimaging Initiative (ADNI) [124], which provides a wealth of imaging and clinical data from Alzheimer's patients; the Autism Brain Imaging Data Exchange (ABIDE) [125], focusing on brain functional imaging data from individuals with autism spectrum disorders; the Human Connectome Project (HCP) [126], aimed at acquiring high-resolution imaging data to map human brain connectivity; the OASIS dataset [127], which contains rich structural and functional imaging information for longitudinal studies of Alzheimer's disease; and the Parkinson's Progression Markers Initiative (PPMI) dataset [128], which offers multimodal imaging data for patients with Parkinson's disease. The COBRE dataset offers resting-state fMRI and structural MRI data for patients with schizophrenia and healthy controls [129]. The NKI-Rockland (NKI) dataset encompasses resting-state fMRI alongside other neuroimaging data derived from the Nathan Kline Institute (NKI) Rockland sample, providing insights into various aspects of brain connectivity [130]. The BNU1 and BNU3 datasets contribute resting-state fMRI data sourced from Beijing Normal University (BNU), facilitating investigations into brain connectivity and its variations across diverse populations [131]. ADHD-200 presents neuroimaging data, inclusive of resting-state fMRI, from individuals with ADHD and control subjects [132]. Additionally, the UK Biobank [133], which integrates genomic and clinical data, provides valuable resources for multidimensional analyses of brain disorders (see Table 11.4 for dataset access links). These feature datasets play a crucial role in hypergraph construction, enabling a more comprehensive characterization of the complex features of brain disorders through the fusion of multi-source information.

2.11.5.2 Tools

In processing these datasets, researchers have developed several widely used open-source tools. For example, Statistical Parametric Mapping (SPM) [134] is a tool developed based on MATLAB for functional and structural MRI analysis and is currently one of the most widely used and comprehensive tools in the field. The FMRIB Software Library (FSL) [135] is mainly utilized for processing fMRI and diffusion tensor imaging (DTI) data. FreeSurfer [136] is primarily used for structural MRI analysis, specializing in brain morphometry and high-quality segmentation. Nilearn [137] is a tool developed in Python for brain imaging and brain network analysis.

To efficiently perform Hypergraph learning, researchers rely on a range of advanced tools and open-source code libraries.

Table 11.4 Neuroimaging datasets and their access links

Dataset Name	Data Access Link
ADNI [124]	adni.loni.usc.edu
ABIDE [125]	nitrc.org/indi/abide
HCP [126]	humanconnectome.org
OASIS [127]	oasis-brains.org
PPMI [128]	ppmi-info.org
COBRE [129]	nitrc.org/indi/retro/cobre.html
NKI-Rockland [130]	nitrc.org/indi/enhanced
BNU1 & BNU3 [131]	nitrc.org/indi/retro/BNU.html
ADHD-200 [132]	nitrc.org/indi/adhd200
UK Biobank [133]	ukbiobank.ac.uk

These tools cover multiple steps, including data preprocessing, hypergraph construction, model training, and evaluation. For instance, PyTorch and TensorFlow are widely used deep learning frameworks that support the construction and training of hypergraph neural networks. Additionally, specialized libraries for graph processing, such as DHG [52], DGL [138], TopoNetX [139], OpenHGNN [140], and PYG [141], offer extensive hypergraph operations, including the generation of hyperedges, attribute management, and advanced network analysis methods. To promote reproducibility and code sharing in research, many teams have made their implemented hypergraph algorithms and models open-source. Researchers [45] proposed a hypergraph neural network (HGNN) framework for data representation learning, capable of encoding high-order data correlations within hypergraph structures. HGNN can learn hidden layer representations considering high-order data structures, providing a universal framework for addressing complex data correlations. They [52] introduced a general high-order multimodal/multitype data association modeling framework called HGNN+ to learn optimal representations within a single hypergraph framework. Subsequently, a new hypergraph convolution scheme is employed in the spatial domain to learn general data representations for various tasks. The authors also released a toolbox named THU-DeepHypergraph [142], which can be utilized for applications such as data classification, retrieval, and recommendation. They [65] proposed HyperGCN, an innovative GCN for self-supervised learning on attributed hypergraphs. Researchers also [143] introduced a novel framework for hypergraph representation learning called HNHN, which combines nonlinear activation functions with normalization schemes to flexibly adjust the importance of high-order hyper-edges and high-degree vertices. They [144] proposed UniGNN, a unified framework for interpreting message-passing processes in graph and hypergraph neural networks. Lastly, researchers [145] developed the Dual-Channel Hypergraph Collaborative Filtering (DHCF)

Table 11.5 Neuroimaging and hypergraph learning tools

Tool Name	Access Link
Neuroimaging Analysis Tools	
Nilearn [137]	nilearn.github.io
FSL [135]	fsl.fmrib.ox.ac.uk
SPM [134]	fil.ion.ucl.ac.uk/spm
BCT [146]	sites.google.com/bctnet
MRtrix3 [147]	mrtrix.org
CONN [148]	conn-toolbox.org
GRETNA [149]	nitrc.org/gretna
BrainNet [150]	nitrc.org/bnv
DPABI [151]	Chaogan-Yan/DPABI
BrainSpace [152]	brainspace.io
Brainlife [153]	brainlife.io
Hypergraph Learning Tools	
DHG [52]	iMoonLab/DeepHypergraph
DGL [138]	docs.dgl.ai
TopoNetX [139]	pyt-team.github.io/toponetx
OpenHGNN [140]	openhgnn.readthedocs.io
PYG [141]	pyg.org
THU-HyperG [142]	iMoonLab/THU-HyperG
HGNN [45]	iMoonLab/HGNN
HGNN+ [52]	iMoonLab/DeepHypergraph/.../hgnnp
HyperGCN [142]	malllabiisc/HyperGCN
HNHN [143]	twistedcubic/HNHN
UniGNN [144]	OneForward/UniGNN
DHCF [145]	iMoonLab/DeepHypergraph/.../dhcf

framework to address the issues of inflexible modeling of users and items as well as insufficient high-order modeling of relationships between subjects.

We summarized some important computational tools in the field of neuroimaging data processing and analysis, as detailed in Table 11.5. These tools encompass multiple levels, from basic image processing to advanced network analysis, providing comprehensive technical support for neuroscience research.

2.11.6 CONCLUSION AND FUTURE DIRECTIONS

This survey provides a systematic review of hypergraph learning in neuroimaging-based brain disorder diagnosis, covering its theoretical foundations, hypergraph construction approaches, and computational frameworks while highlighting its emerging applications and methodological advances in analyzing brain disorders. Research demonstrates that hypergraphs capture intricate higher-order relationships among brain regions and subjects, enabling the construction of sophisticated hypergraph-based brain networks and subject-level representations. This unique capability provides an insightful perspective for understanding individual variations and pathological characteristics of brain disorders, facilitating the exploration of their underlying biological mechanisms. We have systematically compiled essential resources in this field, including commonly used datasets, analytical tools, and open-source implementations for hypergraph-based brain disorder analysis. While significant advances have been made in developing and applying hypergraph learning methods for brain disorder diagnosis, several crucial challenges and opportunities remain unexplored. Accordingly, we identify and discuss promising future research directions to advance this rapidly evolving field.

Firstly, critical challenges in the clinical application of hypergraph learning encompass both interpretability and reproducibility concerns. While contemporary hypergraph algorithmic frameworks predominantly derive biological interpretations through biomarker identification associated with distinct clinical phenotypes, clinical translational research increasingly emphasizes the significance of alterations in inter-regional neural information flow patterns. The limited generalizability of current interpretable models across diverse populations and neuroimaging datasets remains problematic, as these models frequently yield inconsistent interpretations for identical predictive tasks—potentially attributable to demographic heterogeneity, neuroimaging data variation, and model stability constraints. Furthermore, while these models aim to identify clinically relevant biomarkers, their current implementations exhibit high parameter sensitivity and lack robust validation frameworks. In order to address these limitations, a promising avenue involves leveraging multimodal data integration approaches, encompassing neuroimaging, genetic profiles, and behavioral assessments. Recent investigations have demonstrated that such multimodal integration not only improves the accuracy of psychiatric disorder classification but also facilitates the identification of more reliable diagnostic biomarkers, effectively mitigating diagnostic biases arising from individual variability while enabling the detection of more stable and generalizable biomarkers.

Secondly, with the rapid advancement of multi-omics technologies, hypergraph learning in multi-omics data analysis has emerged as a crucial developmental direction in brain disorder research. Contemporary multi-omics data, encompassing genomics, transcriptomics, and proteomics, have assumed paramount importance in brain disorder studies, complementing conventional neuroimaging approaches. The construction of hypergraph models based on multi-omics data enables researchers to elucidate complex higher-order associations among biological molecules, including genes and proteins, and integrate these molecular insights with neuroimaging findings. This sophisticated analytical framework, synthesizing multi-omics and neuroimaging data through hypergraph analysis, facilitates the identification of underlying molecular mechanisms and novel disease biomarkers, thereby providing a more comprehensive understanding of brain disorder pathogenesis. Emerging research has demonstrated the distinctive advantages of hypergraph learning in integrating multidimensional biological data, establishing its utility in advancing our understanding of complex neurological conditions.

Thirdly, a promising direction lies in the development of brain-inspired hypergraph algorithmic frameworks. The human brain, as an intrinsically complex and dynamic system, exhibits mechanisms that current scientific understanding has yet to fully elucidate. While existing hypergraph algorithms typically maintain static configurations throughout their learning processes, they fail to capture the brain's inherent dynamicity, and their initial hypergraph constructions often incorporate spurious connections that may impede effective learning. Developing hypergraph algorithms specifically designed to emulate the brain's distinctive operational mechanisms holds considerable potential for advancing the field. Such biomimetic approaches could not only enhance algorithmic performance but also facilitate a more nuanced analysis of neuroimaging data, ultimately contributing to a deeper comprehension of neural functioning and organization.

A pivotal developmental trajectory lies in integrating large-scale models with medical big-data analytics. Recent advancements in Large Language Models (LLMs) have demonstrated unprecedented capabilities in natural language understanding and generation, garnering substantial attention from the scientific community. The convergence of hypergraph learning with LLMs represents a particularly promising research direction. While LLMs excel in textual data processing, they frequently encounter limitations in capturing the intricate, higher-order structural information inherent in hypergraph data. The synergistic integration of hypergraph computing with LLMs could potentially enhance their capacity to comprehend complex structural relationships, effectively bridging the gap between linguistic understanding and higher-order relational modeling. Furthermore, developing large-scale hypergraph brain network models emerges as another compelling avenue of investigation. Using extensive datasets in model training substantially increases the potential for discovering intricate patterns and correlations, underscoring the imperative for developing comprehensive hypergraph brain network models. These sophisticated models not only serve as robust feature extractors for brain network representation learning but also offer promising solutions to persistent challenges in brain network annotation, model interpretability, and data augmentation through the generation of synthetic brain networks.

REFERENCES

[1] Jin Liu, Min Li, Jianxin Wang, Fangxiang Wu, Tianming Liu and Yi Pan. 2014. A survey of MRI-based brain tumor segmentation methods. Tsinghua Science and Technology. 19(6): 578–595.

[2] Jin Liu, Min Li, Yi Pan, Wei Lan, Ruiqing Zheng, Fang-Xiang Wu, et al. 2017. Complex brain network analysis and its applications to brain disorders: A survey. Complexity. 2017(1): 8362741.

[3] Li Zhang, Mingliang Wang, Mingxia Liu and Daoqiang Zhang. 2020. A survey on deep learning for neuroimaging-based brain disorder analysis. Frontiers in Neuroscience. 14: 779.

[4] Wutao Yin, Longhai Li and Fang-Xiang Wu. 2022. Deep learning for brain disorder diagnosis based on fMRI images. Neurocomputing. 469: 332–345.

[5] Robert W. Brown, Yu-Chung N. Cheng, E. Mark Haacke, Michael R. Thompson and Ramesh Venkatesan. 2014. Magnetic Resonance Imaging: Physical Principles and Sequence Design. John Wiley & Sons.

[6] Susumu Mori, Barbara J. Crain, V. P. Chacko and Peter C. M. Van Zijl. 1999. Three-dimensional tracking of axonal projections in the brain by magnetic resonance imaging. Annals of Neurology. 45(2): 265–269.

[7] Paul M. Matthews and Peter Jezzard. 2004. Functional magnetic resonance imaging. Journal of Neurology, Neurosurgery and Psychiatry. 75(1): 6–12.

[8] Nikos K. Logothetis. 2008. What we can do and what we cannot do with fMRI. Nature. 453(7197): 869–878.

[9] Franco Scarselli, Marco Gori, Ah Chung Tsoi, Markus Hagenbuchner and Gabriele Monfardini. 2008. The graph neural network model. IEEE Transactions on Neural Networks. 20(1): 61–80.

[10] Zonghan Wu, Shirui Pan, Fengwen Chen, Guodong Long, Chengqi Zhang and Philip S. Yu. 2020. A comprehensive survey on graph neural networks. IEEE Transactions on Neural Networks and Learning Systems. 32(1): 4–24.

[11] Alaa Bessadok, Mohamed Ali Mahjoub and Islem Rekik. 2022. Graph neural networks in network neuroscience. IEEE Transactions on Pattern Analysis and Machine Intelligence. 45(5)2: 5833–5848.

[12] Wei Peng, Yanhan Ma, Chunshan Li, Wei Dai, Xiaodong Fu, Li Liu, et al. 2024. Fusion of brain imaging genetic data for Alzheimer's disease diagnosis and causal factors identification using multi-stream attention mechanisms and graph convolutional networks. Neural Networks. 107020.

[13] Junbin Mao, Jin Liu, Xu Tian, Yi Pan, Emanuele Trucco and Hanhe Lin. 2024. Towards integrating federated learning with split learning via spatio-temporal graph framework for brain disease prediction. IEEE Transactions on Medical Imaging. 44(3): 1334–1346.

[14] Jin Liu, Xu Tian, Hanhe Lin, Hong-Dong Li and Yi Pan. 2024. Multi-task learning for Alzheimer's disease diagnosis and mini-mental state examination score prediction. Big Data Mining and Analytics. 7(3): 828–842.

[15] Rui Guo, Xu Tian, Hanhe Lin, Stephen McKenna, Hong-Dong Li, Fei Guo, et al. 2023. Graph-based fusion of imaging, genetic and clinical data for degenerative disease diagnosis. *In*: IEEE/ACM Transactions on Computational Biology and Bioinformatics. 21(1): 57–68.

[16] Jin Liu, Hao Du, Rui Guo, Harrison X. Bai, Hulin Kuang and Jianxin Wang. 2022. MMGK: Multimodality multiview graph representations and knowledge embedding for mild cognitive impairment diagnosis. *In*: IEEE Transactions on Computational Social Systems. 11(1): 389–398.

[17] Jiaxin Wei, Bin Jiao, Xu Tian, Lu Shen and Jin Liu. 2023. Group attention-based multi-wave graph learning for dementia diagnosis. *In*: 2023 IEEE International Conference on Bioinformatics and Biomedicine (BIBM). IEEE. 1531–1536.

[18] Junbin Mao, Hanhe Lin, Xu Tian, Yi Pan and Jin Liu. 2023. FedGST: Federated graph spatio-temporal framework for brain functional disease prediction. *In*: 2023 IEEE International Conference on Bioinformatics and Biomedicine (BIBM). IEEE. 1356–1361.

[19] Yufei Wang, Jin Liu, Yizhen Xiang, Jianxin Wang, Qingyong Chen and Jing Chong. 2022. MAGE: Automatic diagnosis of autism spectrum disorders using multi-atlas graph convolutional networks and ensemble learning. Neurocomputing. 469: 346–353.

[20] Jin Liu, Guanxin Tan, Wei Lan and Jianxin Wang. 2020. Identification of early mild cognitive impairment using multi-modal data and graph convolutional networks. BMC Bioinformatics. 21: 1–12.

[21] Yizhen Xiang, Jianxin Wang, Guanxin Tan, Fang-Xiang Wu and Jin Liu. 2020. Schizophrenia identification using multi-view graph measures of functional brain networks. Frontiers in Bioengineering and Biotechnology. 7: 479.

[22] Jin Liu, Dejiao Zeng, Rui Guo, Mingming Lu, Fang-Xiang Wu and Jianxin Wang. 2021. MMHGE: Detecting mild cognitive impairment based on multi-atlas multi-view hybrid graph convolutional networks and ensemble learning. Cluster Computing. 24: 103–113.

[23] Michel Thiebaut de Schotten and Stephanie J. Forkel. 2022. The emergent properties of the connected brain. Science. 378(6619): 505–510.

[24] Bretto, A. 2013. Hypergraph Theory: An introduction. Series Title: Mathematical Engineering. Cham: Springer. https://doi.org/10.1007/978-3-319-00080-0

[25] Yue Gao, Shuyi Ji, Xiangmin Han and Qionghai Dai. 2024. Hypergraph computation. Engineering. 40: 188–201.

[26] Ju Niu and Yuhui Du. 2023. Applications of hypergraph-based methods in classifying and subtyping psychiatric disorders: A survey. Radiology Science. 2(1): 83–95.

[27] Li Xiao, Junqi Wang, P.H. Kassani, Yipu Zhang, Yuntong Bai, Julia M. Stephen, et al. 2019. Multi-hypergraph learning-based brain functional connectivity analysis in fMRI data. IEEE Transactions on Medical Imaging. 39(5): 1746–1758.

[28] Biao Jie, Chong-Yaw Wee, Dinggang Shen and Daoqiang Zhang. 2016. Hyper-connectivity of functional networks for brain disease diagnosis. Medical Image Analysis. 32: 84–100.

[29] Yanwu Yang, Chenfei Ye, Guoqing Cai, Kunru Song, Jintao Zhang, Yang Xiang, et al. 2024. Hypercomplex graph neural network: Towards deep intersection of multi-modal brain networks. IEEE Journal of Biomedical and Health Informatics. 29(5): 3304–3316.

[30] Zhihua Liu, Lei Tong, Long Chen, Zheheng Jiang, Feixiang Zhou, Qianni Zhang, et al. 2023. Deep learning based brain tumor segmentation: a survey. Complex and Intelligent Systems. 9(1): 1001–1026.

[31] Nathalie Tzourio-Mazoyer, B. Landeau, D. Papathanassiou, F. Crivello, O. Etard, N. Delcroix, et al. 2002. Automated anatomical labeling of activations in SPM

using a macroscopic anatomical parcellation of the MNI MRI single-subject brain. NeuroImage. 15(1): 273–289.

[32] Nikos Makris, Jill M. Goldstein, David Kennedy, S.M. Hodge, Verne S. Caviness, Stephen V. Faraone, et al. 2006. Decreased volume of left and total anterior insular lobule in schizophrenia. Schizophrenia Research. 83(2–3): 155–171.

[33] Lingzhong Fan, Hai Li, Junjie Zhuo, Yu Zhang, Jiaojian Wang, Liangfu Chen, et al. 2016. The human brainnetome atlas: A new brain atlas based on connectional architecture. Cerebral Cortex. 26(8): 3508–3526.

[34] R. Cameron Craddock, G. Andrew James, Paul E. Holtzheimer III, Xiaoping P. Hu and Helen S. Mayberg. 2012. A whole brain fMRI atlas generated via spatially constrained spectral clustering. Human Brain Mapping. 33(8): 1914–1928.

[35] Marc Joliot, Gaël Jobard, Mikaël Naveau, N. Delcroix, Laurent Petit, Laure Zago, et al. 2015. AICHA: An atlas of intrinsic connectivity of homotopic areas. Journal of Neuroscience Methods. 254: 46–59.

[36] Alexander Schaefer, Ru Kong, Evan M. Gordon, Timothy O. Laumann, Xi-Nian Zuo, Avram J. Holmes, et al. 2018. Local-global parcellation of the human cerebral cortex from intrinsic functional connectivity MRI. Cerebral Cortex. 28(9): 3095–3114.

[37] Vince D. Calhoun, T. Adali, G.D. Pearlson and J.J. Pekar. 2001. A method for making group inferences from functional MRI data using independent component analysis. Human Brain Mapping. 14(3): 140–151.

[38] Yuhui Du and Yong Fan. 2013. Group information guided ICA for fMRI data analysis. NeuroImage. 69: 157–197.

[39] Jinglei Lv, Xi Jiang, Xiang Li, Dajiang Zhu, Shu Zhang, Shijie Zhao, et al. 2014. Holistic atlases of functional networks and interactions reveal reciprocal organizational architecture of cortical function. IEEE Transactions on Biomedical Engineering. 62(4): 1120–1131.

[40] Jinglei Lv, Xi Jiang, Xiang Li, Dajiang Zhu, Hanbo Chen, Tuo Zhang, et al. 2015. Sparse representation of whole-brain fMRI signals for identification of functional networks. Medical Image Analysis. 20(1): 112–134.

[41] Qinglin Dong, Ning Qiang, Jinglei Lv, Xiang Li, Tianming Liu and Quanzheng Li. 2020. Spatiotemporal attention autoencoder (STAAE) for ADHD classification. *In*: Medical Image Computing and Computer Assisted Intervention–MICCAI 2020: 23rd International Conference, Lima, Peru, October 4–8. Proceedings, Part VII 23. Springer. 508–517.

[42] Qinglin Dong, Ning Qiang, Jinglei Lv, Xiang Li, Tianming Liu and Quanzheng Li. 2020. Discovering functional brain networks with 3D residual autoencoder (ResAE). *In*: Medical Image Computing and Computer Assisted Intervention–MICCAI 2020: 23rd International Conference, Lima, Peru, October 4–8. Proceedings, Part VII 23. Springer. 498–507.

[43] Mengshen He, Xiangyu Hou, Enjie Ge, Zhenwei Wang, Zili Kang, Ning Qiang, et al. 2023. Multi-head attention-based masked sequence model for mapping functional brain networks. Frontiers in Neuroscience. 17: 1183145.

[44] Junliang Yu, Hongzhi Yin, Jundong Li, Qinyong Wang, Nguyen Quoc Viet Hung and Xiangliang Zhang. 2021. Self-supervised multi-channel hypergraph convolutional network for social recommendation. Proceedings of the Web Conference 2021. 413–424.

[45] Yifan Feng, Haoxuan You, Zizhao Zhang, Rongrong Ji and Yue Gao. 2019. Hypergraph neural networks. *In*: Proceedings of the AAAI Conference on Artificial Intelligence. 33(01): 3558–3565.

[46] Junjie Bai, Biao Gong, Yining Zhao, Fuqiang Lei, Chenggang Yan and Yue Gao. 2021. Multi-scale representation learning on hypergraph for 3D shape retrieval and recognition. IEEE Transactions on Image Processing. 30: 5327–5338.

[47] Yu Zhu, Ziyu Guan, Shulong Tan, Haifeng Liu, Deng Cai and Xiaofei He. 2016. Heterogeneous hypergraph embedding for document recommendation. Neurocomputing. 216: 150–162.

[48] Qingshan Liu, Yubao Sun, Cantian Wang, Tongliang Liu and Dacheng Tao. 2016. Elastic net hypergraph learning for image clustering and semi-supervised classification. IEEE Transactions on Image Processing. 26(1): 452–463.

[49] Taisong Jin, Zhengtao Yu, Yue Gao, Shengxiang Gao, Xiaoshuai Sun and Cuihua Li. 2019. Robust l2-Hypergraph and its applications. Information Sciences. 501: 708–723.

[50] Yonggang Li, Shichao Zhang, Debo Cheng, Wei He, Guoqiu Wen and Qing Xie. 2017. Spectral clustering based on hypergraph and self-re-presentation. Multimedia Tools and Applications. 76: 17559–17576.

[51] Wei He, Xiaohui Cheng, Rongyao Hu, Yonghua Zhu and Guoqiu Wen. 2017. Feature self-representation based hypergraph unsupervised feature selection via low-rank representation. Neurocomputing. 253: 127–134.

[52] Yue Gao, Yifan Feng, Shuyi Ji and Rongrong Ji. 2022. HGNN$^+$: General hypergraph neural networks. IEEE Transactions on Pattern Analysis and Machine Intelligence. 45(3): 3181–3199.

[53] Jie Huang, Xin Liu and Yangqiu Song. 2019. Hyper-path-based representation learning for hyper-networks. *In*: Proceedings of the 28th ACM International Conference on Information and Knowledge Management. 449–458.

[54] Junwei Zhang, Min Gao, Junliang Yu, Lei Guo, Jundong Li and Hongzhi Yin. 2021. Double-scale self-supervised hypergraph learning for group recommendation. *In*: Proceedings of the 30th ACM International Conference on Information and Knowledge Management. 2557–2567.

[55] M. Vijaikumar, Deepesh Hada and Shirish Shevade. 2021. Hypertenet: Hypergraph and transformer-based neural network for personalized list continuation. *In*: 2021 IEEE International Conference on Data Mining (ICDM). IEEE. 1210–1215.

[56] Yicong Li, Hongxu Chen, Xiangguo Sun, Zhenchao Sun, Lin Li, Lizhen Cui, et al. 2021. Hyperbolic hypergraphs for sequential recommendation. *In*: Proceedings of the 30th ACM International Conference on Information and Knowledge Management. 988–997.

[57] Song Bai, Feihu Zhang and Philip HS Torr. 2021. Hypergraph convolution and hypergraph attention. Pattern Recognition. 110: 107637.

[58] Quan Fang, Jitao Sang, Changsheng Xu and Yong Rui. 2014. Topic-sensitive influencer mining in interest-based social media networks via hypergraph learning. IEEE Transactions on Multimedia. 16(3): 796–812.

[59] Dengyong Zhou, Jiayuan Huang and Bernhard Schölkopf. 2006. Learning with hypergraphs: Clustering, classification, and embedding. Advances in Neural Information Processing Systems. 19: 1601–1608.

[60] Yuchi Huang, Qingshan Liu and Dimitris Metaxas. 2009. Video object segmentation by hypergraph cut. *In*: 2009 IEEE Conference on Computer Vision and Pattern Recognition. IEEE. 1738–1745.

[61] Yuchi Huang, Qingshan Liu, Shaoting Zhang and Dimitris N. Metaxas. 2010. Image retrieval via probabilistic hypergraph ranking. *In*: 2010 IEEE Computer Society Conference on Computer Vision and Pattern Recognition. IEEE. 3376–3383.

[62] Yue Gao, Meng Wang, Zheng-Jun Zha, Jialie Shen, Xuelong Li and Xindong Wu. 2012. Visual-textual joint relevance learning for tag-based social image search. IEEE Transactions on Image Processing. 22(1): 363–376.

[63] TaeHyun Hwang, Ze Tian, Rui Kuang and Jean-Pierre Kocher. 2008. Learning on weighted hypergraphs to integrate protein interactions and gene expressions for cancer outcome prediction. *In*: 2008 Eighth IEEE International Conference on Data Mining. IEEE. 293–302.

[64] Yue Gao, Meng Wang, Dacheng Tao, Rongrong Ji and Qionghai Dai. 2012. 3-D object retrieval and recognition with hypergraph analysis. IEEE Transactions on Image Processing. 21(9): 4290–4303.

[65] Naganand Yadati, Madhav Nimishakavi, Prateek Yadav, Vikram Nitin, Anand Louis and Partha Talukdar. 2019. HyperGCN: A new method for training graph convolutional networks on hypergraphs. Advances in Neural Information Processing Systems. 135: 1511–1522.

[66] Daganand Yadati, Madhav Nimishakavi, Prateek Yadav, Vikram Nitin, Anand Louis and Partha Talukdar. 2020. HyperSAGE: Generalizing inductive representation learning on hypergraphs. arXiv preprint arXiv:2010:04558.

[67] Eli Chien, Chao Pan, Jianhao Peng and Olgica Milenkovic. 2021. You are allset: A multiset function framework for hypergraph neural networks. arXiv preprint arXiv:2106: 13264.

[68] Jianwen Jiang, Yuxuan Wei, Yifan Feng, Jingxuan Cao and Yue Gao. 2019. Dynamic hypergraph neural networks. IJCAI. 2635– 2641.

[69] World Health Organization. 2021. Global Status Report on the Public Health Response to Dementia.

[70] Clifford R. Jack Jr., David A. Bennett, Kaj Blennow, Maria C. Carrillo, Billy Dunn, Samantha Budd Haeberlein, et al. 2018. NIA-AA research framework: Toward a biological definition of Alzheimer's disease. Alzheimer's and Dementia. 14(4): 535–562.

[71] Alin Banka, Inis Buzi and Islem Rekik. 2020. Multi-view brain hyperconnectome autoencoder for brain state classification. *In*: Predictive Intelligence in Medicine: Third International Workshop, PRIME 2020, Held in Conjunction with MICCAI 2020, Lima, Peru. Proceedings 3. Springer. 101–110.

[72] Yixin Ji, Yutao Zhang, Haifeng Shi, Zhuqing Jiao, Shui-Hua Wang and Chuang Wang. 2021. Constructing dynamic brain functional networks via hypergraph manifold regularization for mild cognitive impairment classification. Frontiers in Neuroscience. 15: 669345.

[73] Xinlei Wang, Junchang Xin, Zhongyang Wang, Chuangang Li and Zhiqiong Wang. 2022. An evolving hypergraph convolutional network for the diagnosis of Alzheimer's disease. Diagnostics. 12(11): 2632.

[74] Zijian Dong, Joanna Su Xian Chong, Bing Cai Kok and Juan Helen Zhou. 2020. COOP-DHGNN: A Framework for Joint Classification and Prediction of Brain Functional Connectivity Using Sparse Trajectory Dataset with Application to Early

Dementia. *In*: 2022 IEEE International Conference on Big Data (Big Data). IEEE. 4972–4978.

[75] Xinlei Wang, Junchang Xin, Z. Wang, Luxuan Qu, Jiani Li and Zhiqiong Wang. 2024. Graph kernel of brain networks considering functional similarity measures. Computers in Biology and Medicine. 171: 108148.

[76] Xiaoke Hao, Jiawang Li, Mingming Ma, Jing Qin, Daoqiang Zhang, Feng Liu, et al. 2024. Hypergraph convolutional network for longitudinal data analysis in Alzheimer's disease. Computers in Biology and Medicine. 168: 107765.

[77] Xidong Fu, Shengchang Shan, Chun Liu, Yu Lu and Zhuqing Jiao. 2024. Constructing brain functional networks with adaptive manifold regularization for early mild cognitive impairment. International Journal of Imaging Systems and Technology. 34(2): e23053.

[78] Yang Li, X. Gao, Biao Jie, Pew-Thian Yap, Min-jeong Kim, Chong-Yaw Wee, et al. 2017. Multimodal hyper-connectivity networks for MCI classification. *In*: Medical Image Computing and Computer Assisted Intervention-MICCAI 2017: 20th International Conference, Quebec City, QC, Canada. Proceedings, Part I 20. Springer. 433–441.

[79] Junren Pan, Baiying Lei, Yanyan Shen, Yong Liu, Z. Feng and Shuqiang Wang. 2021. Characterization multimodal connectivity of brain network by hypergraph GAN for Alzheimer's disease analysis. *In*: Pattern Recognition and Computer Vision: 4th Chinese Conference, PRCV 2021, Beijing, China. Proceedings, Part III 4. Springer. 467–478.

[80] Qiankun Zuo, Baiying Lei, Yanyan Shen, Yong Liu, Z. Feng and Shuqiang Wang. 2021. Multimodal representations learning and adversarial hypergraph fusion for early Alzheimer's disease prediction. *In*: Pattern Recognition and Computer Vision: 4th Chinese Conference, PRCV 2021, Beijing, China. Proceedings, Part III 4. Springer. 479–490.

[81] Qiankun Zuo, Huisi Wu, C.L. Philip Chen, Baiying Lei and Shuqiang Wang. 2024. Prior-guided adversarial learning with hypergraph for predicting abnormal connections in Alzheimer's disease. IEEE Transactions on Cybernetics. 54(6): 3652–3665.

[82] Biao Jie, Dinggang Shen and Daoqiang Zhang. 2014. Brain connectivity hyper-network for MCI classification. *In*: Medical Image Computing and Computer-Assisted Intervention– MICCAI 2014: 17th International Conference, Boston, MA, USA. Proceedings, Part II 17. Springer. 724–732.

[83] Geng Zhang, Qi Zhu, Jing Yang, Ruting Xu, Zhiqiang Zhang and Daoqiang Zhang. 2022. Functional brain connectivity hyper-network embedded with structural information for epilepsy diagnosis. International Journal of Image and Graphics. 22(04): 2250029.

[84] Yanjiao Ban, Huan Lao, Bin Li, Wenjun Su and Xuejun Zhang. 2023. Diagnosis of Alzheimer's disease using hypergraph p-Laplacian regularized multi-task feature learning. Journal of Biomedical Informatics. 140: 104326.

[85] Hongmin Cai, Zhixuan Zhou, Defu Yang, Guorong Wu and Jiazhou Chen. 2023. Discovering brain network dysfunction in Alzheimer's disease using brain hypergraph neural network. *In*: International Conference on Medical Image Computing and Computer-Assisted Intervention. Springer. 230–240.

[86] Martin Guha. 2014. Diagnostic and Statistical Manual of Mental Disorders: DSM-5 (5th Edition). Reference Reviews. 28(3): 36–37.

[87] Catherine Lord, T.S. Brugha, Tony Charman, James Cusack, Guillaume Dumas, Thomas Frazier, et al. 2020. MW State, et al. 2020. Autism spectrum disorder. Nature Reviews Disease Primers. 6(1): 1–23.

[88] Chen Zu, Yue Gao, Brent Munsell, Minjeong Kim, Ziwen Peng, Yingying Zhu, et al. 2016. Identifying high order brain connectome biomarkers via learning on hypergraph. *In*: Machine Learning in Medical Imaging: 7th International Workshop, MLMI 2016, Held in Conjunction with MICCAI 2016, Athens, Greece. Proceedings 7. Springer. 1–9.

[89] Chen Zu, Yue Gao, Brent Munsell, Minjeong Kim, Ziwen Peng, Jessica R. Cohen, et al. 2019. Identifying disease-related subnetwork connectome biomarkers by sparse hypergraph learning. Brain Imaging and Behavior. 13: 879–892.

[90] Mohammad Madine, Islem Rekik and Naoufel Werghi. 2020. Diagnosing autism using T1-W MRI with multi-kernel learning and hypergraph neural network. *In*: 2020 IEEE International Conference on Image Processing (ICIP). IEEE. 438–442.

[91] Mert Lostar and Islem Rekik. 2020. Deep hypergraph U-net for brain graph embedding and classification. arXiv preprint arXiv:2008(13118).

[92] Junzhong Ji, Yating Ren and Minglong Lei. 2022. FC–HAT: Hypergraph attention network for functional brain network classification. Information Sciences. 608: 1301–1316.

[93] Jie Yang, Fang Wang, Zhen Li, Zhen Yang, Xishang Dong and Qinghua Han. 2023. Constructing high-order functional networks based on hypergraph for diagnosis of autism spectrum disorders. Frontiers in Neuroscience. 17: 1257982.

[94] Mehul Arora, Chirag Shantilal Jain, Lalith Bharadwaj Baru, Kamalaker Dadi and Bapi Raju Surampudi. 2024. HyperGALE: ASD Classification via Hypergraph Gated Attention with Learnable HyperEdges. *In*: 2024 International Joint Conference on Neural Networks (IJCNN). IEEE. 1–8.

[95] Wei Wang, Li Xiao, Gang Qu, Vince D. Calhoun, Yu-Ping Wang and Xiaoyan Sun. 2024. Multiview hyperedge-aware hypergraph embedding learning for multisite, multiatlas fMRI-based functional connectivity network analysis. Medical Image Analysis. 94: 103144.

[96] Zizhao Zhang, Jian Liu, Baojuan Li and Yue Gao. 2021. Diagnosis of childhood autism using multi-modal functional connectivity via dynamic hypergraph learning. *In*: Artificial Intelligence: First CAAI International Conference, CICAI 2021, Hangzhou, China. Proceedings, Part I 1. Springer. 123–135.

[97] Haishuai Wang, Hezi Jing, Jianjun Yang, Chao Liu, Liwei Hu, Guangyu Tao, et al. 2024. Identifying autism spectrum disorder from multi-modal data with privacy-preserving. NPJ Mental Health Research. 3(1): 15.

[98] Xiangmin Han, Jingxi Feng, Heming Xu, Shaoyi Du and Junchang Li. 2024. A hypergraph transformer method for brain disease diagnosis. Frontiers in Medicine. 11: 1496573.

[99] Chen Zu, Yue Gao, Brent Munsell, Minjeong Kim, Ziwen Peng, Yingying Zhu, et al. 2017. Learning Subnetwork Biomarkers via Hypergraph for Classification of Autism Disease. *In*: Proceedings of the International Society for Magnetic Resonance in Medicine. Scientific Meeting and Exhibition. International Society for Magnetic Resonance in Medicine. Scientific Meeting and Exhibition. Vol. 2017. NIH Public Access. 1719.

[100] Yuduo Zhang, Zhichao Lian and Chanying Huang. 2019. A multilayer sparse representation of dynamic brain functional network based on hypergraph theory for

ADHD classification. *In*: Intelligence Science and Big Data Engineering. Big Data and Machine Learning: 9th International Conference, IScIDE 2019, Nanjing, China. Proceedings, Part II 9. Springer. 325–334.

[101] Wenjing Gao, Yuanyuan Yang, Jianrui Wei, Xuntao Yin and Xinhan Di. 2024. Multi-stage graph learning for fMRI analysis to diagnose neuro-developmental disorders. arXiv preprint arXiv:2410(05342).

[102] Sadaf Sadeghian, Xiaoxiao Li and Margo Seltzer. 2024. HyperBrain: Anomaly Detection for Temporal Hypergraph Brain Networks. arXiv Preprint arXiv:2410 (02087).

[103] Jiujiang Guo, Monan Wang and Xiaojing Guo. 2024. Hierarchical Hyperedge Graph Transformer: Towards Dynamic Interactions of Brain Networks for Neurodevelopmental Disease Diagnosis. IEEE Access. 12: 162145–162156.

[104] Wen Li, Biao Jie, Zhaoxiang Wu and Jie Zhou. 2024. Hypergraph attention-based feature extraction method for the classification of brain diseases. *In*: 2024 5th International Conference on Computer Vision, Image and Deep Learning (CVIDL). IEEE. 646–650.

[105] Guangfeng Shen, Weiming Zeng and Jiajun Yang. 2024. Research on migraine classification model based on hypergraph neural network. The Journal of Supercomputing. 80(17): 25403–25423.

[106] Favour Nerrise, Alice Louise Heiman and Ehsan Adeli. 2024. GAMMA-PD: Graph-based Analysis of Multi-Modal Motor Impairment Assessments in Parkinson's Disease. arXiv preprint arXiv:2410(00944).

[107] Ali Behrouz and Farnoosh Hashemi. 2023. Learning Temporal Higher-order Patterns to Detect Anomalous Brain Activity. Machine Learning for Health (ML4H). PMLR. 39–51.

[108] Patrick Luckett, Elena Pavelescu, J. Todd McDonald, Lee Hively and Juan Ochoa. 2018. Hypergraphs in phase-space: A new method for predicting epileptic seizures. SoutheastCon 2018. IEEE. 1–7.

[109] Jingyu Liu, Wenxin Yang, Yulan Ma, Qunxi Dong, Yang Li, Bin Hu, et al. 2024. Effective hyper-connectivity network construction and learning: Application to major depressive disorder identification. Computers in Biology and Medicine. 171: 108069.

[110] Xiaoying Song, Ke Wu and Li Chai. 2023. Brain network analysis of schizophrenia patients based on hypergraph signal processing. IEEE Transactions on Image Processing. 32: 4964–4976.

[111] Ke Wu, Xiaoying Song and Li Chai. 2022. Graph Metrics Based Brain Hypergraph Learning in Schizophrenia Patients. *In*: 2022 China Automation Congress (CAC). IEEE. 3251–3256.

[112] Yuhui Du, Ju Niu and Vince D. Calhoun. 2021. A new hypergraph clustering method for exploring transdiagnostic biotypes in mental illnesses: Application to schizophrenia and psychotic bipolar disorder. *In*: 2021 IEEE 18th International Symposium on Biomedical Imaging (ISBI). IEEE. 971–974.

[113] Lei Wang, Wei Kong and Shuaiqun Wang. 2021. Hypergraph based adaptive sparse multi-view canonical correlation analysis with application to neuroimaging genetics study of Alzheimer's disease. Modern Clinical Medical Research. 4(1): 1–9.

[114] Xia-an Bi, Lou Li, Zizheng Wang, Yu Wang, Xun Luo and Luyun Xu. 2022. IHGC-GAN: influence hypergraph convolutional generative adversarial network for risk prediction of late mild cognitive impairment based on imaging genetic data. Briefings in Bioinformatics. 23(3): bbac093.

[115] Junli Zhuang, Jinping Tian, Xiaoxing Xiong, Taihan Li, Zhengwei Chen, Rong Chen, et al. 2023. Associating brain imaging phenotypes and genetic risk factors via a hypergraph based netNMF method. Frontiers in Aging Neuroscience. 15: 1052783.

[116] Wei Kong, Yufang Xu, Shuaiqun Wang, Kai Wei, Gen Wen, Yaling Yu, et al. 2023. A Novel Longitudinal Phenotype–Genotype Association Study Based on Deep Feature Extraction and Hypergraph Models for Alzheimer's Disease. Biomolecules. 13(5): 728.

[117] Peilun Song, Xue Li, Xiuxia Yuan, Lijuan Pang, Xueqin Song and Yaping Wang. 2024. Identifying frequency-dependent imaging genetic associations via hypergraph-structured multi-task sparse canonical correlation analysis. Computers in Biology and Medicine. 171: 108051.

[118] Wei Shao, Shunian Xiang, Zuoyi Zhang, Kun Huang and Jie Zhang. 2021. Hypergraph based sparse canonical correlation analysis for the diagnosis of Alzheimer's disease from multi-dimensional genomic data. Methods. 189: 86–94.

[119] Xia-An Bi, Yu Wang, Sheng Luo, Ke Chen, Zhaoxu Xing and Luyun Xu. 2022. Hypergraph structural information aggregation generative adversarial networks for diagnosis and pathogenetic factors identification of Alzheimer's disease with imaging genetic data. IEEE Transactions on Neural Networks and Learning Systems. 35(6): 7420–7434.

[120] Angelica I. Aviles-Rivero, Christina Runkel, Nicolas Papadakis, Zoe Kourtzi and Carola-Bibiane Schönlieb. 2022. Multi-modal hypergraph diffusion network with dual prior for Alzheimer classification. *In*: International Conference on Medical Image Computing and Computer-Assisted Intervention. Springer. 717–727.

[121] Meiling Wang, Wei Shao, Shuo Huang and Daoqiang Zhang. 2023. Hypergraph-regularized multimodal learning by graph diffusion for imaging genetics based Alzheimer's Disease diagnosis. Medical Image Analysis. 89: 102883.

[122] Yipu Zhang, Haowei Zhang, Li Xiao, Yuntong Bai, Vince D. Calhoun and Yu-Ping Wang. 2022. Multi-modal imaging genetics data fusion via a hypergraph-based manifold regularization: Application to schizophrenia study. IEEE Transactions on Medical Imaging. 41(9): 2263–2272.

[123] Xia-an Bi, Sheng Luo, Siyu Jiang, Yu Wang, Zhaoxu Xing and Luyun Xu. 2023. Explainable and programmable hypergraph convolutional network for imaging genetics data fusion. Information Fusion. 100: 101950.

[124] Susanne G. Mueller, M.W. Weiner, L.J. Thal, Ronald C. Petersen, Clifford R. Jack, William Jagust, et al. 2005. Ways toward an early diagnosis in Alzheimer's disease: The Alzheimer's Disease Neuroimaging Initiative (ADNI). Alzheimer's and Dementia. 1(1): 55–66.

[125] Adriana Di Martino, C.-G. Yan, Q. Li, E. Denio, F.X. Castellanos, K. Alaerts, et al. 2014. The autism brain imaging data exchange: Towards a largescale evaluation of the intrinsic brain architecture in autism. Molecular Psychiatry. 19(6): 659–667.

[126] David C. Van Essen, Stephen M. Smith, Deanna M. Barch, Timothy E.J. Behrens, Essa Yacoub, Kamil Ugurbil, et al. 2013. The WU-Minn human connectome project: An overview. NeuroImage. 80: 62–79.

[127] Pamela J. LaMontagne, Tammie L. S. Benzinger, John C. Morris, Sarah Keefe, Russ Hornbeck, Chengjie Xiong, et al. 2019. OASIS-3: Longitudinal neuroimaging, clinical, and cognitive dataset for normal aging and Alzheimer disease. Medrxiv. 2019–12.

[128] Kenneth Marek, Danna Jennings, Shirley Lasch andrew Siderowf, Caroline Tanner, Tanya Simuni, et al. 2011. The Parkinson progression marker initiative (PPMI). Progress in Neurobiology. 95(4): 629–635.

[129] Vince D. Calhoun, Jing Sui, Kent Kiehl, J. Turner, E. Allen and Godfrey Pearlson. 2012. Exploring the psychosis functional connectome: aberrant intrinsic networks in schizophrenia and bipolar disorder. Frontiers in Psychiatry. 2: 75.

[130] Kate Brody Nooner, Stanley J. Colcombe, Russell H. Tobe, Maarten Mennes, Melissa M. Benedict, Alexis L. Moreno, et al. 2012. The NKI-Rockland sample: A model for accelerating the pace of discovery science in psychiatry. Frontiers in Neuroscience. 6: 152.

[131] Xi-Nian Zuo, Jeffrey S. Anderson, Pierre Bellec, Rasmus M. Birn, Bharat B. Biswal, Janusch Blautzik, et al. 2014. An open science resource for establishing reliability and reproducibility in functional connectomics. Scientific Data. 1(1): 1–13.

[132] ADHD-200 consortium. 2012. The ADHD-200 consortium: A model to advance the translational potential of neuroimaging in clinical neuroscience. Frontiers in Systems Neuroscience. 6: 62.

[133] Clare Bycroft, Colin Freeman, Desislava Petkova, Gavin Band, Lloyd T. Elliott, Kevin Sharp, et al. 2018. The UK Biobank resource with deep phenotyping and genomic data. Nature. 562(7726): 203–209.

[134] Karl J. Friston, A.P. Holmes, K.J. Worsley, J.-P. Poline, C.D. Frith and R.S.J. Frackowiak. 1994. Statistical parametric maps in functional imaging: a general linear approach. Human Brain Mapping. 2(4): 189–210.

[135] Stephen M. Smith, Mark Jenkinson, Mark W. Woolrich, Christian F. Beckmann, Timothy E. J. Behrens, Heidi Johansen-Berg, et al. 2004. Advances in functional and structural MR image analysis and implementation as FSL. NeuroImage. 23: S208–S219.

[136] Bruce Fischl. 2012. FreeSurfer. NeuroImage. 62(2): 774–781.

[137] Alexandre Abraham, F. Pedregosa, M. Eickenberg, P. Gervais andreas Mueller, Jean Kossaifi, et al. 2014. Machine learning for neuroimaging with scikit-learn. Frontiers in Neuroinformatics. 8: 71792.

[138] Minjie Wang, Da Zheng, Zihao Ye, Quan Gan, Mufei Li, Xiang Song, et al. 2019. Deep Graph Library: A graph-centric, highly-performant package for graph neural networks. arXiv preprint arXiv:1909(01315).

[139] PYT-Team. 2014. TopoX: A Suite of Python Packages for Machine Learning on Topological Domains. arXiv preprint arXiv:2402(02441).

[140] Hui Han, Tianyu Zhao, Cheng Yang, Hongyi Zhang, Yaoqi Liu, Xiao Wang, et al. 2022. Openhgnn: An open source toolkit for heterogeneous graph neural network. *In*: Proceedings of the 31st ACM International Conference on Information and Knowledge Management. 3993–3997.

[141] Matthias Fey and J.E. Lenssen. 2019. Fast Graph Representation Learning with PyTorch Geometric. arXiv preprint arXiv:1903.02428.

[142] Yue Gao, Zizhao Zhang, Haojie Lin, Xibin Zhao, Shaoyi Du and Changqing Zou. 2020. Hypergraph Learning: Methods and Practices. IEEE Transactions on Pattern Analysis and Machine Intelligence. 44(5): 2548–2566.

[143] Yihe Dong, Will Sawin and Yoshua Bengio. 2020. HNHN: Hypergraph networks with hyperedge neurons. arXiv preprint arXiv:2006(12278).

[144] Jing Huang and Jie Yang. 2021. Unignn: a unified framework for graph and hypergraph neural networks. arXiv preprint arXiv:2105(00956).

[145] Shuyi Ji, Yifan Feng, Rongrong Ji, Xibin Zhao, Wanwan Tang and Yue Gao. 2020. Dual channel hypergraph collaborative filtering. *In*: Proceedings of the 26th ACM SIGKDD International Conference on Knowledge Discovery and Data Mining. 2020–2029.

[146] Mikail Rubinov and Olaf Sporns. 2010. Complex network measures of brain connectivity: uses and interpretations. NeuroImage. 52(3): 1059–1069.

[147] J-Donald Tournier, Robert Smith, David Raffelt, Rami Tabbara, Thijs Dhollander, Maximilian Pietsch, et al. 2019. MRtrix3: A fast, flexible and open software framework for medical image processing and visualisation. NeuroImage. 202: 116137.

[148] Susan Whitfield-Gabrieli and Alfonso Nieto-Castanon. 2012. Conn: A functional connectivity toolbox for correlated and anticorrelated brain networks. Brain Connectivity. 2(3): 125–141.

[149] Jinhui Wang, Xindi Wang, Mingrui Xia, Xuhong Liao, Alan Evans and Yong He. 2015. GRETNA: a graph theoretical network analysis toolbox for imaging connectomics. Frontiers in Human Neuroscience. 9: 386.

[150] Mingrui Xia, Jinhui Wang and Yong He. 2013. BrainNet viewer: A network visualization tool for human brain connectomics. PLoS One. 8(7): e68910.

[151] Chao-Gan Yan, Xin-Di Wang, Xi-Nian Zuo and Yu-Feng Zang. 2016. DPABI: Data processing and analysis for (resting-state) brain imaging. Neuroinformatics. 14: 339–351.

[152] Reinder Vos de Wael, Oualid Benkarim, Casey Paquola, Sara Lariviere, Jessica Royer, Shahin Tavakol, et al. 2020. BrainSpace: A toolbox for the analysis of macroscale gradients in neuroimaging and connectomics datasets. Communications Biology. 3(1): 103.

[153] Soichi Hayashi, Bradley A. Caron, Anibal Sólon Heinsfeld, Sophia Vinci-Booher, Brent McPherson, Daniel N. Bullock, et al. 2024. brainlife.io: A decentralized and open-source cloud platform to support neuroscience research. Nature Methods. 21(5): 809–813.

Index

D

E

F

G

U

V

For Product Safety Concerns and Information please contact our EU representative GPSR@taylorandfrancis.com Taylor & Francis Verlag GmbH, Kaufingerstraße 24, 80331 München, Germany